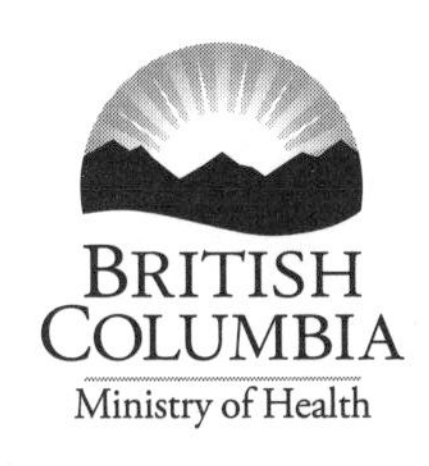

BC Health Guide

Helping you and your family stay healthy

HEALTHWISE® HANDBOOK

Donald W. Kemper, MPH
The Healthwise Staff

Katy E. Magee, Editor
Steven L. Schneider, MD, and A. Patrice Burgess, MD, Medical Editors

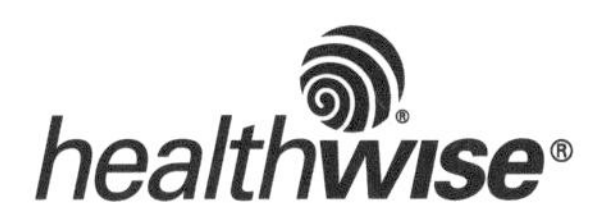

Healthwise, Incorpc
P.O. Box 1989
Boise, Idaho 837

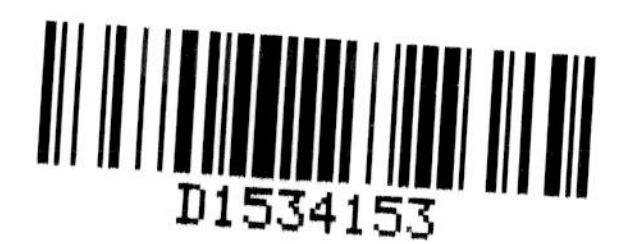

Illustrations by Nucleus Communications

English editions, 2000 and 2005
French edition, 2004

16hwhb/BC-Canada/E-3rd/3-06
ISBN 1-932921-13-3

Printed in British Columbia, Canada.

Table of Contents

About This Book

No book can replace the need for doctors and other health professionals—and no health professional can replace the need for people to care for themselves. The purpose of the *BC HealthGuide* edition of the *Healthwise® Handbook* is to help you and your health professionals work together to manage your health problems.

The *BC HealthGuide* includes basic guidelines on how to recognize and cope with more than 200 of the most common health problems. These guidelines come from evidence-based medical information from reliable medical studies, and we have made every effort to present the information in a way that is unbiased, easy to read, and easy to use.

We recommend that you review pages 1 and 2 right away. Page 1, the Healthwise Self-Care Checklist, is a process you can follow every time a health problem arises. Page 2, the Ask-the-Doctor Checklist, will help you get the most out of every visit to the doctor. You may also wish to read Chapters 1 and 2 before using the rest of the book. Chapter 1, Making Wise Health Decisions, presents basic steps for making health decisions, ways to develop a partnership with your doctor, and information to reduce your health care costs. Chapter 2, Living a Healthy Life, presents information on staying healthy and detecting health problems early. The rest of the book is designed to be used on a topic-by-topic basis whenever a problem or interest develops.

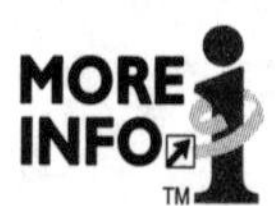

But this is not just a book. This icon is your link to more in-depth information on the Internet. Simply go to the Web site address listed on the back cover and "search" for the underlined text next to the icon. This will link you to more information about the topic.

If you receive professional advice in conflict with this book, please follow your doctor's advice. Because your doctor is able to take your specific history and needs into consideration, his or her recommendations may prove to be the best. Likewise, if any self-care advice fails to provide positive results within a reasonable period, you should consult a health professional.

This book is as good as we can make it, but we cannot guarantee that it will work for you in every case. Nor will the authors or publishers accept responsibility for any problems that may develop from following its guidelines. This book is only a guide; your common sense and good judgment are also needed.

We wish you the best of health!

Disclaimer

This book is intended to provide you with a wide range of medical and health information to assist you in making appropriate health care decisions. Readers should be aware that this publication does not in any way replace consultation with doctors or other health professionals, nor is it intended to act as a substitute for any prescribed treatment. The authors, sponsors, or publishers are not responsible for any problems that may develop from the use or misuse of the information provided in this book. If you suspect that you have a medical condition or problem, or if any self-care advice fails to provide positive results within a reasonable period, please consult a health professional.

About Healthwise

Healthwise is a non-profit organization whose mission is to help people make better health decisions. We create consumer health information that is based on the most current and reliable medical studies available. Expert writers and editors put this medical evidence into user-friendly terms, and a team of nationally recognized medical specialists reviews every word.

Healthwise information reaches more than 20 million families worldwide each year through our self-care handbooks, online content, and nurse call centre resources. Health plans, employers, hospitals, physician groups, community organizations, government agencies, and e-health care companies trust Healthwise to support successful self-care, shared decision making, and Information Therapy™ programs. Healthwise products and consulting services have been shown to help people make better health decisions and to increase their satisfaction with the program sponsor while reducing unnecessary costs.

We publish the *Healthwise® Handbook, La salud en casa: Guía práctica de Healthwise®* (a Spanish translation of the *Healthwise Handbook*), and *Healthwise® for Life* (a medical self-care guide for adults over 50).

This *BC HealthGuide* edition of the *Healthwise Handbook* was edited by Katy Magee. The principal Healthwise medical reviewers were Steven L. Schneider, MD, and A. Patrice Burgess, MD. Jo-Ann Kachigian and Marilyn Allen provided project coordination, editing, and proofreading assistance, while layout and production were provided by Terrie Britton and John Kubisiak.

We also produce the Healthwise® Knowledgebase, which is recognized by many doctors and health organizations as the most comprehensive and reliable source of consumer health information on the Web. The "More Info" icons in this handbook link the basic self-care information in the handbook to in-depth medical information in the Healthwise Knowledgebase. People trust the Healthwise Knowledgebase for evidence-based, commercially unbiased, and referenced information on thousands of health problems, surgeries, medical tests, treatments, medications, and support groups.

Our readers often provide the best ideas for improving this book. If you have a suggestion that will make this book better, please write us at *Healthwise Handbook* Suggestions, c/o Healthwise, P.O. Box 1989, Boise, ID 83701, or e-mail us at moreinfo@healthwise.org. To learn more about our health information programs, products, and services, visit our Web site at www.healthwise.org.

Acknowledgements

This *BC HealthGuide* edition of the *Healthwise® Handbook* reflects an extensive review by provincial health professionals and others, not all of whom can be listed here. Their many helpful comments and suggestions have contributed to a successful adaptation of this book for a British Columbia (BC) audience. This book would not be possible without the extensive help and guidance of health professionals and the helpful input of the dedicated nurses at the BC NurseLine.

Particular thanks go to Brian Winsby, MD, principal reviewer for the BC Medical Association, and Pauline James, RN, MN, principal reviewer for the BC Ministry of Health.

The following provincial organizations generously contributed to the review of previous editions and/or this edition: BC Ministry of Health, BC Ministry of Children and Family Development, BC Medical Association, BC Cancer Agency, BC College of Family Physicians, BC Pharmacy Association, College of Pharmacists of BC, BC Centre for Disease Control, Children's and Women's Health Centre of British Columbia, St. Paul's Hospital, Registered Nurses Association of BC, Victoria Medical Society, Caregivers Association of BC, Arthritis Society (BC and Yukon Division), Canadian Cancer Society (BC and Yukon Division), Canadian Diabetes Association (BC and Yukon Division), Heart and Stroke Foundation of BC and Yukon, BC Lung Association, and Canadian Mental Health Association (North and West Vancouver Branch).

Acknowledgement and gratitude are specifically extended to the following individuals for their role in the review and revision of this book:

Brenda Bains, BA
Margaret Bechard, BA
Wayne Dauphinee, MHA
Judith Delaney, MBA
Andrea Derban, RN, BSN
Valery Dubenko, RN, MBA
Donelda Eve, BJ
Susan Firus, RD
Elaine Gallagher, RN, PhD
Joan Geber, RN, MPA
Tessa Graham, MA
Lori Halls, MPA
Barb Hestrin
Laurianne Jodouin, BScN, MSN
Dianne Kirkpatrick
Janice Linton, RD, MPA
Donna Little, MPA
Kirsten Maier, RCC
Cheryl McIntyre, RN
Linda Mueller, MASA
Del Nyberg, MA
Brian Phillips, MSc
Karen Pielak, MScN
Howard Platt, MD
Heleen Sandvik
Hartaj Sanghara, MA
Vicky Scott, RN, PhD
Margaret Szolnyanszky
Claire Townsend
Konia Trouton, MD
Leslie Wolfe, BSc, CIA, CGA
Eric Young, MD

We wish to thank those health professionals and others who provided review, suggestions and input for previous BC and Canadian editions of the book, which formed the foundation for this edition. We also wish to extend a special thank-you to the residents of BC who provided feedback and suggestions to strengthen this new version. This book is for you, and we wish you the best of health.

The Healthwise® Self-Care Checklist

Step 1. Observe the problem.

- When did it start? What are the symptoms? ______________________________

  ____

  ____

  ____

  ____

- Where is the pain? Dull ache or stabbing pain? Is it constant, or does it come and go? ______________________________

  ____

- Measure your vital signs:

  Temperature: __________ Pulse: __________/minute

  Breaths: _______/minute Blood Pressure: ______/______

- Think back:

  Have you had this problem before? Yes ______ No ______

  What did you do for it? ______________________________

  ____

  Any changes in your life (stress, medications, food, exercise, etc.)?

  ____

  ____

  Does anyone else at home or work have these symptoms?

  ____

Step 2. Learn more about it.

- *BC HealthGuide* (note page number): ______________________________
- BC HealthGuide OnLine (www.bchealthguide.org) topic:

  ____

- Other books or articles: ______________________________
- Advice or opinions of others (lay or professional): ______________________________

  ____

  ____

Step 3. Make an action plan.

- What do you think is wrong? ______________________________
- What have you decided to do about it? ______________________________

  ____

  ____

  ____

Step 4. Evaluate your progress.

- Are you getting better or worse? ______________________________

  ____

  ____

  ____

Ask-the-Doctor Checklist

Before the visit:

- Complete the Healthwise Self-Care Checklist on page 1 and take it with you.
- Take a list of any medications you are currently taking. If you have seen a doctor before for a similar problem, take the record from the visit with you.

During the visit:

- State your main problem first.
- Describe your symptoms (use page 1).
- Describe past experiences with the same problem.

After the visit, write down:

- What is wrong: ______________________________
- What might happen next: ______________________________
- What you can do at home: ______________________________

____

For drugs, tests, and treatments, you may want to ask:

- What is its name? ______________________________
- Why is it needed? ______________________________
- What are the risks? ______________________________
- Are there alternatives? ______________________________
- What if I do nothing? ______________________________
- (For drugs) How do I take this? ______________________________
- (For tests) How do I prepare? ______________________________

At the end of the visit, ask:

- Am I to return for another visit? ______________________________
- Am I to phone in for test results? ______________________________
- What danger signs should I look for? ______________________________
- When do I need to report back? ______________________________
- What else do I need to know? ______________________________

____

____

Doctors, hospitals, and medical devices support us when we are ill; the job of keeping healthy is one where we, as individuals, have a big role to play.
Dr. Perry Kendall,
Provincial Health Officer,
British Columbia

1

Making Wise Health Decisions

Throughout your life you will have to make health decisions for yourself and your family. The decisions you make will influence your overall well-being as well as the quality and cost of your care. In general, people who work with their doctors to make health decisions are happier with the care they receive and the results they achieve.

Why should you help make decisions with your doctor? Aren't you trusting him or her to know what to do? Well, the choices aren't always black and white. There are often several approaches to diagnosing and treating a health problem, and you are more likely to feel better about the chosen approach if it is the one best suited to your needs and values.

The best way to make health decisions is to combine the most reliable medical facts with your personal values. Among your personal values are your beliefs, fears, lifestyle, and experiences. They all play a role in helping you make decisions about your health. Put more simply:

Medical Information + Your Information = Wise Health Decisions

Skills for Making Wise Health Decisions

The following are some simple steps for you to follow when you have a health decision to make. Depending on the decision, the process may take a few minutes, a few hours, or several weeks. Take as much time as you need to make the decision that is right for you.

1. What are your choices? Tell your doctor that you want to share in making a decision. Ask your doctor to clearly state the decision that needs to be made and what your choices are.

2. Get the facts. Learn all about each option by using resources like the library, the Internet, and your doctor. Make sure the information you collect is based on sound medical research, not the results of a single study or facts published by a company that will profit by your using its product.

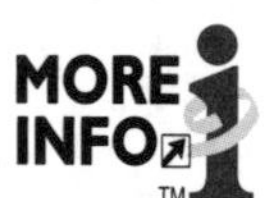
In this book, a special icon marks some of the health problems for which more information will help you make better decisions about your care. Read the back cover of this book to learn more about where you can find reliable health information.

3. What do you think? Think about your own needs and values and what you hope for as the best possible outcome. Talk with family members and others who will be affected by your decision. Then sort out the information you've gathered into a list of pros and cons as you see them for each option. You may want to share your list with your doctor to make sure you have all the information you need.

4. Try on a decision. Write down what you expect will happen if you choose a particular option. Ask your doctor if what you expect is reasonable. Ask again about the side effects, pain, recovery time, or long-term outcomes of that option. Then see if you still feel it's the best choice for you.

5. Make an action plan. Once you and your doctor have made a decision, find out what you can do to make sure that you will have the best possible outcome. Write down the steps that you need to take next. Think positively about your decision, and do your part to ensure success by following your doctor's advice. Remember, when you share in making a decision, you share the responsibility for the outcome.

Work in Partnership With Your Doctor

Your relationship with your doctor greatly influences your ability to make wise health decisions. It will also affect the outcome of your care. Tell your doctor that you want to be a partner in making decisions about your health. Chances are, your doctor will be happy to know that you are interested in taking an active role in your health. Common goals, shared effort, and good communication are the basis of successful doctor-patient partnerships.

Skills for Becoming a Good Partner

You can hold up your end of the doctor-patient partnership by doing the following:

1. Take good care of yourself. Many health problems can be prevented if you protect yourself and your family by getting immunizations, being screened for health problems, and making healthy lifestyle choices.

MORE INFO For more information, see the back cover.

See Living a Healthy Life starting on page 15 for information about how you can have more control over your health.

2. Practise medical self-care. You can manage a lot of minor problems on your own. All it takes is for you to trust your common sense and monitor how well your efforts are working. Use this book, your own experience, and advice from others to create a self-care plan.

- Use the Healthwise Self-Care Checklist on page 1 to record your self-care plan. Note whether home treatment seems to help. If you do end up calling your doctor or a nurse, he or she will want to know what your symptoms are; what you've tried to do for the problem; and how well your self-care worked.
- Plan a time to call a health professional if the problem continues. If the problem seems to be getting more severe, don't wait too long before calling for help.

3. Prepare for office visits. Most medical appointments are scheduled to last only 10 to 15 minutes. The better organized you are, the more value you can get from the visit.

- Prepare an Ask-the-Doctor Checklist like the one on page 2 and take it with you.
- Complete a self-care checklist like the one on page 1 and take it with you.

Calling Your Doctor

Is it okay to call your doctor? Of course it is. Often a phone call to the doctor is all you need to manage a problem at home or determine if an appointment is needed. Here's how to get the most from every call:

Prepare for your call.
Write down a one-sentence description of your problem. Then list two or three questions you have about the problem.

Have your symptom list handy.

Have your calendar handy in case you need to schedule an appointment.

Leave a clear message.
Tell your one-sentence description to the person who answers and ask to talk with your doctor.

If your doctor is not available, ask the receptionist to relay your message and have someone call you back. Ask when you might expect the return call.

Follow through.
When the doctor calls back, briefly describe your problem, ask your questions, and describe any major symptoms.

Some doctors are willing to answer their patients' questions through e-mail. If e-mail is convenient for you, check with your doctor to see if he or she accepts e-mail from patients.

- Write down your hunches or fears about what is wrong. These are often helpful to your doctor.
- Write down the three questions that you most want to have answered. There may not be time to ask a long list of questions.

4. Be an active participant in every medical visit.

- Be honest and straightforward. If you don't intend to take a prescribed medication, say so. If you are getting complementary treatment, such as acupuncture or chiropractic treatments, or taking herbal supplements, let your doctor know. To be a good partner, your doctor has to know what's going on.
- If your doctor recommends a drug, test, or treatment, get more information about the risks and benefits, other alternatives, and the likely outcomes before agreeing to follow the recommendation.
- Take notes. Write down the diagnosis, treatment and follow-up plan, and what you can do at home. Then read your notes back to the doctor to make sure you have it right. If you think it will help, take a friend along to write down what the doctor says so you can concentrate on listening.

5. Learn all you can about your health problem. Throughout this book, a special icon marks topics for which more information will help you make better decisions about your care. The information you gather—whether you get it from your doctor, the library, or the Internet—is a powerful tool for helping you make wise health decisions.

If you have a complicated problem or want to know more about your health options:

- Start by asking your doctor if he or she has information about your problem that you could take home. Some doctors offer video- or audiotapes, brochures, or reprints from medical journals.
- Call the BC NurseLine (see the back cover of this book). The nurses can give you more details about your health concern and options and can direct you to other resources.
- If you use the Internet to find health information, start with BC HealthGuide OnLine at www. bchealthguide.org, or visit the Web site of the Canadian Health Network at www.canadian-health-network.ca or the site for the BC Centre for Disease Control at www.bccd.org. See Health Information at Home on page 415 for tips on finding reliable information.
- The back cover of this book offers tips to help you get more information about health problems and your testing and treatment choices.

If you have questions or concerns about the information you find, discuss them with your doctor.

BC NurseLine

British Columbians have 24-hour, toll-free access to registered nurses specially trained to provide confidential health information and advice on the telephone. A telephone service is available for BC residents who are deaf or hard of hearing, and translation services are available on request in 130 languages.

British Columbians can also access a pharmacist to get answers to their medication-related questions. Pharmacists are available by calling the BC NurseLine between the hours of 5 p.m. and 9 a.m. every day.

BC NurseLine nurses can give you the information you need to make sound health decisions for you and your family. The nurses will help you understand and manage your health problems, provide information on medically sound treatment options, and advise when to see a health professional. They will answer your questions about various health topics, tests, and procedures and help you learn what other resources might exist in your community.

- Within Greater Vancouver, call 604-215-4700.
- Elsewhere within BC, call toll-free 1-866-215-4700.
- If deaf or hearing-impaired, call toll-free throughout BC 1-866-889-4700.

Finding a Doctor Who Will Be a Partner

A primary care doctor or family doctor who knows and understands your needs can be your most valuable health partner. A host of specialists who work on separate health problems may not see your whole health picture or get a good understanding of what's important to you. In choosing a doctor, there are lots of questions to ask, but these three matter the most:

- Is the doctor well trained and experienced?
- Will the doctor be available when needed?
- Will the doctor work in partnership with me?

Training and Experience

Most family doctors have broad knowledge about many common medical problems. Some have additional training or experience in particular areas. For example, some family doctors may take a special interest in sports medicine, maternity, or environmental illnesses, to name a few. If you have a particular health concern or interest, it is worth finding more information on the doctors in your community. This kind of information can be learned by asking your friends and family, looking in the phone directory under Physicians and Surgeons, or contacting the BC College of Family Physicians.

Availability

Because health problems rarely develop at convenient times, it helps to have a doctor who can be contacted whenever he or she is needed. Before you select a doctor, call or visit his or her office. Tell the clinic receptionist that you are looking for a new doctor. Ask these questions:

- Is the doctor accepting new patients?
- What are the office hours?
- If I called right now for a routine visit, how soon could I be seen?
- How much time is allowed for a routine visit?
- If I cancel an appointment, will I be charged for it?
- Will the doctor discuss health problems over the phone or by e-mail?
- Who fills in for the doctor when he or she is not available?
- What hospitals does the doctor use?

Partner Potential

During your first visit, tell your doctor that you would like to share in making treatment decisions.

Pay attention to how you feel during the visit.

- Does the doctor listen well?
- Does the doctor speak to you in terms you can understand?
- Does the doctor spend enough time with you?
- Do you think you could build a good working relationship with the doctor?

If the answers are no, look for another doctor. It may take more than one visit for you to decide if you will be able to work with a doctor.

Is It Time for a Change?

If you are unhappy with how your doctor treats you, it may be time for a change. Before you start looking for a new doctor, tell your current doctor how you would like to be treated. Your doctor will probably be pleased to work with you as a partner if you tell him or her that's what you want. If you don't make your wishes known, your doctor may think that you, like many people, want him or her to do all the work.

Skills for Ensuring Quality Care

Making wise health decisions can help ensure that you get just the care you need, nothing more, and certainly nothing less.

It is likely that you will be faced with one or more of the following health decisions at some time. Use the Skills for Making Wise Health Decisions described on pages 3 and 4 to help you decide if the services or treatments in question are right for you.

1. Should I see a doctor about a health problem? If your symptoms and the guidelines in this book suggest that you should see a doctor, don't put it off. Ignoring problems often leads to complications that are more difficult to treat.

2. Should I have a test (X-rays, blood test, CT or MRI scan, etc.) to diagnose my health problem? Don't agree to any medical test until you understand how it will help you. See page 11 for more information. The only good reason to do a test is because the benefits to you outweigh the risks. No test can be done without your consent.

3. Should I take medication to treat my health problem? Always ask your doctor about any medication he or she prescribes for you. Ask what would happen if you chose not to take a medication and whether there are alternatives to taking medication. See page 12 for more information.

4. Should I have surgery to treat my health problem? Review the questions to ask about surgery on page 13. Get as much information about the surgery as you can and consider your needs and values. If you are not convinced that the benefits to you outweigh the risks, don't have the surgery.

5. Do I need to go to the emergency room? In life-threatening situations, modern emergency services are vital. However, emergency rooms cost two to three times more for routine services than a doctor's office would. They are not set up to care for routine illnesses, and they do not work on a first-come, first-served basis. During busy times, people with minor illnesses may wait for hours. Also, your records may not be available, so emergency room doctors have no information about your medical history.

Use good judgment in deciding when to use emergency medical services. Whenever you feel you can apply home treatment safely and wait to see your regular doctor, do so. Whenever you are not sure what to do, call your doctor or the BC NurseLine for help.

Skills to Use in the Hospital

When you need to be in the hospital, there are things you can do to improve the quality of the care you receive. However, if you are very sick, ask your spouse or a friend to help watch out for your best interests.

- Ask "why?" Don't agree to anything unless you have a good reason. Agree only to those procedures that make sense for you.
- Provide an extra level of quality control. Check medications, tests, injections, and other treatments to see if they are correct. Your diligence can improve the quality of the care that you receive.

6. Do I need to be hospitalized? A large amount of health care dollars are spent on hospitalizations. A stay in a hospital costs far more than a vacation to most luxury resorts, and hospitals are a lot less fun.

Don't check in to the hospital just for tests. Ask your doctor if the tests can be done on an outpatient basis. If you agree to control your diet and activities, your doctor will usually support your request.

If you need in-patient care, get in and out of the hospital as quickly as possible. This will reduce costs and your risk of hospital-acquired infections.

Try to avoid additional days in the hospital by bringing in extra help at home. Ask about home nursing services to help while you recover.

If you have a terminal illness, know that hospitalization is not your only choice. Many people choose to spend their remaining time at home with the people they know and love. Special arrangements can be made through hospice care programs in most communities. Look up Hospice in the phone directory, or ask your doctor.

7. Should I see a specialist about my health problem? Specialists are doctors who have in-depth training and experience in a particular area of medicine. For example, a cardiologist has years of special training to deal with heart problems.

When your primary care doctor refers you to a specialist, a little preparation and good communication can help you get the most from your visit. Before you go see a specialist:

- Know your diagnosis or expected diagnosis.
- Learn about your basic treatment options.
- Make sure that any test results or records on your case are sent to the specialist.
- Know what your primary care doctor would like the specialist to do (take over the case, confirm the diagnosis, conduct tests, etc.).

Wise Medical Consumers:

- Ask to be spoken to in words that they understand.
- Ask to have their medical problems explained to them.
- Ask to read their medical records.
- Ask about the benefits and risks of any treatment and its alternatives.
- Ask what treatments or tests will cost them, if anything.
- Share in all treatment decisions.
- Know they can refuse any medical procedure.

Shared Decisions About Medical Tests

Medical tests are important tools, but they have limits. Informed consumers know that some medical tests have costs and risks as well as benefits.

Learn the facts:

- What is the name of the test, and why do you need it?
- If the test is positive, what will the doctor do differently?
- What could happen if you don't have the test?

Consider the risks and benefits:

- How accurate is the test? How often does it indicate a problem exists when there is none (false positive)? How often does it indicate there is no problem when there is one (false negative)?
- Is the test painful? What can go wrong?
- How will you feel afterward?
- Are there less risky alternatives?

Ask about the costs:

- Will the test cost you anything? If so, is it really necessary, or is there a less expensive test that might give the same information?

If a test seems costly, risky, or not likely to change the recommended treatment, ask your doctor if you can avoid it. Try to agree on the best approach. No test can be done without your permission, and you have the right to refuse to have a test.

Let your doctor know:

- Your concerns about the test.
- What you expect the test will do for you. Ask if that is realistic.
- Any medications you are taking (prescription and non-prescription).
- Whether you have other medical conditions.
- Whether you prefer to accept or decline the test.

If you agree to a test, ask what you can do to reduce the risk of errors. Should you restrict food, alcohol, exercise, or medication before the test? After the test, ask to review the results. Take notes for your home records. If the results of the test are unexpected and the error rate of the test is high, consider redoing the test before basing further treatment on the results.

Shared Decisions About Medications

The first rule of medications is to know why you need each drug before you use it.

Learn the facts:

- What is the name of the medication and why do you need it?
- How long does it take to work?
- How long will you need to take it?
- How and when do you take it (with food, on an empty stomach, etc.)?
- Are there non-drug alternatives?

Consider the risks and benefits:

- How much will this medication help?
- Are there side effects or other risks?
- Could this medication interact with other medications or herbal supplements that you currently take?

Ask about costs:

- How much does the medication cost? Is it covered by PharmaCare?
- Is a generic form of the medication available and appropriate for you?
- Is there a similar medication that will work almost as well and be less expensive?
- Can you start with a prescription for a smaller quantity to make sure the medication agrees with you?

Let your doctor know:

- Your concerns about the medication.
- What you expect the medication will do. Ask if that is realistic.
- What other medications you are taking (prescription and non-prescription).
- Whether you prefer to take the medication or try other ways of treating the problem.

If you need professional advice or more information about your prescription or over-the-counter medications after hours, call the BC NurseLine to speak with a pharmacist between 5 p.m. and 9 a.m. every day.

Shared Decisions About Surgery

Every surgery has risks. Only you can decide if the benefits are worth the risks.

Learn the facts:

- What is the name of the surgery? Get a description of the surgery.
- Why does your doctor think you need the surgery?
- Are there other options besides surgery?
- Is this surgery the most common one for this problem? Are there other types of surgery?

Consider the risks and benefits:

- How many similar surgeries has the surgeon performed? How many surgeries like this are done at this hospital?
- What is the success rate? What does success mean to your doctor? What would success mean to you?
- What can go wrong? How often does this happen?
- How will you feel afterward? How long will it be until you are fully recovered?
- How can you best prepare for the surgery and the recovery period?

Ask about costs:

- Will the surgery cost you anything?
- Can it be done on an outpatient basis?

Let your doctor know:

- How much the problem really bothers you. Are you willing to put up with symptoms to avoid surgery?
- Your concerns about the surgery.
- Whether or not you want to have the surgery at this time.
- If you want a second opinion. Second opinions are helpful if you have any doubt that the proposed surgery is the best option for your problem. If you want a second opinion, ask your primary care doctor or your surgeon to recommend another specialist. Ask that your test results be sent to the second doctor. Consider getting an opinion from a doctor who is not a surgeon and who treats similar problems.

If I'd known I was going to live this long, I'd have taken better care of myself.
Eubie Blake

2

Living a Healthy Life

Most of this book focuses on helping you deal with health problems. This chapter is meant to be used as a guide to help you prevent illness and injury by making wise health and lifestyle choices.

These basic health habits are the foundation of lifelong health and well-being:

- Stay up to date with immunizations and health screenings.
- Be physically active.
- Eat right.
- Maintain a healthy body weight.
- Be tobacco-free.
- Avoid drugs and excess alcohol.
- Manage stress.
- Take care of your teeth.
- Practise safety.
- Pursue healthy pleasures.
- Help to make a healthier world.

Maintaining these health habits will give you the best chance of staying healthy and active and feeling good about yourself throughout your life. If you have health problems, good health habits are even more important. It's never too late to make lifestyle changes that may help you recover faster or make living with a chronic disease easier.

Immunizations

Immunizations help your immune system recognize and quickly attack organisms that can cause diseases before those organisms can cause problems. Some immunizations are given in a single shot or oral dose, while others require several doses over a period of time.

Schedule your child's immunizations according to the chart on page 16. There is no need to delay immunizations because of colds or other minor illnesses. Record immunizations in your "Child's Health Passport" available from your public health unit. Your child will need it at school entry.

British Columbia's Immunization Program — Routine Immunization Schedule by Age Groups

Vaccine → Age Group ↓	Diphtheria, Pertussis, Tetanus, Polio, *Haemophilus Influenzae* type b (DaPT/IPV/Hib)	Pneumococcal Conjugate Children born on or after July 1, 2003, are eligible	Hepatitis B Children born on or after January 1, 2001, are eligible	Measles, Mumps, Rubella (MMR)[a]	Meningococcal C Conjugate Vaccine	Varicella (Chicken Pox) Vaccine If susceptible (have not had chicken pox)	Diphtheria, Pertussis, Tetanus, Polio (DaPT/IPV)	Tetanus, Diphtheria, Pertussis (TdaP)	Tetanus, Diphtheria (Td) Booster Every 10 years[b]	Influenza Vaccine[c]	Pneumococcal Polysaccharide Vaccine
2 months	✔	✔	✔								
4 months	✔	✔	✔								
6 months	✔	✔	✔								
12 months				✔	✔ For those born on or after July 1, 2002	✔ For those born on or after January 1, 2004					
18 months	✔	✔		✔							
4–6 years						✔ Began September 2004	✔				
Grade 6			✔ Began in 1992		✔ Began September 2003	✔ Began September 2004					
Grade 9					✔ Catch-up program for 2004 to 2006			✔			
Adults				✔					✔		
65 and older									✔	✔ (annual)	✔ (one time only)
High Risk Program*		✔*	✔*		✔*	✔*				✔*	✔*

[a] Children under 18 years of age are eligible for two doses, if not previously immunized. Adults 18 years of age and older born after 1957 are eligible for one dose free of charge.

[b] A person with a deep, dirty wound or bite may needed additional tetanus protection after 5 years.

[c] Annual influenza vaccination is recommended for: people 65 and over, health care workers, emergency responders, people with chronic health conditions, infants 6 to 23 months of age, household contacts and caregivers of infants 0 to 23 months of age, and pregnant women in their 3rd trimester who will deliver during the flu season.

* High Risk Program: British Columbia has a number of high risk programs that provide vaccines free of charge for specific groups within the population, such as people with chronic illness or weakened immune systems. For more information about high risk programs, call your doctor, public health unit, or the BC NurseLine.

Note: The vaccine schedule can change. Talk to your doctor, public health nurse, or the BC NurseLine if you have questions.

Immunization table developed by the Ministry of Health Services in collaboration with the BC Centre for Disease Control, January 2005.

If you are considering not having your child immunized, talk with your health professional. There are few valid reasons for not having your child immunized.

The need for immunizations does not end with childhood. Thousands of people are hospitalized, and many die, as the result of influenza and other diseases that can be prevented by immunization. If you are in one of the high-risk groups for whom the influenza or pneumococcal vaccine is recommended (see page 19), make sure you get immunized.

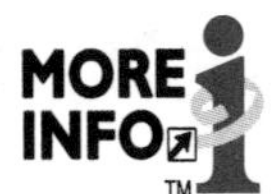

Medical experts are constantly reviewing the effectiveness of immunization programs. Therefore, immunization recommendations change periodically. Your family doctor or local public health unit can provide the most up-to-date information about immunizations.
If you have not been able to follow the recommended immunization schedules (see page 16), talk to your doctor. Alternative schedules are usually available.

Diphtheria, Pertussis, and Tetanus (DaPT and TdaP)

Diseases like diphtheria and pertussis caused many deaths before a vaccine was developed to prevent them. This vaccine also protects against tetanus ("lockjaw"), which can result from bacterial infection of a deep cut or wound.

Childhood immunizations for these diseases consist of a series of shots and boosters starting at age 2 months. The first and only tetanus, diphtheria, and pertussis (TdaP) booster is given between ages 14 and 16 years. After that, a tetanus and diphtheria (Td) booster is needed every 10 years. A person with a deep, dirty wound or bite may need additional tetanus protection if it has been 5 years or longer since the last booster. See your public health nurse or family doctor. Follow the guidelines on page 16 for DaPT, TdaP, and Td.

Reactions to Immunizations

Temporary, mild reactions to immunizations are common. Babies may develop a fever after the DaPT shot, and the area where the shot was given may become sore, red, or swollen. A child may develop a rash or fever 1 to 2 weeks after receiving a dose of MMR vaccine. The rash will go away without treatment and is not contagious.

The hepatitis B vaccine may cause pain at the injection site as well as a mild fever.

- Acetaminophen may soothe the discomfort and relieve fever caused by immunizations. Also see page 278.
- Keep written notes about any reactions you observe.
- Tell your health professional if you think the reactions are excessive.

Polio

Polio is a viral illness that can lead to paralysis. It is rare today because of the polio vaccine. The first dose of vaccine is given at age 2 months, and the immunization series gives lifelong protection (immunity).

Adults who have not been immunized need immunization only if they are travelling to a part of the world where new cases of polio still occur.

Haemophilus influenzae Type b (Hib)

Haemophilus influenzae type b does not cause the flu. It is a bacterial infection that can cause meningitis, pneumonia, skin and bone infections, and other serious illnesses in young children. Every child between 2 months and 5 years of age should be immunized against Hib. Older children and adults need immunization if they have medical conditions that put them at high risk for infection.

Meningococcal Infection

Meningococcal bacteria can infect the blood (bacteremia) or the covering of the brain (meningitis), causing permanent disabilities, such as hearing loss, or death. There are several types, or serogroups, of meningococcal bacteria; in recent years group C bacteria have caused most of the outbreaks in Canada. Vaccination against meningococcal C is provided at age 12 months for all infants born on or after July 1, 2002. Immunization is also offered to all Grade 6 and Grade 9 students who have not already been immunized and to people of any age who have medical conditions that put them at high risk for infection.

Vaccination against meningococcal disease may be considered for other groups, including military recruits, students who live in dormitory housing, and people travelling to areas where meningococcal disease is common. Talk with your doctor or local public health unit about whether you need to be immunized.

Measles, Mumps, and Rubella (MMR)

Measles (rubeola), mumps, and rubella (German measles) were once common childhood illnesses. Today they are quite rare, thanks to the MMR vaccine. Two shots, one given at 12 to 15 months and another given at 18 months, provide lifelong immunity.

If there is a measles outbreak in your area and your baby has not been immunized, call your doctor or local public health unit to discuss an early MMR shot. If your child receives the vaccine before he or she is 12 months old, 2 additional doses are still required.

If you don't have records showing that you received 2 doses of MMR vaccine and you did not have these illnesses as a child, discuss your need for immunization with your doctor.

Women who are planning to get pregnant need to make sure they have been vaccinated. Rubella contracted during pregnancy, especially during the first few months, increases the risk of miscarriage, stillbirth, and severe birth defects.

Varicella Virus (Chicken Pox)

The varicella vaccine is recommended at age 12 months for babies born on or after January 1, 2004. It is also recommended for children in kindergarten or Grade 6. Babies and children who have had chicken pox do not need the vaccine.

Hepatitis B Virus (HBV)

The hepatitis B virus (HBV) infects liver cells and can destroy them. Over time, chronic HBV infection can lead to serious, sometimes fatal liver disease. Vaccination prevents HBV infection and its possible complications. See page 122.

It is recommended that all children be vaccinated against HBV. Immunization is also recommended for adults at risk for exposure to the virus. See page 334.

Influenza Virus

Annual influenza vaccinations are recommended for: all adults age 65 and over; residents of long-term care facilities; people under 65 who have chronic diseases; health care workers and emergency responders; babies age 6 to 23 months; and household contacts and caregivers of babies 0 to 23 months. A flu shot is also recommended for pregnant women in their third trimester who are expected to deliver during flu season. The vaccine can be given to anyone older than 6 months of age. The vaccine is given in the autumn, before the start of the flu season.

Pneumococcal Infection

In addition to infecting the lungs (pneumonia), pneumococcal bacteria can infect the blood (bacteremia) or the covering of the brain (meningitis). The pneumococcal conjugate vaccine (PCV) is recommended for all infants. The first of 4 doses should be given at age 2 months. This vaccine is also recommended for children between 2 months and 5 years of age who have medical conditions that put them at high risk for infection.

A one-time-only dose of pneumococcal polysaccharide vaccine is recommended for people age 65 and older. Younger people who have chronic diseases should also get the pneumococcal polysaccharide vaccine.

Hepatitis A Virus (HAV)

Unlike other types of hepatitis, infection with the hepatitis A virus (HAV) usually does not cause long-term problems. However, it is very contagious and can cause serious illness in some cases. The vaccine series is extremely effective.

Vaccination against hepatitis A is recommended for individuals at risk for exposure to the hepatitis A virus.

Other Immunizations

Contact your local public health unit to find out which other immunizations you need. Immunization may be needed in certain disease outbreak situations or for international travel.

Health Screenings

Another way to protect your health is to detect disease early, when it may be easier to treat. You can do this in two ways: by having appropriate screening tests when recommended by a health professional and by becoming a good observer of changes in your own body.

Periodic Medical Examinations and Screening Tests

The schedule on page 21 will help you decide which examinations and tests are right for you and your family and how often you should have them. The most appropriate schedule of preventive examinations is one you and your doctor agree upon, based on your age, your risk factors for disease, how healthy you are, and how important periodic health screening is to you.

The recommendations on page 21 apply to people of average risk in each age group. You may be at higher risk for certain diseases and may therefore need more frequent examinations and tests. Factors that may help your doctor determine your level of risk include your overall health, your family history (whether your close relatives have had certain diseases), and lifestyle factors, such as whether you use tobacco, how often you exercise, and your sexual history.

Self-Examinations

Periodic self-examinations are also an important part of staying healthy. See the breast self-examination on page 299, the genital self-examination for women on page 302, and the testicular self-examination on page 328. Turn to page 259 to learn how to look for changes in your skin that may be early signs of skin cancer.

Other Recommended Tests and Examinations

Birth to 10 years

Well-baby visits are recommended at 2 weeks and at 2, 4, 6, 9, 12, 15, 18, and 24 months of age. Your doctor may recommend a different schedule. Babies at high risk for hearing problems may be tested during this time.

Discuss the frequency of visits for a child older than 2 years with your health professional. A vision test is recommended at age 3 to 4 years. Some childhood immunizations are given at 4 to 6 years. See page 16.

Regular blood pressure checks are recommended after age 3 years and may be done during visits for other reasons.

Health Screening Schedule			
Assessment	**Birth–10 years**	**11–24 years**	**25–64 years**
Height and Weight	Growth chart plotted during office visit from birth on.	Periodically.	Periodically. See Body Mass Index on p. 23.
Vision Screening	Screening between ages 3 and 4 years.		Periodically. More often if you have diabetes.
Hearing	Universal screening of infants for hearing impairment before age 3 months.		Periodically if you are regularly exposed to loud noise.
Blood Pressure, p. 290	Screening during any office visit starting at age 3 years.	Every 2 to 5 years.	Every 2 to 5 years.
Breast Cancer Screening, pp. 297 and 299			Ages 40 to 49: mammography every 1 to 2 years or counselling on benefits of mammography, based on risk factors. From age 40: annual clinical examination. From age 50: mammography every 1 to 2 years.
Cervical Cancer Screening Test (Pap test), p. 302		Every 1 to 3 years for any female who has ever had sexual intercourse.	Every 1 to 3 years for any female who has ever had sexual intercourse.
Chlamydia, p. 333		Routine for sexually active females or people at high risk.	Routine for sexually active females or people at high risk.
Cholesterol, p. 292			Periodically. Discuss with health professional.
Diabetes, p. 285			Every 3 years after age 45.
Prostate Cancer Screening, p. 325			Risk increases with age starting at age 50; discuss with health professional.

11 to 24 years
A tetanus, diphtheria, and pertussis (TdaP) booster is recommended at 14 to 16 years of age. After age 21, periodic blood pressure checks are recommended and may be done during any doctor visit.

Pap tests are recommended every 1 to 3 years for any female who has ever had sexual intercourse.

25 to 64 years
The Health Screening Schedule on page 21 can help you decide which tests are valuable for you and how often you should have them.

Pregnant Women
Discuss the frequency of visits and testing with your doctor. During the first prenatal visit, blood tests, urinalysis, blood pressure measurement, and screening for hepatitis B virus and HIV infection are recommended. Additional tests are needed throughout the pregnancy.

Tuberculin Test
A tuberculin test is done to determine if you have been infected with the organisms that cause tuberculosis (TB). See page 187.

Whether you need to be tested depends on how common TB is in your area and your risk of coming in contact with TB-causing organisms. If you think you may have been exposed to TB and wish to be tested, contact your doctor or local public health unit.

Be Physically Active

Every body needs regular physical activity. Along with a positive attitude and a healthy diet, your fitness level plays a major role in how well you feel, what illnesses you avoid, and how much you enjoy life. Regular physical activity:

- Lowers your risk of premature death and death caused by heart disease.
- Reduces your risk of developing diabetes, high blood pressure, colon cancer, and osteoporosis.
- Helps lower high cholesterol and blood pressure levels.
- Improves your mood, relieves stress, and promotes a sense of well-being.
- Helps build and maintain healthy bones, muscles, and joints.
- Helps you maintain a healthy body weight.

If you already make regular physical activity a part of your life, keep up the good work. If you aren't physically active, there is good news.

The latest research shows that exercise doesn't have to be vigorous to improve your health. Many everyday activities raise your heart rate and, if done regularly, will keep your heart and lungs healthy, make your muscles stronger, and improve your flexibility. For more specific information about designing your personal fitness plan and staying motivated, see Fitness starting on page 343.

Eat Right

How and what you choose to eat affects many aspects of your health. Your diet plays an important role in helping you:

- Meet your nutritional needs and maintain a healthy weight.
- Have regular bowel movements.
- Prevent diseases such as heart disease, diabetes, and certain cancers.
- Treat diseases such as diabetes and high blood pressure.

Another important aspect of your diet is how carefully you prepare and handle foods. You need good food preparation and food handling habits in order to avoid food-borne illnesses. For more information about food safety, see Stomach Flu and Food Poisoning on page 133.

For more information about how you can evaluate and improve your diet, see Nutrition starting on page 351.

Maintain a Healthy Body Weight

Healthy bodies come in a variety of shapes and sizes. Weight is not the only measurement of health. In fact, your weight may say very little about your health. No matter what your shape or body size, you can improve your health by eating a balanced diet, getting regular exercise, and learning to feel good about your body.

Body Mass Index (BMI)

Your body mass index (BMI) is based on your height and weight. A healthy BMI for an adult is between 19 and 25. Disease risk increases both above and below this BMI range. A person is said to be obese when his or her BMI is 30 or higher.

Use the following table to look up the upper and lower limits of weight for your height. The height is given in centimetres (and inches) and the weight in kilograms (and pounds).

Height	Healthy weight based on a BMI range from 19 to 25
cm (inches)	kg (lb)
147.3 (58)	40–53 (90–119)
149.9 (59)	42–56 (93–124)
152.4 (60)	43–58 (96–128)
154.9 (61)	44–59 (99–132)
157.5 (62)	46–61 (103–136)
160.0 (63)	48–63 (106–141)
162.6 (64)	49–65 (109–145)
165.1 (65)	51–67 (113–150)
167.6 (66)	53–70 (117–155)
170.2 (67)	54–71 (120–159)
172.7 (68)	56–74 (124–164)
175.3 (69)	57–76 (127–169)
177.8 (70)	59–78 (131–174)
180.3 (71)	61–80 (135–179)
182.9 (72)	62–83 (139–184)
185.4 (73)	64–85 (143–189)
188.0 (74)	66–87 (147–194)
190.5 (75)	68–90 (151–200)
193.0 (76)	70–92 (155–205)

Heredity plays a big role in your body shape and what you weigh. It would be impossible for most of us to look like fashion models or world-class athletes, but we can all learn to appreciate our bodies and treat them well to maximize our health and self-esteem.

What Is a Healthy Weight?

The Body Mass Index (see page 23) provides an estimate of your total body fat, which influences your risk for certain diseases. However, your health is determined by more than just your weight. Other measurements of health include:

- Your fitness level.
- The quality of your diet and your eating habits.
- The presence of disease indicators such as high cholesterol.
- The presence of diseases such as high blood pressure, heart disease, and diabetes.
- How fat is distributed on your body.
- Your self-esteem and body image.

You can improve your health without changing your weight. The amount you weigh now could be, or could become, a healthy weight for you.

If you think that your current weight puts you at risk for health problems, talk to your health professional about different ways you can manage your weight. Most people are concerned about being overweight, but for some people being underweight is a health concern. Being **obese** (having a body mass index of 30 or greater) can increase your risk of developing high blood pressure, high cholesterol, heart disease, type 2 diabetes, sleep apnea, some cancers, and other long-term illnesses. Losing as little as 5 percent to 10 percent of your body weight can lower your blood pressure, reduce other risk factors for heart disease, and improve your blood sugar levels.

Set Realistic Goals

Before you start a weight management program, think about your goals, your expectations, and your readiness to make lifestyle changes. A realistic weight management program should focus on the following:

- Reducing your risk of health problems.
- Increasing your fitness level by becoming more physically active.
- Making positive lifestyle changes that will become lifelong habits.
- Coming to accept the size and shape of your body.

Tools for Change

Set your body in motion

Regular physical activity makes you feel stronger and more energetic. It also improves your overall health. Physical activity makes your body burn more calories, not just while you're exercising, but throughout the day. So if you exercise regularly and eat a healthy diet, you will find it easier to manage your weight. In addition, regular exercise builds muscle. Increasing the amount of muscle in your body (lean muscle mass) is healthier for you and will make your body look more toned. For tips on making regular physical activity a part of your healthy lifestyle, see Fitness starting on page 343.

Plan your meals

People who eat regular meals find it easier to maintain a healthy weight than do people who overeat, skip meals, or snack. Meals that are planned are usually more nutritious than those that are grabbed at the last minute. Taking time to plan what you will eat will improve your diet and can help you control your weight. Skipping meals usually leads to feelings of deprivation, which can lead to overeating at the next meal or eating a less-than-nutritious snack.

Focus on reducing fat

Eat a variety of nutritious, low-fat foods. Rather than counting calories, focus on eating more fruits and vegetables and less fat.

A low-fat diet (less than 35 percent of total calories from fat) will help you control your weight and reduce your risk of developing heart disease, high blood pressure, cancer, and other diseases. For tips on how to cut fat from your diet, see page 355.

Enjoy your food

You can enjoy all the foods you love and still control your weight. The key is to be sensible about how much you eat and to balance calorie intake with calorie burn-off (exercise). Here are some tips:

- Enjoy your steak (or cake) twice as much: eat half in the restaurant and take the rest home to enjoy the next day.
- Have one helping of your favourite food and enjoy every bite.
- Craving an ice cream cone? Walk to the ice cream shop, have a single dip, and walk home.

All foods can fit into a healthy diet; the proper balance of those foods is what's most important.

Be Tobacco-Free

It's never too late to quit using tobacco, even if you've been doing it for 20 or 30 years. Quitting smoking or chewing tobacco is the most important thing you can do to improve your own health and the health of those around you. Quitting is not easy. If you have already tried to quit, you know how difficult it is. But don't give up—with the right attitude and enough help, you will eventually succeed.

Tobacco use increases your risk for many health problems, including cancer, heart disease, and stroke. Your tobacco use also puts others at risk. Children who are exposed to tobacco smoke in the home have more ear infections and are prone to other health problems such as asthma. Perhaps the greatest risk to your children is that they will learn from you. Children whose parents use tobacco are more likely to use tobacco themselves.

When you stop using tobacco, it doesn't take long for your body to start to heal and for your risk of developing other health problems to decrease.

- When you quit smoking, your risk of heart attack is cut in half within 1 year after quitting. Five years after quitting, your risk is about the same as that of a person who never smoked.
- While the lung damage that smoking causes is not reversible, quitting smoking prevents more lung damage from occurring. Shortness of breath and cough will decrease.
- When you give up tobacco products, damage to your lips, tongue, mouth, and throat is reduced. Your risk for mouth and throat cancer decreases.
- If you have asthma, you will have fewer and less severe attacks after you quit smoking.
- After quitting smoking, a man may have fewer problems getting and maintaining erections.

Cigars and Smokeless Tobacco

Cigars have become popular in recent years. Many people who smoke cigars feel it is safe because they do not inhale the cigar smoke. However, holding cigars and cigar smoke in your mouth increases your risk for cancers of the mouth, tongue, throat, and larynx.

Smokeless tobacco, or snuff, can be chewed, inhaled, or held in your cheek. There is a direct link between using these products and developing mouth and throat cancer.

Facts you should know about cigars and smokeless tobacco:

- They contain nitrosamines, which cause cancer.
- They contain nicotine, which raises your heart rate and blood pressure.
- They may produce leukoplakias (wrinkled, thick, white patches) on the inside of the mouth. Leukoplakias can develop into mouth cancer.

Tips for Quitting

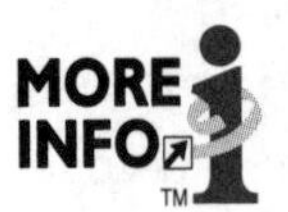

No one can tell you when or how to quit smoking or chewing tobacco. Only you know why you use tobacco and what will be most difficult as you try to stop. The important thing is that you try. Believe that you will succeed, if not the first time, then the second time, or twenty-second time.

MORE INFO For more information, see the back cover.

Smoking Cessation Aids

Nicotine replacement products can help you break the habit of using tobacco and prevent nicotine withdrawal symptoms. The products deliver nicotine to the bloodstream without the dangerous tars, carbon monoxide, and other chemicals released by tobacco and smoke. You gradually reduce the amount of nicotine you give yourself until your body is no longer dependent on nicotine.

In BC, nicotine replacement treatment comes in two forms: chewing gum and skin patches.

All nicotine replacement products can cause side effects. You may need to try more than one product before you find the one that works best for you.

Using a nicotine replacement product works best if you also enroll in a tobacco cessation program. Such programs help you deal with the habit of smoking or chewing tobacco, while the replacement product helps you overcome your addiction to nicotine.

A medication that does not contain nicotine is now available to help control irritability and cravings when you quit using tobacco. The medication is available only with a doctor's prescription. First try to stop using tobacco without the medication. Many people succeed without it.

Preparation

- List your reasons for quitting: for your own health and your family's health, to save money, to prevent wrinkles, or whatever. Read through your list daily for 1 month, and your chances of success will increase.
- Figure out why you smoke. Do you use tobacco to pep yourself up? To relax? Do you like the ritual of smoking or chewing? Do you use tobacco out of habit, often without knowing why you are doing it? If specific situations trigger your desire to smoke or chew tobacco, changing your routine may help you stop.
- Decide how and when you will quit. About half of ex-tobacco users quit "cold turkey." The other half cut down more slowly.
- Find a healthful alternative that can replace what smoking or chewing does for you. For example, if you like to have something to do with your hands, pick up something else: a coin, worry beads, pen, or pencil. If you like to have something in your mouth, substitute sugarless gum or minted toothpicks.
- Plan a healthful reward for yourself for when you have stopped using tobacco. Take the money you save by not buying tobacco and spend it on yourself.

- Plan things to do for when you get the urge to smoke or chew. Urges don't last that long: take a walk, brush your teeth, have a mint, drink a glass of water, or chew gum.
- Choose a reliable 24/7 tobacco cessation program like Quitnow.ca or Quitnow by Phone. Quitnow.ca is a free online service, and Quitnow by Phone gives confidential access to a counsellor. Both services offer expert advice, peer support, and tools to help you quit. Visit www.quitnow.ca, or call 1-877-455-2233 to speak to a cessation counsellor.

Action

- Set a quit date and stick to it. Choose a time that will be busy but not stressful.
- Remove ashtrays and all other reminders of using tobacco. Choose non-smoking sections in restaurants. Avoid alcohol. Do things that reduce the likelihood of using tobacco, like taking a walk or going to a movie.
- Ask for help and support. Choose a trusted friend, preferably another former tobacco user, to give you a helping hand over the rough spots.
- Know what to expect. The worst will be over in just a few days, but physical withdrawal symptoms may last 1 to 3 weeks. After that, it is all psychological. See page 386 for relaxation tips.
- Keep low-calorie snacks handy for when the urge to munch hits. Your appetite may perk up, but most people gain fewer than 4.5 kilograms (10 lb) when they quit using tobacco. The health benefits of quitting outweigh a few extra kilograms. The information in the Nutrition chapter starting on page 351 can help you plan healthy meals and snacks.
- Get out and exercise. It will distract you, help keep off unwanted weight, and release tension. See Fitness starting on page 343.
- Don't be discouraged by slip-ups. It often takes several tries to quit using tobacco for good. If you do slip up and smoke or chew, forgive yourself and learn from the experience. You will not fail as long as you keep trying.
- Good luck!

Avoid Drugs and Excess Alcohol

When you say no to drugs and limit the amount of alcohol that you drink, you prevent accidents and several diseases and avoid a lot of other problems for yourself and your family. Even if you drink moderately, never drink then drive. If problematic substance use affects you or someone close to you, now is the time to seek help. For more information about drug and alcohol problems, see page 366.

Manage Stress

Stress is practically unavoidable, but it doesn't have to have a negative impact on your health and well-being. By learning how to deal with stress in ways that make you feel more in control, you may be able to improve your health, your relationships, your job or school performance, and your outlook on life.

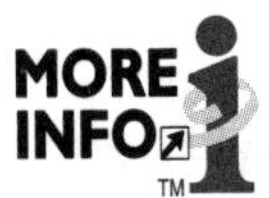

It shouldn't surprise you that some of the key factors in helping you manage stress are eating a healthy diet, getting regular exercise and enough sleep, avoiding drugs and tobacco, and drinking alcohol only in moderation. All these lifestyle factors work together.

For more information about how stress can affect your health and how you can identify and deal with the sources of stress in your life, see Mental Health, Addictions, and Mind-Body Wellness starting on page 365.

Take Care of Your Teeth

Your teeth will last a lifetime if you care for them properly. Brushing and flossing regularly, eating a mouth-healthy diet, and visiting your dentist for regular checkups will help keep your teeth healthy.

Brushing

- Brush at least twice a day for 3 to 5 minutes each time.
- Use a fluoride toothpaste (young children should use only a pea-sized dab). Tartar-control toothpastes may help slow the formation of hard mineral buildup (tartar) on the teeth.
- Brush your tongue. Plaque buildup (a sticky film made of bacteria) on the tongue can cause bad breath.

Start brushing your child's teeth as soon as they come in. Brush your child's teeth for the first 4 to 5 years, until your child seems able to do it alone. A good teaching method is to have your child brush in the morning and you brush at night until your child masters the skill.

If your local water supply does not contain enough fluoride, your child may need a fluoride supplement. Discuss this with your dentist.

Flossing

Flossing properly once a day is the best way to remove plaque from below the gums and between the teeth.

Start flossing your child's teeth as soon as they touch each other. As with brushing, you will have to help with flossing until the child is old enough to manage it alone.

Diet

- Avoid high-sugar foods and drinks, especially sticky, sweet foods like taffy and suckers. The longer sugar stays in touch with your teeth, the more damage it will do.
- Choose healthy and nutritious snacks.
- Be sure to brush before bed. Food is more likely to cause cavities at night because saliva doesn't clean the mouth as well at night.
- Mozzarella and other cheeses, peanuts, yogourt, milk, and sugar-free chewing gum (especially gum that contains xylitol) are good for your teeth. They help clear the mouth of harmful sugars and reduce plaque formation.

Dental Checkups

Choose a dentist as carefully as you choose any other doctor. See page 7 for tips on finding a dentist who meets your needs and is concerned about preventive care.

Most people who do not have serious problems with their teeth need to visit the dentist at least once a year. During a dental checkup the dentist will examine your teeth and gums for signs of tooth decay and gum disease. X-rays of your teeth are taken when required. If you don't have any active tooth decay or gum disease, changes in your brushing and flossing habits probably won't be necessary.

A dentist or dental hygienist will clean your teeth. He or she will scrape hard mineral buildup (tartar) off of your teeth with a small metal tool; floss your teeth thoroughly; and use a polishing compound to help clean and polish your teeth. Cleanings may be uncomfortable but usually aren't painful. Other procedures (application of sealants to prevent cavities or fluoride treatments) may be done during a routine office visit if needed.

The Canadian Dental Association recommends that your child see a dentist by the time he or she is about 1 year of age.

See your dentist if you have any of the following problems:

- Gums that bleed when you press on them or often bleed when you brush your teeth.
- Teeth that are loose or moving apart or changes in the way your teeth fit together when you bite down.
- Very red, swollen, or tender gums or pus oozing from your gums.
- A toothache. Toothaches can have many causes—from tooth decay to sinus infection. Tooth pain may go away temporarily, but the problem will not go away until it is treated. Take Aspirin, ibuprofen, or acetaminophen for pain relief until you can see your dentist. Do not give Aspirin to anyone younger than 20. Placing a cold pack on your jaw may also help relieve tooth pain.

Practise Safety

Taking safety precautions is one of the most important things you can do to protect yourself and your family from accidents and injuries. Let common sense and these partial lists be your guides.

At Home

- Post emergency telephone numbers near telephones.
- Have an emergency plan in case of accidents, fire, or injury. Practise the plan with your family.
- Install smoke and carbon monoxide detectors in your home, and check them twice a year to make sure they work.
- Keep a working fire extinguisher in your home. Make sure everyone in the house (including the babysitter) knows how to use it.
- Keep all medications, cleaning and automotive supplies, and other hazardous products securely stored and out of the reach of children.
- Turn off appliances after use. Unplug small appliances and put them away after they have cooled.
- Prevent falls by securing rugs that slip, keeping stairs and hallways clear of clutter, and turning on lights.
- Practise safer sex. See page 336.
- Store firearms unloaded and securely, out of the reach of children. Store ammunition separately.

When On the Move

- Don't drink and drive any vehicle (car, boat, bicycle, or machinery).
- Don't drive if any medications or herbal products you are taking may cause drowsiness.
- Make sure everyone in your car is wearing a safety belt. See Automobile Seat Restraints on page 32.
- Obey traffic laws and speed limits.
- Keep your car, bike, skateboard, skis, and other recreational gear in good operating condition.
- Wear helmets and sport-specific padding when bicycling, in-line skating, playing baseball or hockey, etc. Wear eye protection when playing racquet sports.
- Never let children play unattended near water.

At Work

- Follow your employer's safety guidelines.
- Wear clothing and protective equipment that is appropriate for your job (hard hat, gloves, goggles, earplugs, etc.).
- Protect yourself against smoke, dangerous fumes, and exposure to chemicals.
- Know the location of fire extinguishers, first aid equipment, and emergency exits nearest your workstation.

Automobile Seat Restraints

Wearing seat belts saves lives and prevents injuries. No one is strong enough to brace themselves against a sudden impact in a motor vehicle, even at very low speeds. Seat belts reduce the risk of serious injury and death.

- Wear your seat belt every time you are in a vehicle. Always use both the lap and shoulder belts. Position the lap belt low over your hip bones and the shoulder belt over your shoulder and across your chest (never under your arm or behind your back). Pregnant women should position the lap belt below the developing baby.
- Seat belts are necessary even if your car is equipped with air bags. Air bags inflate from the steering wheel or dashboard of your car in the event of sudden impact. They are very effective in protecting front-seat riders, but they must be used with seat belts. Infants in car seats and children and adults under 142 cm (4 feet 8 inches) in height should not sit in front of an air bag.
- Children younger than 12 years of age should sit in the back seat. Use child car seats for infants, children under 4, and those weighing less than 18 kg (40 lb). See Child Car Seats on page 266.

Pursue Healthy Pleasures

Give yourself permission to make yourself happy. The good things in life make it easier to deal with the things that aren't so good. If it's been a while since you've indulged yourself in something pleasurable, try this exercise:

- Make a list of 10 (or more) things that give you pleasure.
- Do at least 1 of the things on your list every day for 1 week.
- Enjoy and repeat!

Help to Make a Healthier World

Do what you can to make your home, your community, and your world a better place. Support a cause that is working to make positive changes. Recycle. Mentor. Tutor. Volunteer. And remember, peace on Earth begins at home: seek non-violent ways to resolve conflicts at home, at school, at work, and in your community. See pages 369 and 379.

Healthy aging is my grandma making plans for her future.
Granddaughter

3

Healthy Aging

FOR SENIORS

You will find information helpful to older adults throughout this book. Colds, headaches, back pain—everyone has to deal with these problems from time to time, and seniors are no exception. To find topics aimed specifically at older adults, however, look for the "For Seniors" icon. You can also look in the index under "Senior health concerns" for items of special interest.

This chapter focuses on two key issues for seniors:

- Staying healthy as you age.
- Caregiving. If you take care of an ill or disabled spouse, family member, or friend, the information in this section can help you feel good about the care you give and help you take care of yourself too. See page 42.

Healthy lifestyle choices can help you feel your best for all the years to come. There is no doubt that your body changes as you age, but those changes don't have to lead to health problems. Even if certain health problems run in your family, you may be able to prevent them or keep them from getting worse by making healthy lifestyle choices.

Healthy aging also means more than just staving off disease. It means having energy and enthusiasm for daily activities, maintaining relationships, contributing to your community, and nourishing your spirit. Even if you have a chronic illness like diabetes or heart disease, you can make lifestyle choices that may help you maintain your vigor, your independence, and your zest for life.

Perhaps the most important message is that your body will benefit from healthy lifestyle choices no matter when you make them. With the right attitude and enough support, you can develop new habits that will have a positive effect on your health and well-being. It's never too late to get started.

Keys to Healthy Aging

There is no magic to vitality and health in old age. The best approach to good health at any age is to develop good health habits and stick with them. Let these keys be your general guide.

Keep Your Body Moving

Keeping physically fit may be the single most important thing you can do to maintain your health as you age. Find an activity that you enjoy, such as walking, swimming, or dancing, and do it regularly. Many everyday activities, such as gardening and housework, raise your heart rate and, if done regularly, will keep your heart and lungs healthy, make your muscles stronger, and improve your flexibility. For more specific information about staying fit, see Fitness starting on page 343.

Eat Right

What you choose to eat affects many aspects of your health. Your diet plays an important role in helping you:

- Get the nutrition your body needs.
- Maintain a healthy weight.
- Prevent problems such as constipation, heart disease, diabetes, and certain cancers.
- Treat diseases such as diabetes and high blood pressure.

For more information about how you can evaluate and improve your diet, see Nutrition starting on page 351.

Maintain a Healthy Body Weight

What is a healthy weight? Healthy bodies come in all shapes and sizes. If you think that your current weight puts you at risk for health problems, talk to your health professional about different ways you can manage your weight.

Most people are concerned about being overweight, but for some people being underweight is a health concern. Being **obese** (having a body mass index of 30 or greater; see the chart on page 23) can increase your risk of developing joint problems, high blood pressure, high cholesterol, heart disease, type 2 diabetes, sleep apnea, some cancers, and other long-term illnesses. Losing as little as 5 to 10 percent of your body weight can do good things for your health, such as lowering your blood pressure, reducing other risk factors for heart disease, and lowering your blood sugar level if you have diabetes.

For more information about weight management, see page 24.

Do Not Use Tobacco

In addition to exercising regularly and eating a healthy diet, being tobacco-free is one of the most important things you can do to improve your own health and the health of those around you. Tobacco use increases your risk for many health problems, including cancer, heart disease, and stroke. Your tobacco use puts others at risk as well. Second-hand smoke (the smoke other people breathe from your burning cigarettes and exhaled smoke) causes lung and other cancers, heart disease, and a long list of other health problems in non-smokers.

It's never too late to quit. No matter how much tobacco you use or how long you've been using it, once you stop, it doesn't take long for your body to start to heal and for your risk of developing other health problems to decrease.

See pages 25 to 28 to learn more about the benefits of quitting, and how to do it.

Use Alcohol and Drugs Wisely

Alcohol and drug use can be very hard on your body. Alcohol, in particular, increases your risk for accidents and injuries by impairing your mental alertness, judgment, memory, and physical coordination. What's more, many of the prescription and non-prescription medications that older adults take increase the intoxicating effect of alcohol.

Long-term overuse of alcohol increases your risk for many illnesses, including liver disease, high blood pressure, and certain cancers. It can also put your relationships and livelihood in jeopardy.

Limit your consumption of alcoholic beverages to no more than one drink per day. One drink equals 360 ml (12 fl oz) of beer, 150 ml (5 fl oz) of wine, or 44 ml (1.5 fl oz) of hard liquor.

Never use prescription or non-prescription medications along with alcohol.

Many medications, even as they are doing good, also have some risks. Go over your list of medications with your doctor regularly. Review all the prescription and non-prescription medications you take, and determine whether they are necessary. However, don't stop taking a medication unless your doctor tells you it is all right to do so.

If problematic substance use affects you or someone close to you, now is the time to seek help. For more information about alcohol and drug problems, see page 366.

Keep Up With Shots and Screenings

Immunizations provide protection against many serious diseases. Chances are, you have been immunized against the major childhood illnesses, or you are immune because you had the diseases when you were a child.

However, there are several immunizations that need to be updated throughout your life or given for the first time later in life. If your doctor does not suggest them to you, make a note to mention them at your next visit.

Tetanus

Tetanus (lockjaw) is a bacterial infection that can be fatal. The bacteria enter the body through a deep cut or puncture wound. The only sure protection against tetanus is immunization. Many cases of tetanus occur in adults over age 50 who have forgotten to keep their tetanus immunizations up to date.

Routine boosters are recommended every 10 years throughout your life to maintain immunity. If you are age 50 or older and have not had boosters every 10 years, now is a good time to talk to your doctor about updating your tetanus boosters. If you suffer a puncture wound or deep cut, get a booster shot if you haven't had one in the past 5 years.

Influenza

Older people are more likely to develop complications of influenza (flu), such as pneumonia and dehydration.

To protect yourself, get a flu shot each autumn if any one of the following applies to you:

- You are age 65 or older.
- You have a chronic lung disease, such as asthma or emphysema.
- You have heart disease.
- You have diabetes.
- You have sickle cell anemia or another red blood cell disorder.
- You have an illness that has weakened your immune system or are taking medication that weakens the immune system.
- You have frequent contact with people who could develop complications if they caught the flu from you (for example, nursing home residents, people over age 65, and people who have weakened immune systems).
- You want to reduce your risk of getting the flu.

Side effects of the flu shot, such as a low-grade fever and minor aches, are usually mild and do not last long. Don't get a flu shot if you are allergic to eggs: the virus in the vaccine is grown in eggs, and you may develop an allergic reaction.

Pneumococcal Infection

Most people think of pneumococci as the bacteria that cause pneumonia, but pneumococci can also infect the blood (bacteremia) or the covering of the brain (meningitis). Older people have a higher risk than younger people of developing pneumonia and other pneumococcal infections.

A one-time-only dose of the pneumococcal vaccine is recommended for people age 65 and older. You can get the pneumococcal vaccine at the same time as your yearly flu shot. Get a pneumococcal vaccine if:

- You are healthy, over 65, and have never received the shot.
- You have a chronic illness, such as cancer, an immune system disorder, diabetes, or heart, lung, or kidney disease.

If you received the pneumococcal vaccine before age 65 and it has been more than 5 years since you last had the shot, ask your doctor if you need a booster shot.

Side effects of the shot often include mild swelling and pain at the injection site.

Other Immunizations

Contact your local public health unit to find out which other immunizations you need. Immunization may be needed in certain disease outbreak situations or for international travel.

Periodic Medical Examinations and Screening Tests

Another way to protect your health is to detect diseases early, when they may be easier to treat. You can do this in two ways: by getting periodic medical examinations from a health professional and by becoming a good observer of changes in your own body.

The Health Screening Schedule for Older Adults on pages 38 and 39 will help you decide which tests are right for you and how often you should have them. Recommended immunizations are also listed. The recommendations apply to people of average risk in each age group. If you are at high risk for certain diseases, you may need more frequent examinations and tests. Factors that may help your doctor determine your level of risk include your overall health, your family history (whether your close relatives have had certain diseases), and lifestyle factors, such as whether you use tobacco, how often you exercise, and your sexual history.

The most appropriate schedule of preventive examinations is one you and your doctor agree upon, based on your age, your risk factors for disease, how healthy you are, and how important periodic health screening is to you.

Practise Safety

Accidents do happen, but they don't have to happen to you. Many older adults are injured in car accidents, fires, and falls. Follow these safety precautions to reduce the risk of fire in your home and to make the roads safer for you and your fellow drivers.

For tips on preventing falls, see page 80.

Health Screening Schedule for Older Adults

Recommended Time Intervals Between Preventive Services
(For more information about this chart, see Periodic Medical Examinations and Screening Tests starting on page 37.)

Preventive Service	Age 50–64	Age 65+	Comments
Blood pressure, p. 290	1–2 years	1–2 years	More often if your blood pressure is high.
Cholesterol, p. 292	5 years	5 years	More often if you have risk factors for heart disease (see p. 292). Talk with your doctor about screening after age 65 even if your cholesterol levels have been normal.
Colorectal cancer screening, p. 131			Screening may involve one or more of these tests. Talk with your doctor about which tests and screening schedules are most appropriate for you. More frequent screening with flexible sigmoidoscopy or colonoscopy is recommended if you have risk factors for colorectal cancer (see p. 131).
• Blood in stool test (fecal occult blood test)	1 year	1 year	
• Flexible sigmoidoscopy	3–5 years	3–5 years	
• Colonoscopy	10 years (5 if high-risk)	10 years (5 if high-risk)	
Hearing test	Assess during other regular visits.		
Vision test	2–5 years	1–2 years	More often for people who have eye diseases or diabetes.
Glaucoma test	Usually done as part of regular eye examinations.		
Dental examination	6 months	6 months	
Men Only			
Prostate cancer screening, p. 325	1 year	1 year	May include digital rectal examination (DRE) or prostate-specific antigen (PSA) test. Talk with your doctor to determine whether screening is appropriate for you.

Health Screening Schedule for Older Adults

Recommended Time Intervals Between Preventive Services
(For more information about this chart, see Periodic Medical Examinations and Screening Tests starting on page 37.)

Preventive Service	Age 50–64	Age 65+	Comments
Women Only			
Clinical breast examination, p. 299	1–2 years	1–2 years	Discuss appropriate frequency with your doctor.
Mammogram, p. 297	1–2 years	1–2 years	Discuss appropriate frequency and whether to discontinue the examination after age 70 with your doctor.
Pelvic examination, p. 302	1 year	1 year	
Pap test, p. 302	1–3 years	1–3 years	May discontinue after age 65 if prior examinations were normal and you have no significant risk factors for cervical cancer. If you have had a hysterectomy, talk to your doctor about whether and how often you need a Pap test.
Immunizations			
Tetanus booster, p. 17	10 years	10 years	Recommended after 5 years if you get a deep, dirty wound or bite.
Flu shot, p. 19	1 year	1 year	Given in fall. Recommended before age 65 if you have chronic lung disease, heart disease, diabetes, or an impaired immune system.
Pneumococcal vaccine, p. 19		Once	Recommended before age 65 if high-risk. Booster may be needed if high-risk.

Fire Safety

- Post emergency telephone numbers near telephones.
- Have an emergency exit plan in case of fire. Practise the plan.
- Install smoke detectors in or near every bedroom and on every level of your home. Test the alarms once a month, and change the batteries at least once a year.
- Keep multi-purpose fire extinguishers in the kitchen and near fireplaces or woodstoves. Shake the extinguisher once a month to make sure the chemicals don't settle to the bottom. Have the extinguisher inspected yearly. Practise using the fire extinguisher in a non-emergency situation, and have it recharged after you use it.
- Turn off appliances after use. Replace frayed or damaged electrical cords on appliances.
- Don't run electrical cords under rugs or furniture. Keep cords away from bathtubs, showers, and sinks.
- Install special safety outlets in your bathroom. Ask for a ground fault circuit interrupter.
- Never smoke in bed or when you are sleepy.
- Don't tuck in electric blankets, and don't cover them with other blankets. Turn the temperature down before you go to bed.
- Avoid using electric, kerosene, and propane heaters. If you must use them, keep them away from curtains, rugs, and furniture.
- Clean woodstove and fireplace chimneys at least once a year.
- Keep objects such as kitchen towels and paper wrappers away from the stove top. Roll up loose long sleeves when cooking.
- Select a stove with controls that clearly show when the burners are on.
- If your clothing catches fire:
  - Do not run, because running will fan the flames. Stop, drop, and roll on the ground to smother the flames. Or, you can smother the flames with a blanket, rug, or coat.
  - Use water to douse the fire and cool your skin.

Automobile Safety

- Always wear a seat belt, especially if your car has air bags.
- Never drink and drive.
- Check with your doctor or pharmacist about driving while on medications, especially if you take insulin or an oral diabetes medication. Medications, including some non-prescription drugs, can cause dizziness, drowsiness, impaired judgment, and balance problems.
- Be sure that your car is properly tuned and equipped with emergency supplies.
- Consider updating your driving skills by taking a driver's safety course.

- Have your vision checked regularly, and always wear prescription eyewear when driving.
- Wear high-quality sunglasses to reduce glare.
- If your night vision is limited, don't drive at night.
- If your hearing is limited, keep a window open and the radio volume low.

Stay Mentally Active

The "use it or lose it" approach definitely applies to brain power. Memory loss and decreased mental function are not inevitable aspects of aging. The brain benefits from exposure to stimulating environments and activities, and this stimulation can help you retain your memory and stay sharp.

Learn something new every day. Take classes or read books about new subjects. Read, write, talk, and think about what interests you.

Nurture the Ties That Bind

People who have many social ties are healthier than people with few social connections. Examples of social ties are being married, having contact with friends and relatives, belonging to a church or social group, and volunteering to help others.

Create a support network of family and friends who will help see you through a crisis. Find a friend you can confide in. Be a confidant for someone else.

Combine physical and social health by joining a walking group or exercise class.

Know Where Your Help Is

The best way to stay independent is to know when to ask for help. Become familiar with your community's support services for seniors, such as transportation, financial counselling, and Meals on Wheels. Contact your local health authority for information on available services.

Accentuate the Positive

The pictures we have in our minds and the verbal messages or self-talk we give ourselves affect both our minds and bodies.

Expect good things to happen. Count your blessings and express thanks. Add humour, laughter, and fun into every day. Also see Mental Health, Addictions, and Mind-Body Wellness starting on page 365.

Celebrate Your Wisdom

Victor Hugo said, "One sees a flame in the eyes of the young, but in the eyes of the old, one sees light." More than anything else, the world needs wisdom. Recognize your purpose for living. Think about your values and beliefs. Help others to gain wisdom too. Consider becoming a mentor. You could be the one to make all the difference in the world to someone else.

Caregiver Tips

Many people are caring for a chronically ill or disabled spouse, parent, or other family member. Caregiving can be a rewarding experience, especially when you know that your care makes a positive difference. However, caregiving can be difficult. There are three keys to being a good caregiver:

- Take care of yourself first.
- Don't help too much.
- Don't do it alone.

This section will tell you more about these tips and how they can help you and the person you are caring for.

Caregiver Tip No. 1: Take Care of Yourself First

If you want to give good care, you have to take care of yourself first. Caregivers tend to deny their own needs. This strategy may work fine for short-term caregiving. For long-term caregiving, however, it is sure to lead to problems.

Several things happen when caregivers don't take good care of themselves:

- They become ill.
- They become depressed.
- They "burn out" and stop providing care altogether.

These things are bad for both the caregiver and the person receiving the care.

Planning for Caregiving

- Learn as much as you can about the person's illness. Talk to his or her health care providers and find out how the illness may progress, how it is being treated, and what the expected results of treatment are. Know what medications the person is taking, what side effects to expect, and whether he or she has any drug allergies. Find out what kind of problems might come up and what additional health care services might be needed (for example, home nursing, hospitalization, or residential care facility).
- Work with the person's case manager or a social worker to review his or her financial situation. If financial assistance may be needed to pay for long-term care expenses, find out how and when to apply for such assistance. Find out about Power of Attorney and Representation Agreements for yourself and your family member so that you can manage his or her finances and ensure his or her health care decisions are respected.
- Talk to your family member about his or her after-death wishes. Does he or she want a funeral or memorial service? To be buried or cremated? Does he or she own a burial plot? Has money been set aside for these expenses? If not, it may be possible for you to establish a fund for these needs. Discuss this matter with a funeral director.

On the other hand, when caregivers take time to care for themselves, good things happen:

- They avoid health problems.
- They feel better about themselves.
- They have more energy and enthusiasm for helping others and can continue giving care.

When you take on the task of caregiving, time becomes your most important resource. Caregiving requires a large time commitment, perhaps all of the extra time you have for yourself. If that happens, problems can develop.

The best way to prevent the depression, frustration, and resentment that cause caregiver burnout is to hold back some time out of every day for yourself. If you wait until all of your chores and caregiving tasks are done before doing things for yourself, you will wait a very long time. Instead, decide on the minimum amount of time you need each day to meet your basic personal needs. Carve that time out of your schedule. Then figure out how the chores will get done.

Elder Abuse and Neglect

Abuse and neglect of an older adult may include any or all of the following:

- Physical or sexual abuse. This may include hitting, shaking, shoving, pinching, or burning a person, or performing sexual acts with the person without his or her consent.
- Psychological abuse. This may include verbal assault, threats, intimidation, humiliation, harassment, or isolating the person from his or her family, friends, or usual activities.
- Financial exploitation. This may include the improper or illegal use of a person's funds, assets, or properties without the person's consent.
- Abandonment of an older adult by his or her caregivers.
- Self-neglect. This occurs when an older person's behaviour threatens his or her own health and safety.

The reasons why elder abuse and neglect occur are complex. The overwhelming amount of stress that comes with taking care of an older person—especially one who has severe health problems—is often a factor. Elder abuse is committed most often by family members, although it can occur at the hands of hired caregivers and employees of care facilities.

If you suspect elder abuse or neglect, contact the Home and Community Care office of your local health authority.

Here are some important things that you need to find time to do—just for yourself:

1. Get regular exercise, even just a few minutes several times a day. Exercise can be a good energizer for both physical and emotional health.

2. Maintain a healthy diet. When you are busy giving care, it may seem easier to eat fast food than to prepare healthy, low-fat meals. However, healthy meals are easy to prepare, and a good diet will give you more energy to carry you through each day.

3. Make time for an activity you enjoy—reading, listening to music, painting or doing crafts, playing an instrument—even if you can only do it for a few minutes each day. If you like to participate in church activities or take classes, ask a friend or another family member to stay with the person in your care for an hour or two once or twice a week so you can do those things.

4. Recognize stress and take steps to manage it. Your need for relaxation increases during periods of caregiving. For more information about recognizing and managing stress, see Stress and Distress on page 384.

5. Recognize and deal with signs of depression. Depression is common in caregivers. Maintaining a positive self-image is the most important thing you can do for yourself. Use self-care and ask for extra support when the earliest signs of depression appear. If that doesn't work, seek professional help. Also be on the lookout for signs of depression in the person you are caring for. Depression is common in older adults, especially those who have chronic diseases or who are disabled. Encouraging the person to seek treatment for depression will make your job easier in the long run. See Depression on page 372.

6. Deal with important issues in your life and maintain supportive relationships. Being a caregiver adds another dimension to your life, but it does not mean you have to put the rest of your life on hold. Issues involving your family and other relationships, your finances, your job, and other responsibilities still need to be addressed. Taking time to deal with issues as they arise and planning for the future are an important part of taking care of yourself. Make a conscious effort every day to stay connected with family, friends, and others in your support system.

7. Let go of guilt. The best way to let go of guilt is to accept the fact that you just can't be everything to everyone all of the time. Acknowledge your limitations, and do only what is most important. Tell yourself that you are doing a good job at a very difficult task, and ask for help. Feeling guilty is often a sign that you need a break from your caregiving schedule. Ask your friends and family to pitch in.

Your Rights as a Caregiver

As a caregiver you have the right:

- To take care of yourself. This is not an act of selfishness. It will allow you to take better care of your family member.
- To seek help from others even though your family member may object. Recognize the limits of your endurance and strength.
- To maintain parts of your life that do not include the person you care for, just as you would if he or she were healthy.
- To get angry, be depressed, and express other difficult feelings occasionally.
- To reject any person's attempt (either conscious or unconscious) to manipulate you through guilt, anger, or depression.
- To receive consideration, affection, forgiveness, and acceptance from your family member as long as you offer these qualities in return.
- To take pride in what you are accomplishing and to applaud your courage in the sometimes difficult task of caregiving.
- To protect your individuality and make a life for yourself that will sustain you when your relative no longer needs your full-time help.
- To expect and demand that as new strides are made in finding resources to aid people with physical or mental disability, similar strides will be made toward aiding and supporting caregivers.

Adapted from the AARP's "Caregiver's Bill of Rights."

Caregiver Tip No. 2: Don't Help Too Much

The biggest mistake most caregivers make is providing too much care. Even if they don't admit it, people like to help themselves. Every time you do something for a person that the person could have done alone, there is a double loss. First, your effort may have been wasted. Second, the person has missed an opportunity to help him- or herself.

As a caregiver, your highest goal is to give the person you are caring for the power and the permission to be in control of his or her own life (as much as possible). Every act your family member or friend makes to maintain independence is a victory for you as a caregiver.

Here are some things you can do to empower the person you are caring for to do things independently:

1. Expect more. People respond to expectations. If you expect the person to get dressed, care for house-plants, or prepare simple meals, the person often will.

2. Limit your availability to help. If you are not always there to help, the person will be forced to do more on his or her own.

3. Simplify. If you are caring for a person who has mild dementia, divide complex tasks into simpler parts for him or her: first, get out the cereal box; next, get out the milk and the bowl, etc.

4. Make it easy. One of the most productive things a caregiver can do is to make modifications to the person's home and provide tools that will allow the person to do things without help.

5. Allow for mistakes and less-than-perfect results. The hardest thing about letting someone do something alone is knowing that you could do it better or faster. Mistakes are okay.

6. Reward both the effort and the result. Help the person feel good about doing things independently.

7. Let the person make as many decisions as possible, such as what to wear, what to eat, or when to go to bed. Help the person retain as much control as possible.

8. Give the person responsibility to care for something. Studies show that nursing home residents who are asked to care for pets or plants live longer and become more independent.

9. Match tasks with abilities. Identify the person's skills, and try to match them with tasks that the person can do independently.

10. Take acceptable risks. A few broken dishes or a few bruises are a small price to pay for letting someone explore what he or she can do. You can't eliminate all risks without eliminating all opportunities.

Caregiver Needs for Respite

If you can answer yes to any of the following questions, it's time to get more help.

- Do I feel overworked and exhausted?
- Do I feel dissatisfied with myself?
- Do I feel isolated?
- Do I feel depressed, resentful, angry, or worried?
- Do I feel that I have no time for myself?
- Do I lack time for exercise and rest?
- Do I lack time for fun with people outside of my family?

Caregiver Tip No. 3: Don't Do It Alone

Some caregivers live under the impression that they are the only available source of help. However, there are often other sources of assistance available that can make your caregiving easier. If you want to be a good caregiver, know where to find help when you need it. The more support you have, the more successful you are likely to be. Examples of services that may be useful to caregivers are discussed in this section.

Respite care may be the most important service for caregivers. Respite services provide someone who will stay with the person so you can take a break for a few hours. If the person you are caring for needs routine medical and nursing care, you may be able to arrange to have the person stay in a residential care facility for a few days while you get away for a break.

Adult day centres are "drop-off" sites where a person who does not need individual supervision can stay during the day. This service is usually offered during working hours and may or may not be available on weekends. Meals, personal and health care services, and social activities are provided.

Adult group homes are private homes where older adults receive around-the-clock personal care, supervision, and meals. BC requires group homes serving more than three adults to be licensed.

Family care homes are single-family residences that provide supportive accommodation for up to two people. A family care home can be an alternative to a care facility for some individals.

Residential care facilities provide 24-hour professional nursing care and supervision in a protective, supportive environment for people who have complex care needs and can no longer be cared for in their own homes. Some facilities have special units for people with dementia.

End-of-life care programs provide social, personal, nursing, medical, and other professional services for people nearing end of life who wish to spend their remaining time at home or in a less formal environment than that of a hospital or residential care facility.

Hospice is a residential home-like setting where supportive and professional care services are provided for people of any age who are in the end stages of an illness or preparing for death.

Support groups give you an opportunity to discuss problems or concerns about caregiving with other caregivers.

Ten Ways to Make Extra Time for Yourself

Five Ways That Don't Cost Money

- Trade one morning or afternoon "off" each week with another caregiver.
- Ask several relatives, friends, church members, or neighbours if each would relieve you for a few hours per week on a regular schedule.
- Sign up for respite services. Some are available for no cost or for a voluntary donation.
- Barter for services: offer a loaf of bread, a casserole, or errands in exchange for an hour of care.
- Plan some time each day to be alone, perhaps during a time when the person you care for doesn't need your attention.

Five Ways That Can Cost Money

- Hire a teenager or older adult to stay with the person for a few hours each day.
- Sign up for homemaker or chore services. By saving a few hours of housekeeping, you might have more time and energy for more important caregiving tasks.
- Sign up for a home-delivered meal service.
- Enroll the person in an adult day centre. Even a part-time placement for several hours per week can be helpful to both you and the person you are caring for.
- Hire a home support worker or personal care assistant.

How to Access Caregiver Services

There are two provincial gateways to caregiver information and services in British Columbia.

- The Home and Community Care office of your local Community Health Centre offers access to services provided by the Medical Services Plan. In most cases, an intake worker will arrange to visit you at your home to discuss your situation and help identify which services you need. Then a case manager will work with you and your family member to make any needed referrals and set up the services. Call your local Community Health Centre for more information. Also see page 422.
- The Caregivers Association of BC (CABC), a non-profit organization, provides information, referrals, and support for family caregivers in BC. You can contact the CABC toll-free at 1-800-833-1733, or the BC NurseLine.

Take Pride

Now that you know the three keys to caregiving, you can see that there is nothing magical or mysterious about being a good caregiver.

- Care for your own needs first. Your physical and mental health depend on it. Give yourself as much special attention as you give the person you are caring for.
- Help the person you care for to be independent. This is a gift to both of you.
- Recognize when you need extra help, and know where you can get it. A helping hand at the right time can make all the difference.

Take pride in being a caregiver. It is not easy, and those who do it are special people. Using these tips for caregiving can help you feel good about yourself and the care you give.

Home and Community Care

Home and Community Care services provide a range of health care and support services for eligible residents who have acute, chronic, palliative, or rehabilitative health care needs. These services are designed to complement and supplement, but not replace, the efforts of individuals to care for themselves with the help of family, friends, and community.

In-home services for eligible individuals include home care nursing, community rehabilitation, home support (including a self-managed option), and palliative care. Community-based services include adult day programs, meal programs, assisted living, residential care services, and hospice care. Case management services are also provided.

Home and Community Care:

- Helps people remain independent and in their own homes for as long as possible.
- Provides services at home to people who would otherwise require admission to hospital or would stay longer in hospital.
- Provides assisted living and residential care services to those who can no longer be supported in their homes.
- Helps support people who are nearing the end of life, and their families, at home or in a hospice.

To learn more about Home and Community Care in BC, contact your local health authority.

Hope for the best, and prepare for the worst.
Common sense

4

Disasters and Public Health Threats

Earthquakes, slides, pandemic flu and other disease outbreaks, and accidents or exposures involving hazardous substances are real or potential health threats to individuals and communities. They can affect air quality, cause shortages of safe water and food, and cut off your access to electricity, gas, telephone, medications, and other services. Family members may be separated. Hospitals and other health services may be overwhelmed during public health emergencies. While such incidents are difficult to prepare for, there are steps you can take to protect your health and well-being.

So, what can you do to be prepared?

1. Learn how specific public health threats might affect you and what you can do to reduce the risk to your health and safety. This chapter explains how harmful bacteria and viruses, dangerous chemicals, and other health hazards can spread through a community and how you can limit your exposure to them.

2. Create an emergency plan and supplies kit to provide for yourself and your family during a community emergency. See Get Organized on page 56.

3. Always refer to local authorities and health experts for specific, up-to-date information for your community. Follow their advice, even if it differs from this book. You can also rely on the BC Centre for Disease Control (www.bccdc.org), the BC NurseLine (see phone numbers on the back cover), and the World Health Organization (www.who.int/en) for current information about specific health emergencies.

We hope this information helps you feel better prepared for any type of natural disaster or public health emergency that you may face.

Emergency Food and Water Supplies

Having a supply of food and water can be helpful in any kind of extended emergency. If you are unable to leave your home, if the local water supply becomes contaminated, or if access to food and water is limited or unavailable, your family may be able to live on emergency supplies until the emergency has passed.

The question of how long you should plan for your supplies to last does not have an easy answer. It's impractical for most people to maintain large reserves of food and water, and it's unlikely that you will ever need them. Having a short-term supply, however, may make sense. The Red Cross recommends that you have enough food and water to last from several days to 2 weeks.

Water is the most important part of any emergency supplies kit. Without it, your body will not be able to function. Most people need to drink about 2 litres of water per day. Including the water needed for hygiene and cooking as well as drinking, a reasonable guideline is to store 4 litres of water per person per day. So, a family of 4 that wanted to keep a 1-week supply of water on hand would need to store 112 litres (4 litres per day per person, times 4 people, times 7 days). A 3-day supply for 4 people would be 48 litres.

Remember that water and most food supplies have to be replaced periodically.

- Replace bottled water that has remained sealed and unopened once a year.
- Replace water that you have opened or filled yourself every 6 months.
- Visit the Web site of the Red Cross (www.redcross.org) for information on how often to replace food supplies. Some may need replacing every few months; others may remain safe to eat for much longer.

Health Threats in Your Community

Chemicals, fumes, viruses, bacteria, low-level radiation, and other potentially harmful substances are common in the environment. When these substances are released in large quantities or get out of our control, they can become immediate public health threats. Guidelines for how to prepare for and avoid a problem often depend on how the particular agent is spread.

In general, a health threat may spread through a community:

- Through the air.
- Through the water supply or through food.
- From human to human.
- From animal or insect to human.

Air Contamination

Chemicals are the most likely source of air contamination. An accident at a plant or factory might release large amounts of a hazardous chemical into the air, for instance. If bacteria or viruses causing diseases such as anthrax, pneumonic plague, smallpox, or tularemia were released in an aerosol form, anyone who inhaled the substance could be affected.

While air itself does not become radioactive, release of radiation into the environment can create radioactive dust and dirt (fallout) that can make the air unsafe.

What to do

If a hazardous substance is released into the environment:

- Get out of the immediate area if possible. If the release has occurred outdoors, go inside; if it has occurred indoors, go outside. Move out of low-lying spots to higher ground—most chemicals released into the environment are heavier than air and will sink.
- Tune in to a local radio or TV station for instructions from public health and emergency officials. (Phone lines are likely to be overwhelmed during a public health emergency, so do not try to call for instructions.) Depending on the kind of release, authorities may advise you to shelter in place (see page 57), or simply to stay indoors. You do not need to leave your community unless local authorities tell you to.
- If you are directly exposed to radioactive dust, dirt, or other fallout, follow the steps for personal decontamination on page 58.
- Do not take potassium iodide (KI) pills unless local authorities tell you to. These pills are effective against radioactive iodine only, and they can be harmful if taken improperly.

Water and Food Contamination

Chemicals, heavy metals like lead and mercury, and living organisms such as bacteria and viruses can all be threats to a safe water supply. These substances can also contaminate food.

Unintentional contamination of water as a result of chemical leaks or spills, natural disasters, and other causes has been a much bigger problem than deliberate contamination. Likewise, accidental food contamination by botulinum toxin (the agent that causes botulism), *E. coli*, and other harmful organisms during the storage or preparation of food is much more likely than intentional food poisoning.

How to prepare

With the exception of a known accident (such as a chemical spill into the water supply), you probably would not know you had consumed contaminated water or food unless you developed symptoms.

To reduce your risk of consuming contaminated food or water and to be better prepared for public health emergencies affecting the water supply:

- Don't eat food or drink water or any other beverage that looks or smells suspicious. In general, it's not a good idea to eat or drink something when you don't know who has prepared or provided it or where it has come from.
- When shopping, avoid food or beverage items that look like they may have been tampered with—for instance, if the seal is broken or you suspect the container may have been opened.
- Remember that most cases of food poisoning happen by accident. See the prevention tips in Food Poisoning on page 133.
- Know generally where your household water comes from. Is it from the city water supply? Most public water supplies are carefully monitored and treated to guard against contamination. Does a private well supply your water? Private water supplies are unlikely to be targets of intentional contamination, but they can become contaminated accidentally and may not be as closely monitored as city water supplies.
- Consider storing emergency water and food supplies. See page 52.
- Learn how to purify water, and make sure you include the supplies it requires in your emergency kit. See Safe Drinking Water on page 55. Knowing how to purify water is useful in any situation where you have to rely on untreated water.

What to do

If there is an emergency affecting the water supply:

- Follow all instructions from local authorities about purifying your water (commonly called "boil orders") or using other water sources. Authorities will notify your community when it is safe to drink from the regular water supply again.
- Do not strictly ration emergency drinking water supplies. Try not to waste any water, but drink what you need. On average a person needs about 2 litres of water a day. (Individual water needs vary depending on age, health, diet, and climate.) Learn the signs of dehydration in children and adults so you know what to watch for. See Dehydration on page 118.
- Use the safest water you have first before turning to other water sources.
- If you know or suspect that your skin has come in direct contact with water that has been contaminated by a hazardous chemical or radiation fallout, follow the steps for personal decontamination on page 58.

Safe Drinking Water

Having water that is safe to drink is essential to your health and survival during a long emergency. Knowing how to purify water can help you if your regular water supply becomes contaminated or if you are in a place where clean water is not available. Even if you have stored clean water to use in an emergency, you may run out before the emergency situation has ended.

Water purification can greatly reduce your chance of getting sick from bacteria, viruses, and other living organisms in the water. You can disinfect water using one of the following methods:

- Boil the water for 3 to 5 minutes. This is the most effective purification method but may be impractical if you need large quantities of water. It also requires a heat source, which may not be available in some emergency situations.
- Use an eyedropper to add 4 drops of household liquid bleach per litre of water. Stir, and let it stand for 30 minutes. If the water does not smell slightly like bleach after 30 minutes, add 4 more drops of bleach and let it stand for another 15 minutes. You should notice a bleach smell.
- Use iodine or chlorine purification tablets or drops. These are available at stores that sell camping equipment and at some drugstores. Follow the instructions on the package. Purification tablets are not as effective as boiling or disinfecting with bleach, but they do eliminate some types of organisms.
- Water filters can get rid of some micro-organisms and improve the taste of water. There are many different types of filters, so be sure you know which organisms your filter can remove.

None of the purification methods described above eliminates heavy metals, salts, chemicals, or radioactive dust or dirt (fallout) from water. Many of these substances can be removed by distilling water, a more complicated method of purifying water. Radioactive fallout can also be minimized using a homemade filter:

1. Punch holes in the bottom of a bucket, and cover the bottom with 4 cm of gravel. Cover the gravel with a towel.

2. Place the bucket over a larger container, and pour the water into the bucket so that it filters through the towel and gravel and drains into the container below.

3. Disinfect the water by boiling, adding chlorine bleach, or using purification tablets as described above.

4. Replace the gravel after every 50 litres of water.

Disease Transmission from Humans, Animals, and Insects

Some bacteria, viruses, and other biological agents can be spread from person to person, or from animals or insects to people. The ease of international travel has made many of these health threats more difficult to contain. Recent health threats such as SARS (severe acute respiratory syndrome), the West Nile virus, and monkeypox have made people more aware of how easily disease can spread not just within a community but from one community to the next.

The BC Centre for Disease Control and the World Health Organization have current, reliable information on communicable diseases and health concerns throughout the world. Visit their Web sites at www.bccdc.org and www.who.int/en for updates on specific health emergencies.

What to do

To reduce your chances of being infected with or spreading a contagious disease:

- Wash your hands with soap and water frequently.
- Do not share bedding, towels, utensils, or other items with someone who is sick. If you are sick, do not share these items with anyone else.
- Avoid exposure to disease-carrying animals and insects if you are in an area where these are a problem. Use DEET to reduce insect bites (see page 209).
- Follow the advice of local health authorities if there has been a disease outbreak in your community or in an area where you are travelling. It is especially important to follow health experts' instructions if you live or work with someone who becomes sick. For instance, you may be advised to wear a properly fitted surgical mask if you are in close contact with someone who has a serious contagious illness.
- If there is an outbreak of a contagious disease in your area, do not leave the area unless authorities tell you to. If you have already been infected, you could spread the disease. Leaving the area may also cause a delay in your diagnosis or treatment.

Get Organized

A little organization can go a long way toward helping you feel ready to handle the unexpected. Having an emergency plan and an emergency supplies kit for your household can help you and your family be better prepared for any kind of disaster.

Develop an emergency plan

Putting together an emergency plan is easy:

- Choose a friend or relative as a contact person for family members to call if they are separated during a disaster. It is best to choose an out-of-province contact. Make sure every member of your household has the contact's phone number. E-mail may also be a good way to get in touch.

- Pick a place to meet outside your neighbourhood in case you cannot return home. Make sure every member of your household has the address and phone number. Also designate a place to meet just outside your home—a neighbour's front yard, for instance—in case there is a fire in your home.
- Write down where and how to turn off the water, gas, and electricity to the house. Make sure you have any special tools this requires.
- Discuss what you would do if you had to leave your home and the area. Include your pets in your plans. Most emergency shelters and health facilities will not accept animals.

You may have other things you want to include in your plan, especially if you have children in school or if anyone in your household has special needs. Review your plan yearly, and make sure that phone numbers, e-mail addresses, and other items are still current.

Assemble an emergency supplies kit

The essentials of an emergency kit are the same no matter what the situation: water, food, first aid supplies and medications, blankets and clothing, special needs items (such as baby formula), and certain tools and household items, including a battery-powered radio, a flashlight, and extra batteries.

Sheltering in Place

In many types of public health emergencies, the safest thing to do is simply to stay indoors. If the air is unsafe because of hazardous chemicals, radiation, or an aerosol release of a biological agent, local authorities may advise you to "shelter in place," which limits your exposure to the outside air. To shelter in place:

1. Make sure all family members and pets that are at home are inside. Then close and lock all doors and windows.

2. Turn off air conditioners, fans, and furnaces. Close vents and fireplace dampers.

3. Move to an inner room, preferably at or above ground level and without windows. (If the incident involves radiation, authorities may tell you to take shelter in a basement.) If you have an emergency supplies kit, take it with you. At the very least, make sure you have a battery-powered radio and plenty of drinking water.

4. If local authorities advise you to do so, use duct tape to secure plastic sheeting around door and window frames.

5. Stay tuned in to the local news, and stay inside until local authorities say that it is safe to come out.

Use the checklist on page 59 as you gather supplies. Store everything in one place, preferably a cool, dark location. Consider putting together a smaller version of your emergency kit that you could take if you had to leave your home.

Once you've assembled your emergency supplies, remember to check and replace them periodically:

- Bottled water that has remained sealed and unopened needs to be replaced once a year. Water in containers that you filled yourself or have opened needs to be replaced every 6 months.
- Follow Red Cross guidelines (www.redcross.org) on how often to replace food supplies. Even "non-perishable" items may need to be replaced occasionally.
- Remember that both non-prescription and prescription medications have expiration dates.

Personal Decontamination

Your skin can be contaminated by contact with dangerous chemicals, including some common household and lawn products; biological agents such as anthrax powder; or dust, dirt, or other substances that contain radioactive fallout. In many cases, immediately removing all traces of the harmful substance from your skin can minimize any damage.

Watering or burning eyes and stinging or burning skin are signs that you may have been exposed to something harmful. If you know or suspect a hazardous exposure has occurred, take immediate action:

1. Remove clothing, jewellery, eyeglasses, and other items that have come in contact with the substance. Seal the items in a plastic bag.

2. If you wear contact lenses, wash your hands with soap and water, and then remove your contacts.

3. Use soap and water to wash any areas of your skin that may have been contaminated—in some cases this may mean your whole body. A shower works best, but you can also use water from a faucet, a garden hose, or another source. Flush eyes with lots of water. A faucet with a hand-held sprayer works well.

4. Call Poison Control or emergency services to find out what to do next. Further medical assistance may or may not be necessary.

These are general guidelines for removing contaminants and are appropriate for many—but not all—hazardous substance exposures. Poison Control or other local authorities may have more specific instructions for you depending on what you were exposed to.

Disaster Supplies Checklist

Use this checklist to prepare a disaster supplies kit for your household. Remember to replace water, food, batteries, medications, outgrown clothing, and other items periodically. Visit the Web site of the Red Cross at www.redcross.org for more information.

Water

- ❑ 4 litres of water per person per day

Food

- ❑ Ready-to-eat canned meats, fruits, and vegetables
- ❑ Canned juices, milk, and soup (if powdered, store extra water)
- ❑ Sugar, salt, pepper, and other staples
- ❑ High-energy foods (peanut butter and jelly, crackers, granola bars)
- ❑ Vitamins
- ❑ Comfort foods (cookies, hard candy, instant coffee, tea bags)

First aid kit

- ❑ Adhesive bandages, gauze pads, and tape
- ❑ Scissors
- ❑ Safety pins
- ❑ Tweezers
- ❑ Cold pack
- ❑ Moist towelettes
- ❑ Antiseptic
- ❑ Thermometer
- ❑ Tube of petroleum jelly or other lubricant
- ❑ Soap or cleanser
- ❑ Latex gloves
- ❑ Sunscreen
- ❑ Non-prescription drugs (Aspirin and non-Aspirin pain relievers, antidiarrheals, antacids, laxatives)
- ❑ Activated charcoal (for use if advised by Poison Control Centre)

Clothing and bedding (per person)

- ❑ Sturdy shoes or work boots
- ❑ Rain gear
- ❑ Blankets or sleeping bag
- ❑ Hat and gloves
- ❑ Thermal underwear
- ❑ Sunglasses

Tools and supplies

- ❑ Battery-operated radio and extra batteries
- ❑ Flashlight and extra batteries
- ❑ Mess kits, or paper cups and plates and plastic utensils
- ❑ Emergency preparedness manual
- ❑ Cash or traveller's cheques, change
- ❑ Non-electric can opener or utility knife
- ❑ Fire extinguisher
- ❑ Pliers
- ❑ Duct tape
- ❑ Compass
- ❑ Matches in a waterproof container
- ❑ Aluminum foil
- ❑ Plastic storage containers, bags, and sheeting
- ❑ Signal flare
- ❑ Paper and pencils
- ❑ Needles and thread
- ❑ Medicine dropper
- ❑ Shut-off wrench to turn off household gas and water
- ❑ Whistle
- ❑ Map of the area

Sanitation

- ❑ Toilet paper and towelettes
- ❑ Soap and liquid detergent
- ❑ Feminine supplies
- ❑ Personal hygiene items
- ❑ Plastic garbage bags and ties
- ❑ Plastic bucket with tight lid
- ❑ Disinfectant
- ❑ Household bleach

Family documents (stored in a waterproof, portable container)

- ❑ Wills, insurance policies, deeds, etc.
- ❑ Passports and identification
- ❑ Bank account numbers
- ❑ Credit card account and phone numbers
- ❑ Immunization records
- ❑ Birth, marriage, and death records

Special items for babies

- ❑ Formula
- ❑ Diapers
- ❑ Bottles
- ❑ Powdered milk
- ❑ Medications

Special items for older children and adults

- ❑ Prescription medications (for asthma, diabetes, high blood pressure, etc.)
- ❑ Contact lens supplies
- ❑ Extra eyeglasses
- ❑ Denture needs

From "Disaster Supplies Kit" developed by the Federal Emergency Management Agency and the American Red Cross.

It is by presence of mind in untried emergencies that the native metal of man (or woman) is tested.
James Russell Lowell

5

First Aid and Emergencies

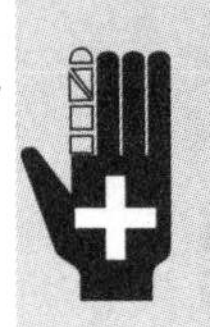

This chapter covers both serious medical emergencies and minor first aid situations. Review this chapter before you need it. Then, when you are faced with an emergency or injury, you will know where to turn. Your confidence in dealing with both major and minor emergencies will be reassuring to an injured person.

Some of the medical emergencies covered in this chapter include:

- Bleeding, see Cuts on page 76.
- Breathing emergencies, page 66.
- Head injuries, page 85.
- Heart attack, page 86.
- Poisoning, page 96.
- Shock, page 103.
- Stroke, page 108.
- Unconsciousness, page 110.

Dealing With Emergencies

Take a deep breath. Count to 10. Tell yourself you can handle the situation.

Assess the danger. Protect yourself and the injured person from fire, explosions, or other hazards. If you suspect a spinal injury, do not move the person unless the danger is great.

If the person is unconscious or unresponsive, check the ABCs: Airway, Breathing, Circulation. If the person is not breathing, see Rescue Breathing and CPR on page 68.

Try to survey the situation as a whole. Identify and prioritize the injuries. The most obvious problem is not always the most serious. Treat the most life-threatening problems, like bleeding or shock, first. Check for broken bones and other injuries.

If you need emergency assistance, call 911 or other emergency services, such as the local fire department, police, or hospital. The BC NurseLine is also available 24 hours a day, 7 days a week, if you do not think emergency care is needed but are not sure what to do. See the phone numbers on the back cover.

Legal Protection

If you are needed in an emergency, give what help you can. Most provinces have a Good Samaritan law to protect people who help in an emergency. You cannot be sued for giving first aid unless it can be shown that you are guilty of gross negligence.

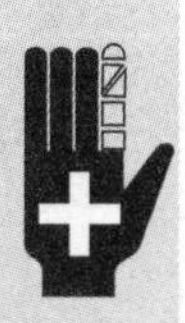

Accidental Tooth Loss

If a permanent tooth is knocked out, a dentist may be able to reimplant it. Baby teeth need to come out anyway, so they are not usually reimplanted.

A chipped tooth can be repaired. A blow that was hard enough to chip a tooth may have moved several teeth out of alignment or broken the portion of bone that holds the tooth in place.

Home Treatment

If a permanent tooth is knocked out:

- Call your dentist immediately for an emergency visit. Reimplanting a tooth works best when it is done within 30 minutes. After 2 hours, it is unlikely the procedure will be successful.

Prepare for the Emergency Room

- If possible, call ahead to let emergency room staff know you are coming.
- Call your doctor, if possible. He or she may meet you at the emergency room or call in important information.
- If you think you may have to wait to be seen by a doctor, take this book and your medical records with you. While you are waiting you can:
  - Use page 1, the Healthwise Self-Care Checklist, to help you think through the problem and report symptoms to the doctor.
  - Use page 2, the Ask-the-Doctor Checklist, to organize questions for the doctor.
  - Review the medical test checklist on page 11.
  - Use your home medical records to prepare to discuss your medications, past test results, or treatments. Information about your allergies, medications, and health conditions may be critical.

- Rinse the tooth gently and place it back in the socket, between the gum and cheek (use care not to swallow the tooth), or in a small container of milk. Use tap water if milk is not available.

When to Call a Health Professional

- If a permanent tooth is knocked out or chipped.
- If a baby tooth is accidentally knocked out, schedule an appointment within 2 weeks to determine if a spacer is needed until a permanent tooth comes in.

Animal and Human Bites and Scratches

After being bitten or scratched by an animal, most people want to know if they need a rabies shot. The main wild animal carriers of rabies in Canada and the United States are bats, raccoons, skunks, and foxes. Pet dogs, cats, and ferrets that have been vaccinated rarely have rabies. However, many stray animals have not been vaccinated. Rabies is quite rare, but it can be fatal if you are not vaccinated within 48 hours after exposure. The vaccination is no more painful than a typical injection. Report all wild animal bites to your doctor and the local public health unit or animal control department.

Bites and scratches that break the skin can cause infections. Cat and human bites or scratches are particularly prone to bacterial infection. You can get tetanus from any bite or scratch if your tetanus shots are not up to date. See page 17.

Prevention

- Vaccinate all pets against rabies. Do not keep wild animals as pets.
- Do not disturb animals—not even your pets—while they are eating.
- Teach children not to approach or play with stray animals.
- Do not touch wild animals or provoke them to attack. Do not handle sick or injured animals.

Home Treatment

- Scrub the wound immediately with soap and water. Treat it as a puncture wound. See page 98.
- If you are bitten or scratched by a pet dog, cat, or ferret, find out whether the animal has been vaccinated for rabies.
- A healthy pet that has bitten or scratched someone should be confined and observed for 10 days by a veterinarian to see if the pet develops symptoms of rabies. If you cannot locate the pet's owner, contact the local public health unit.
- If you are bitten or scratched by a wild animal, contact your doctor and the local public health unit. The public health unit can tell you

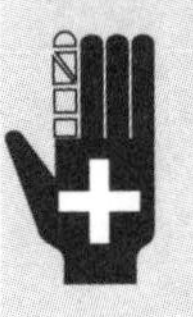

whether that animal is a rabies carrier in your area, and whether treatment is needed.

When to Call a Health Professional

- If the bite or scratch is from a bat or other wild animal.
- If the bite or scratch is from a human or a cat.
- If the bite or scratch is from a dog, cat, or ferret that is acting strangely or foaming at the mouth, or if the animal attacked for no apparent reason.
- If the bite or scratch is from a pet whose owner cannot be found or cannot confirm that the animal has been vaccinated for rabies.
- If there is a loss of feeling or function below the wound.
- If the wound is severe and may need stitches or if it is on your face, hand, or foot, or over a joint. If stitches are needed, they usually should be done within 8 hours.
- If signs of infection develop. See page 100.

Blood Under a Nail

Fingernails and toenails often get crunched, bashed, or smashed. These injuries usually aren't too serious, but if there is bleeding under the nail, the pressure can be very painful. The only way to relieve the throbbing and pain is by making a hole in the nail to drain the blood. Draining is helpful only if you have severe, throbbing pain (you can feel the pulse beating under the nail) that keeps you from sleeping. This procedure is not necessary or recommended unless you are having severe pain.

Home Treatment

- Apply ice and elevate the injured area as soon as possible to minimize swelling and relieve pain. Acetaminophen or ibuprofen will also ease discomfort.
- If you have severe, throbbing pain, make a hole in the nail to relieve the pressure. (Do not do this unless you are in pain and you are confident you can do it without burning yourself. Do not do this if you have diabetes or circulation problems.) Follow these steps:
  - Straighten a paper clip and heat the tip in a flame until it is red-hot.

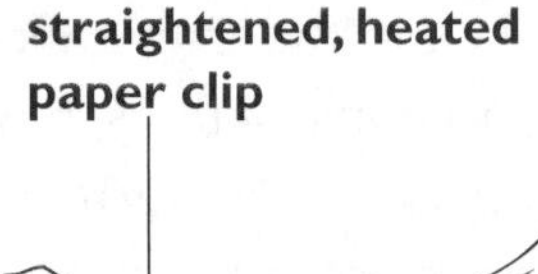

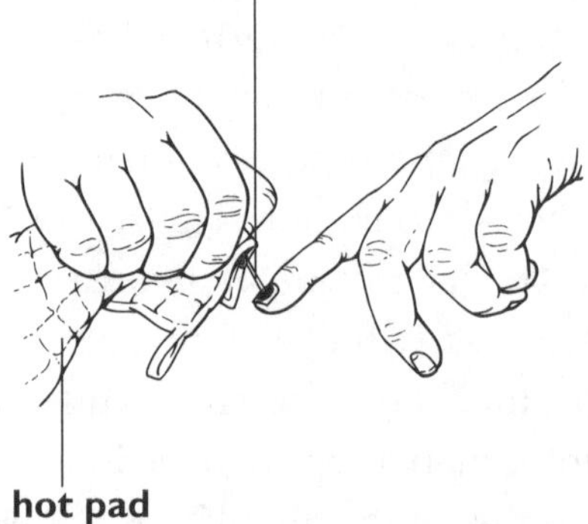

Use a red-hot paper clip to relieve the pain caused by blood under a fingernail or toenail.

- Place the tip of the paper clip over the area with blood and let it melt through. You do not need to push. This will not be painful, because the nail has no nerves. Go slowly and reheat the clip as necessary. A thick nail may take several tries.
- As soon as the hole is complete, blood will escape and the pain should be relieved. Pain and pressure that are not relieved by this procedure may indicate a more serious injury, such as a broken finger or toe or a deep cut. In this case, you should see your doctor.
- Soak the finger twice a day for 15 minutes in warm, soapy water. Apply an antibiotic ointment and cover the nail with an adhesive bandage.
- If the pressure builds up again in a few days, repeat the procedure, using the same hole.

When to Call a Health Professional

- If blood under a nail is causing severe pain and you are not willing to drain the blood from the nail yourself.
- If you drained the blood from under the nail, but your fingertip or the tip of your toe still hurts a lot.
- If you smashed your toenail and you have a condition that decreases blood flow to the feet, such as diabetes or peripheral vascular disease.
- If signs of infection develop. See page 100.
- If your nail has torn or separated from the nail bed and you need help removing it.

Blunt Abdominal Wounds

Blunt abdominal wounds caused by a blow to the stomach can cause severe bruising of the abdominal wall and bleeding from the internal organs. Such injuries are often caused by automobile, bicycle, sledding, or skiing accidents, when the victim is thrown into an object or to the ground.

An abdominal injury may cause the abdomen to become tender or rigid. The injured person may become confused and may not be able to remember what caused the injury. Signs of shock (faintness, weakness, drowsiness, confusion, and cool, clammy skin) may also develop.

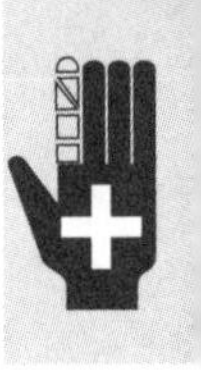

Home Treatment

- Monitor the injured person's pulse and respiration rate. See pages 89 and 103. If possible, monitor the person's blood pressure as well. A rapid, weak pulse, very rapid or very slow breathing, or falling blood pressure may indicate internal bleeding. If these signs develop, **call 911** or take the person to the emergency room immediately.

- Have the injured person lie down with the feet elevated above the heart. Loosen the person's clothing and cover him or her with a blanket for warmth. Do not give the person anything to eat or drink, even though he or she may be thirsty.
- Watch for signs of shock (see page 103).

When to Call a Health Professional

- If the abdominal pain is severe.
- If signs of shock or internal bleeding (see page 103) develop. These may develop up to 48 hours after an abdominal injury.
- If there is bleeding from the rectum, blood in the urine, or unexpected vaginal bleeding following a blow to the abdomen.
- If the injury causes nausea, vomiting, heartburn, or loss of appetite.
- If the abdomen is swollen and hard, or if pressing on the abdomen causes severe pain.
- If an abdominal wound is deeper than a scratch.

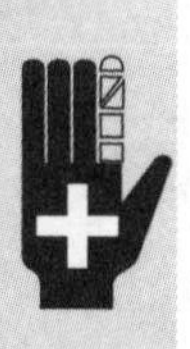

Breathing Emergencies

Who needs to be trained to help a person who is having a breathing emergency? You do. If you have children, drive a car, shop at the mall, or go anyplace where a person may be in a life-threatening situation, you need to know how to respond. An added benefit is the confidence you will have when you know you can help a person when it matters most.

The guidelines presented in this book are not meant to replace formal training from a certified instructor. They are here for you to use to refresh your memory between trainings or to read aloud to a person who is performing a rescue procedure. (Note, however, that your first responsibility as a helper is to call 911 or other emergency services and to make the area safe for the victim and the rescuer.)

Choking Rescue Procedure (Heimlich Manoeuvre)

Choking is usually caused by food or an object stuck in the windpipe. A person who is choking cannot talk, cough, or breathe, and may turn blue or dusky. The Heimlich manoeuvre can help dislodge the food or object.

WARNING: Do not begin the choking rescue procedure unless you are certain that the person is choking.

Adult or child older than 1 year:

- Stand behind the person and wrap your arms around his or her waist. If the person is standing, place one of your feet between his or her legs so you can support the person's body if he or she loses consciousness.

- Make a fist with one hand. Place the thumb side of your fist against the person's abdomen, just above the navel but well below the breastbone (sternum).

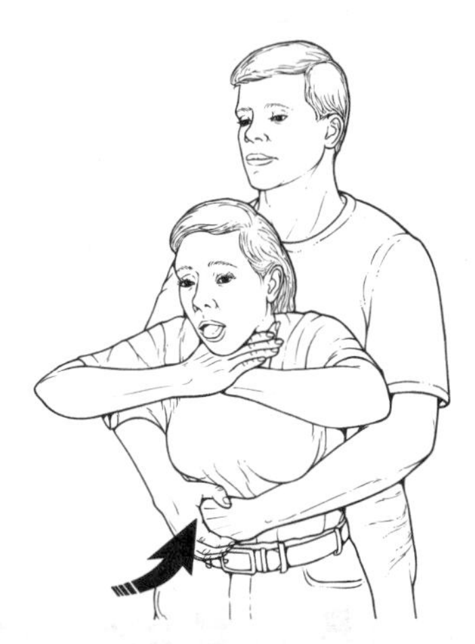

Heimlich Manoeuvre: Give quick upward thrusts to dislodge the object.

- Grasp your fist with the other hand. Give a quick upward thrust into the abdomen. This may cause the object to pop out. Use less force for a child.
- Repeat thrusts until the object pops out or the person loses consciousness.
- **If you choke while you are alone**, do abdominal thrusts on yourself, or lean over the back of a chair and press forcefully to pop out the object.

If the person loses consciousness, gently lower him or her to the ground. **Call 911 or other emergency services.**

- Begin standard CPR (cardiopulmonary resuscitation), including chest compressions. See page 68.
- Each time the airway is opened during CPR, look for an object in the mouth or throat. If you see an object, remove it.
- Do not perform blind finger sweeps.
- Do not perform abdominal thrusts, such as the Heimlich manoeuvre.
- Continue performing CPR until the person is breathing on his or her own or until an ambulance arrives.

Preventing Choking

- Don't drink too much alcohol before eating. It may dull your senses, and you might not chew food properly or might try to swallow too large a portion of food.
- Take small bites. Cut meat into small pieces. Chew your food thoroughly.
- Do not give popcorn, nuts, or hard candy to children younger than 3, and supervise older children when they eat these foods. Cut hot dogs and grapes lengthwise.
- Do not allow children younger than 3 to play with small objects or toys that have very small parts that could be swallowed.
- Keep balloons and plastic bags away from any child who may put them in his or her mouth.

See the Choking Rescue Procedure on page 66, or visit the Web site for the BC Children's and Women's Health Centre to read about choking prevention at www.cw.bc.ca/safestart.

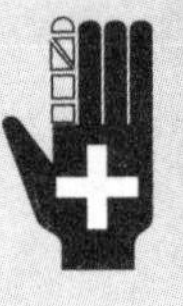

Infant (younger than 1 year):

- Put the baby face down on your forearm so the baby's head is lower than his or her chest.
- Support the baby's head in your palm, against your thigh. Don't cover the baby's mouth or twist his or her neck.

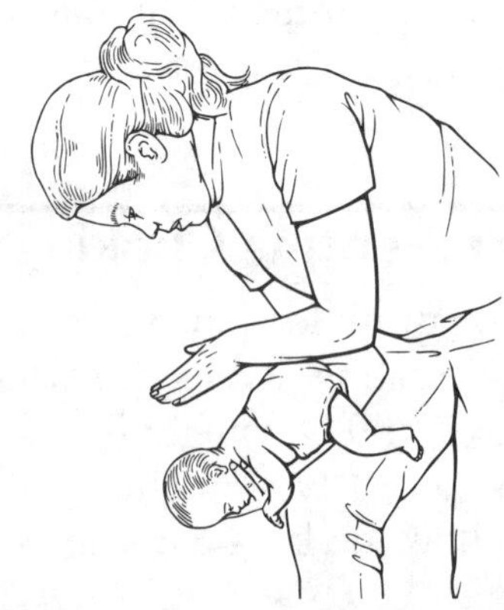

To help a baby who is choking, use the heel of your hand to give back blows between the baby's shoulders.

- To dislodge the object, use the heel of one hand to give up to 4 back blows between the baby's shoulder blades.
- If the airway remains blocked, support the infant's head and turn him or her face up on your thigh with his or her head pointing toward the floor.
- Place 2 or 3 fingers on the lower part of the baby's breastbone, and give up to 5 upward thrusts.
- Look for the object in the infant's mouth. If you can see it, remove it with your finger. Then give 2 rescue breaths (see page 70).
- If the back blows and chest thrusts do not dislodge the object, **call 911 or other emergency services** and begin rescue breathing (see page 70).
- Continue with back blows, chest thrusts, looking for the object, and rescue breaths until the infant coughs up the object and starts breathing on his or her own, or until help arrives.

Rescue Breathing and CPR

WARNING: CPR (cardiopulmonary resuscitation) that is done improperly or on a person whose heart is still beating can cause serious injury. Do not perform CPR unless:

1. The person has stopped breathing.
2. The person does not have signs of circulation, such as normal breathing, coughing, or movement in response to rescue breathing.
3. No one with more training in CPR is present.

For basic life support, think **ABC: A**irway, **B**reathing, and **C**irculation, in that order. You must give rescue breaths before you can begin the chest compressions, which will help circulate blood for a person whose heart has stopped beating.

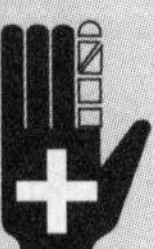

CPR Ready Reference			
	Adults	**Children Age 1 through 8**	**Infants Under 1 Year**
If the person is not breathing, begin rescue breathing:	Give 2 full breaths.	Give rescue breaths for 1 full minute.	Give rescue breaths for 1 full minute.
If the person does not breathe or show signs of circulation in response to rescue breaths, locate the compression land-mark:	Trace the ribs into the sternal notch; place 2 fingers on the sternum. See illustration on p. 71.	Same as for an adult.	1 finger-width below nipple line.
Do chest compressions with:	2 hands stacked; heel of 1 hand on sternum	Heel of 1 hand on sternum	2 or 3 fingers on sternum
Rate of compressions per minute:	100	100	100
Compression depth:	4 to 5 cm	2.5 to 4 cm	1 to 2.5 cm
Ratio of compressions to breaths:	15:2	5:1	5:1
Guidelines from the American Heart Association			

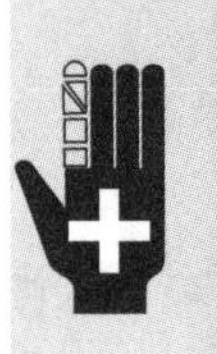

Step 1: Check for consciousness. Tap or gently shake the person and shout, "Are you okay?" If you suspect a neck or spinal injury, do not shake the person.

If the person does not respond:

- **Adult (age 9 and older): Call 911 or other emergency services immediately** (have someone else make the call if possible). Then proceed to Step 2.
- **Infant or child through 8 years:** Check to see if the infant or child is breathing (see Step 2). If the infant or child is not breathing, give rescue breaths for 1 full minute (see Step 3).

Then **call 911 or other emergency services**. If the child is small enough, carry him or her to the telephone with you so you can continue to give rescue breaths. Keep the child's head and neck steady.

Step 2: Check for breathing. Look, listen, and feel for breathing for 5 seconds. Kneel next to the person with your head close to his or her head.

- Look to see if the person's chest rises and falls.
- Listen for breathing sounds, wheezing, gurgling, or snoring.
- Put your cheek near the person's mouth and nose to feel whether air is moving out.

If the person is not breathing (or if you can't tell), roll the person onto his or her back. If he or she may have a spinal injury, gently roll the person's head, neck, and shoulders together as a unit until the person is on his or her back.

Step 3: Begin rescue breathing.

- Place your hand on the person's forehead and pinch the person's nostrils shut with your thumb and forefinger. With your other hand, tilt the chin upward to keep the airway open.

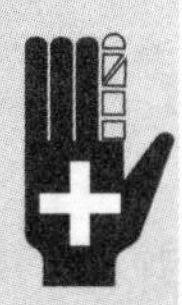

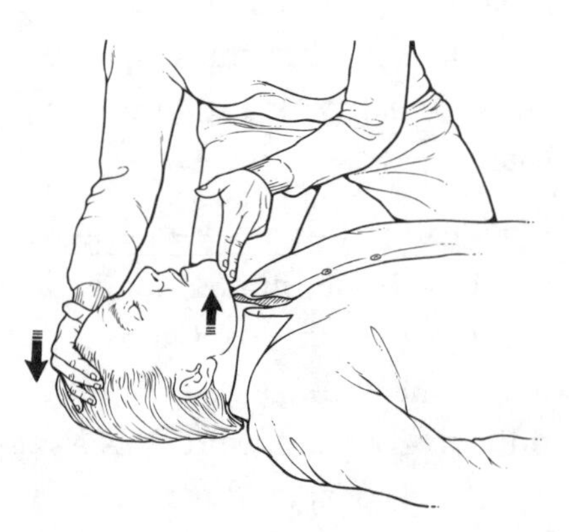

Airway: Position the head to open the airway.

- Take a deep breath and place your mouth over the person's mouth, making a tight seal. For an infant, place your mouth over the baby's mouth and nose. As you slowly blow air into the person, watch to see if his or her chest rises.

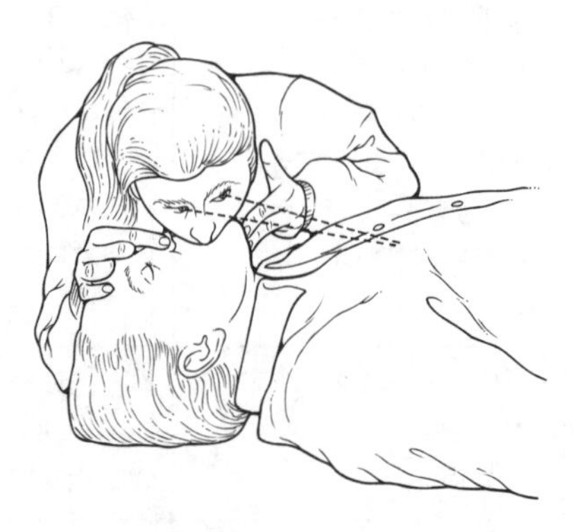

Breathing: Blow air in slowly; look to see if chest rises.

- If the first breath does not go in, try tilting the person's head again and give another breath.
- Slowly blow air in until the person's chest rises. Take 1½ to 2 seconds to give each breath. Between rescue breaths, remove your mouth from the person's mouth and take a deep breath. Allow his or her chest to fall, and feel the air escape.
- Give the person 2 full breaths. Then check for circulation.

Step 4: Check for circulation. Look for signs of circulation, such as breathing, coughing, or movement in response to rescue breathing.

If there are **no signs of circulation**, begin chest compressions. See Step 5.

If there are signs of circulation, continue to give rescue breaths until help arrives or until the person starts breathing on his or her own. If the person starts breathing again, he or she still needs to be seen by a health professional.

Give rescue breaths:

- Adult (age 9 and older): 2 breaths every 15 seconds
- Infant or child through 8 years: 1 breath every 3 seconds

Step 5: Begin chest compressions. Adult (age 9 and older):

- Kneel next to the person. Use your fingers to locate the end of the person's breastbone (sternum), where the ribs come together. Place 2 fingers at the tip of the sternum. Place the heel of the other hand directly above your fingers (on the side closest to the person's face).

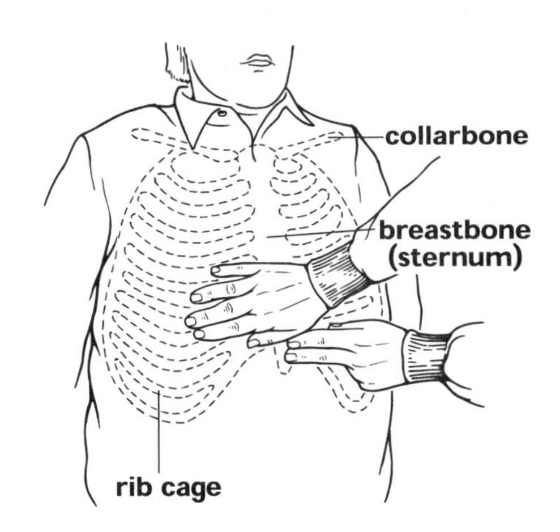

Put your hand 2 fingers'-width above the bottom of the breastbone.

- Place your other hand on top of the one that you just put in position. Lock the fingers of both hands together, and raise the fingers so they don't touch the person's chest.
- Straighten your arms, lock your elbows, and centre your shoulders directly over your hands.

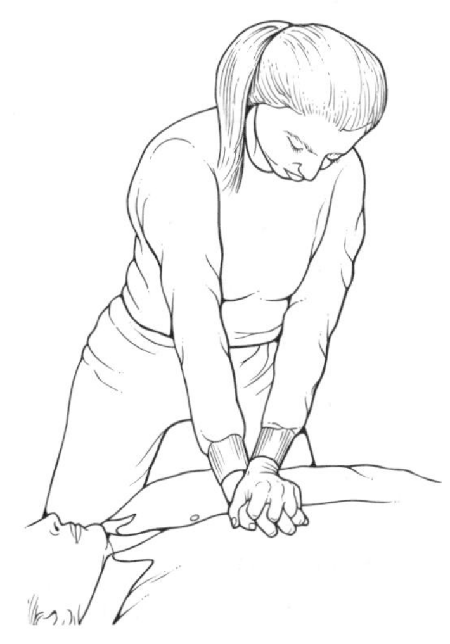

Chest Compressions: Keep your shoulders directly over your hands with your elbows straight as you give chest compressions.

- Press down in a steady rhythm, using your body weight and keeping your elbows locked. The force from each thrust should go straight down onto the sternum, compressing it 4 to 5 cm. It may help to count "one and two and three and four . . .," giving 1 downward thrust each time you say a number. Lift your weight, but not your hands, from the chest each time you say "and." Give 15 compressions.

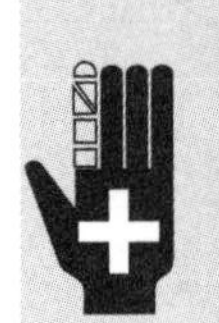

- After 15 compressions, give 2 full, slow breaths.
- Repeat the 15 compressions/ 2 breaths cycle 4 times; then check again for signs of circulation. If there are still no signs of circulation, continue to give chest compressions and rescue breaths until help arrives or until signs of circulation are present and breathing is restored.

Child (age 1 through 8 years):

- Position the heel of one hand 2 fingers'-width above the tip of the sternum. Press with less force than you would for an adult, compressing the sternum 2.5 to 4 cm.
- Give 5 chest compressions. Then give 1 rescue breath. Repeat the 5 compressions/1 breath cycle 12 times; then check again for signs of circulation, such as normal breathing, coughing, or movement in response to rescue breaths. If there are still no signs of circulation, continue to give chest compressions and rescue breaths until help arrives or until signs of circulation are present and breathing is restored.

Infant (younger than 1 year):

- Place 2 fingers on the baby's sternum, about 1 finger-width below an imaginary line connecting the nipples. Press with gentle force, compressing the sternum about 1 to 2.5 cm.
- Give 5 chest compressions. Then give 1 rescue breath. Repeat the 5 compressions/1 breath cycle 12 times; then check again for signs of circulation. If there are still no signs of circulation, continue to give chest compressions and rescue breaths until help arrives or until signs of circulation are present and breathing is restored.

Bruises

Bruises (contusions) occur when small blood vessels under the skin rupture or tear. Blood seeps into the surrounding tissues, causing the black-and-blue colour of a bruise.

Bruises usually develop after a bump or fall. People who take Aspirin or blood thinners (anticoagulants) may bruise easily. A bruise may also develop after blood is drawn.

A black eye is a type of bruise. If you have a black eye, apply home treatment for a bruise and inspect the eye for blood. If there is any loss of vision or change in vision or if you cannot move your eye in all directions, see a doctor.

Home Treatment

- Apply ice or cold packs for 10 minutes several times a day. Do this for the first 48 hours to help blood vessels constrict and to reduce swelling. The sooner you apply ice, the less bleeding and swelling there will be.

- If possible, elevate the bruised area above the level of your heart. Blood will leave the area and there will be less swelling.
- Rest the injured area so you don't injure it further.
- If the area is still painful after 48 hours, apply heat with warm towels, a hot water bottle, or a heating pad.

When to Call a Health Professional

- If signs of infection develop. See page 100.
- If pain increases or if your ability to use or move the bruised body part decreases.
- If a blow to the eye causes:
  - Blood in the coloured part of the eye or blood in the white part of the eye (see page 211).
  - Loss of or change in vision.
  - Inability to move the eye normally in all directions.
  - Severe pain.
- If you suddenly begin to bruise easily, or if you have unexplained recurrent or multiple bruises.

Burns

Burns are classified as first-, second-, third-, or fourth-degree depending on their depth, not on the amount of pain or the extent of the burn. A first-degree burn involves only the outer layer of skin. The skin is dry, painful, and sensitive to touch. A mild sunburn is an example of a first-degree burn.

A second-degree burn involves several layers of skin. The skin becomes swollen, puffy, weepy, or blistered.

A third-degree burn involves all layers of skin and may include any underlying tissue. The skin is dry, pale white or charred black, and swollen and sometimes breaks open. Nerves are destroyed or damaged, so there may be little pain except on the edges of the burn, where there may be second-degree burns.

A fourth-degree burn extends through the skin to injure muscle and bone.

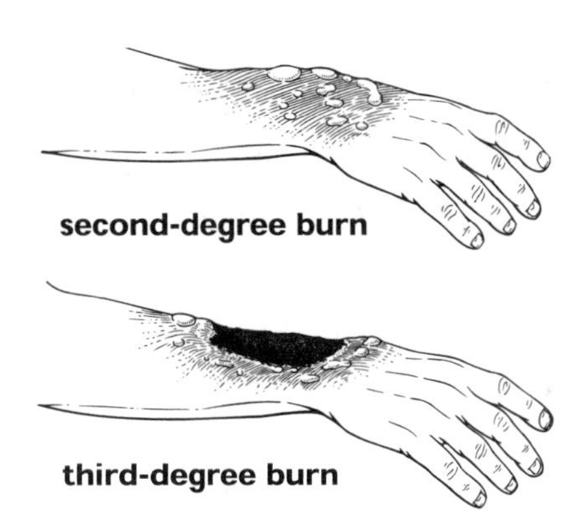

A second-degree burn will cause skin to swell and blister, and it may also weep fluid. A third- or fourth-degree burn may cause skin to look pale white or charred black.

Prevention

- Install smoke detectors on each story of your home. Check and replace the batteries regularly.

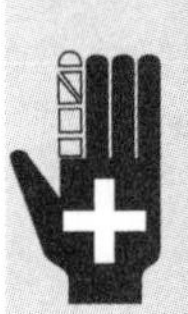

- Keep a fire extinguisher near the kitchen. Have it inspected yearly.
- Set your water heater at 50°C or lower to avoid burns.
- Supervise children closely, especially in the kitchen.
- Don't smoke in bed.
- Use caution around campfires and hot appliances.

If your clothing catches fire:

- Do not run, because running will fan the flames. Stop, drop, and roll on the ground to smother the flames, or smother the flames with a blanket, rug, or coat.
- Use water to douse the fire and cool the skin.

To avoid kitchen burns:

- Use caution when handling hot foods and beverages.
- Turn pot handles toward the back of the stove.
- Smother burning food or grease with a pot or pot lid.

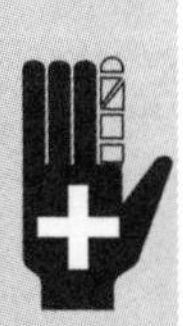

Home Treatment

Third-degree and fourth-degree burns require immediate medical treatment. Call a health professional and apply home treatment:

- Make sure the source of the burn has been extinguished.
- Have the person lie down to prevent shock.
- Cover the burned area with a clean sheet.
- Do not apply any ice, salve, or medication to the burn.

First- and second-degree burns can be treated at home as follows:

- Run cool tap water over the burn until the pain stops (15 to 30 minutes). Cool water is the best immediate treatment for minor burns. The cold lowers skin temperature and lessens the severity of the burn. Do not use ice or ice water, because it may further damage the injured skin.
- Remove rings, jewellery, or clothing from the burned limb. Swelling may make these items difficult to remove later, and if left on, they may damage nerves or blood vessels.
- Clean the burned area with mild soap and water. If the burned skin or blisters have broken open, a bandage is needed. Otherwise, don't cover the burn unless clothing rubs on it. If clothing rubs the burned area, cover the burn with a non-stick gauze pad taped well away from the burn. Do not encircle a hand, arm, or leg with tape. Keep the bandage clean and dry. Change it once a day and anytime it gets wet.
- Do not put salve, butter, grease, or oil on a burn. They increase the risk of infection and don't help the burn heal.

- After 2 to 3 days of healing, apply aloe to soothe minor burns.
- If the burn causes blisters to form, do not break blisters. If blisters break, clean the area by running tap water over it and applying a mild soap. Cover the burn with a non-stick sterile dressing. Don't touch the burned area with your hands or any unsterile objects. Remove the dressing every day, clean the burned area with mild soap, and cover it with a new dressing.
- Take ibuprofen or acetaminophen to help relieve pain. Aspirin is not recommended because it can affect the swelling and bleeding in the burned area.

When to Call a Health Professional

- For all third- and fourth-degree burns.
- If you are in doubt about the extent of a burn or aren't sure whether it is a second- or third-degree burn.
- If a second-degree burn involves the face, ears, eyes, hands, feet, genitals, or a joint.
- If the burn encircles an arm or leg, or if it covers more than 25 percent of the body part involved.
- If the pain lasts longer than 48 hours.
- If signs of infection develop. See page 100.
- If a child younger than 5, an older adult, or a person with a weakened immune system or a chronic health problem (such as cancer, heart disease, or diabetes) is burned.
- If there is a chance the burn was caused on purpose.

Chemical Burns

Chemical burns occur when something caustic, such as a cleaning product, gasoline, or turpentine, is splashed into an eye or onto the skin.

The vapours or fumes of strong chemicals can also burn or irritate the eyes, the skin, the respiratory passages, and the lungs.

A chemically burned eye becomes red and watery and may be sensitive to light. If the damage is severe, the eye will look whitish. Chemically burned skin may become red, blistered, or blackened, depending on how strong the caustic material is.

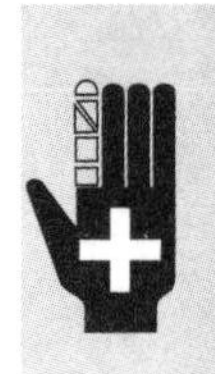

Prevention

Wear safety glasses, goggles, or a face shield when working with chemicals. Know the location of the nearest sink or shower.

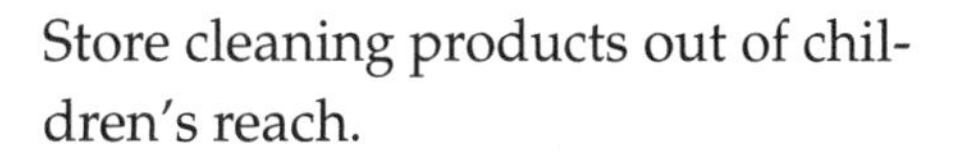

Store cleaning products out of children's reach.

Home Treatment

- Call Poison Control for specific advice. Have the chemical's container or label available.

- Immediately flush your eye or skin with a large amount of water. Use a cold shower for skin burns. For eye burns, fill a sink or dishpan with water, immerse your face in the water, and open and close your eyelids with your fingers to force the water to all parts of the eye. Or flush your eye under a running faucet or shower. A sink with a sprayer also works well.
- Continue flushing for 30 minutes or until the pain stops, whichever takes longer.

When to Call a Health Professional

Call 911 or other emergency services:

- If a strong chemical such as acid or lye is splashed into your eye.
- If you have swallowed a chemical that may cause burning or be poisonous.

Call your doctor or Poison Control if any of the following occurs:

- A large area of skin (more than 25 percent of any part of the body) or the face is exposed to a strong acid, such as battery acid, or to a caustic substance, such as lye or drain cleaner.
- A chemically burned eye still hurts after 30 minutes of home treatment.
- A chemically burned eye appears to be damaged. Symptoms include:
  - Pain.
  - Persistent redness.
  - Discharge or watering.
  - Any vision problems, such as double vision, blurring, or sensitivity to light.
  - A grey or white discolouration over the coloured part of the eye.
- Your skin shows signs of a chemical burn (see page 75).

Cuts

When you see a cut (laceration), the first steps are to stop the bleeding and determine whether medical evaluation is needed.

If the cut is bleeding heavily or spurting blood, see Stopping Severe Bleeding on page 77.

Bleeding from minor cuts will usually stop on its own or after you apply a little direct pressure.

To decide whether stitches are needed, see Are Stitches Necessary? on page 78.

If stitches are needed, apply home treatment and seek medical care as soon as possible. Most cuts that need stitches should be sutured within 6 to 8 hours. If stitches are not needed, you can clean and bandage the cut at home.

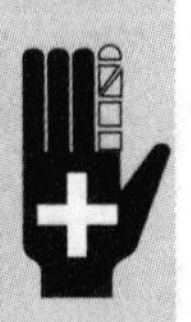

Stopping Severe Bleeding

- Elevate the site that is bleeding.
- Wash your hands well with soap and water. Put on medical gloves or place several layers of fabric or plastic bags between your hands and the wound.
- Remove any visible objects from the surface of the wound. Do not attempt to clean out the wound.
- Press firmly on the wound with a clean cloth or the cleanest material available. If there is an object deep in the wound, apply pressure around the object, not directly over it. Do not try to remove the object.
- Apply steady pressure for a full 15 minutes. Don't peek after a few minutes to see if bleeding has stopped. If the bleeding has not slowed down or stopped after 15 minutes, **call 911 or other emergency services** and continue to apply pressure to the wound. If blood soaks through the cloth, apply another cloth without lifting the first one.
- If bleeding decreases after you apply pressure for 15 minutes, but minimal bleeding starts again once you release the pressure, apply direct pressure to the wound for another 15 minutes. Direct pressure may be applied up to 3 times (total of 45 minutes) for minimal bleeding. If bleeding (more than just oozing small amounts of blood) continues after 45 minutes of direct pressure, call a health professional.
- Watch for signs of shock. See page 103.

Home Treatment

- Stop any bleeding by applying direct, continuous pressure over the wound for 15 minutes.
- Wash the cut well with soap and water. Treat an animal bite like a puncture wound. See page 98.
- If you think the cut may need stitches, see a health professional (see page 78). If the cut does not need stitches, proceed with home treatment.
- Consider bandaging the cut, especially if it is in an area that may get dirty or irritated.
- Apply antibiotic ointment (such as Bacitracin or Polysporin) to keep the cut from sticking to the bandage. Do not use rubbing alcohol, hydrogen peroxide, iodine, or Mercurochrome, which can harm tissue and slow healing.

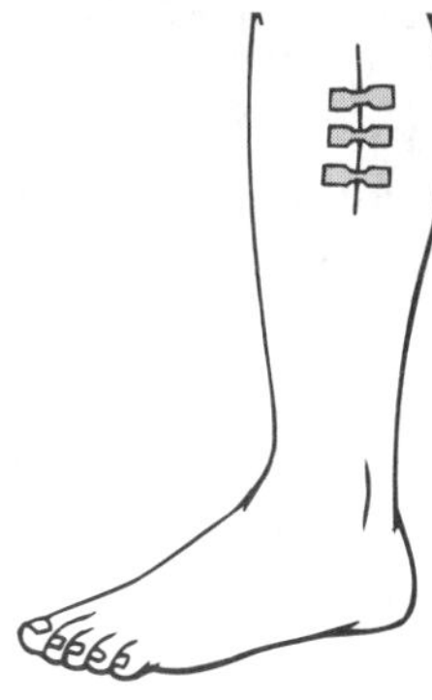
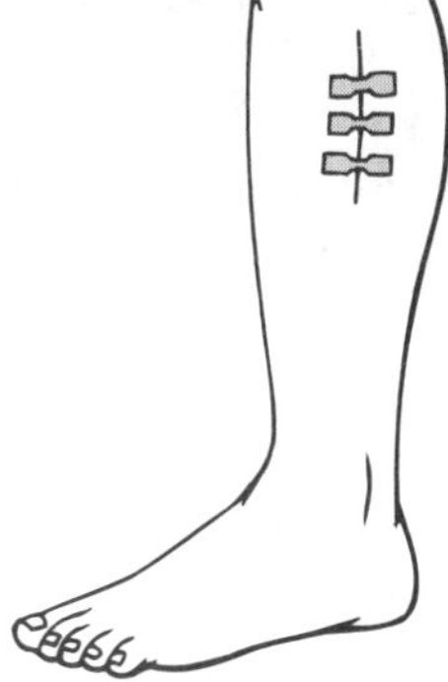

Butterfly bandages are best for closing a long cut.

- Use an adhesive bandage to provide continuous pressure and to protect the cut from further irritation. Always put an adhesive bandage across a cut rather than

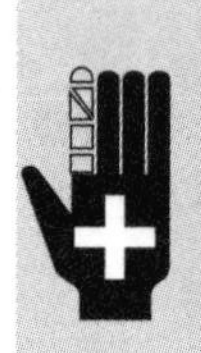

lengthwise. Butterfly bandages (see the illustration on page 77) can help hold cut skin edges together. Small cuts that are not in easily irritated locations may be bandaged or left uncovered.

- Apply a clean bandage at least once a day, or whenever the old bandage gets wet or dirty.

When to Call a Health Professional

- If a person has signs of shock, even if bleeding has stopped. See Shock on page 103.
- If a cut continues to bleed through bandages after you apply direct pressure for 15 minutes.
- If the skin near the wound is blue, white, or cold; if you have numbness, tingling, or loss of feeling; or if you are unable to move a limb normally below the wound.
- If the cut has removed all the layers of skin.
- If the cut contains, or might contain, foreign objects such as wood, glass, or gravel.
- If the cut needs stitches (see page 78). Stitches usually need to be done within 8 hours.
- If you have been cut and your tetanus shots are not up to date. See page 17. If you need a tetanus booster, you should have it within 2 days of being injured.
- If signs of infection develop. See page 100.

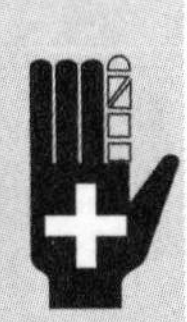

Are Stitches Necessary?

For best results, cuts that need stitches should be sutured within 6 to 8 hours. Wash the cut well with soap and water and stop the bleeding; then pinch the sides of the cut together. If it looks better, you may want to consider stitches. If stitches are needed, avoid using an antibiotic or antiseptic ointment until after a health professional has examined the cut.

Stitches may be needed for:

- Deep cuts (more than 0.6 cm deep) that have jagged edges or gape open.
- Deep cuts on a joint, such as an elbow, knuckle, or knee.
- Deep cuts on the hands or fingers.
- Cuts on the face, eyelids, or lips.
- Cuts in any area where you are worried about scarring.
- Cuts that go down to the muscle or bone.
- Cuts that continue to bleed after you have applied direct pressure for 15 minutes.

Cuts like these that are sutured usually heal with less scarring than similar cuts that are not sutured.

Stitches may not be needed for:

- Cuts with smooth edges that tend to stay together during normal movement of the affected body part.
- Shallow cuts that are less than 0.6 cm deep and less than 2.5 cm long.

Electrical Burns

Electrical burns are a medical emergency. An electrical burn may look minor on the outside, but electricity can cause serious internal damage, including burns and heart rhythm disturbances.

Prevention

- Keep electrical cords out of the reach of small children and pets. Plug bare electrical sockets with plastic inserts.
- Replace frayed power cords on electric appliances.
- Unplug lamps before replacing lightbulbs. Turn off the power at the circuit breaker when replacing bulbs in ceiling or wall lights.
- Unplug all appliances (including your computer) when making minor repairs.
- Keep appliances away from water.
- During a lightning storm, take cover inside a car, large building, or house, or seek low ground. Do not stand under a tree during a lightning storm. Get out of the water and get off boats. Stay away from metal objects.

Home Treatment

- Do not approach a victim who has been electrocuted until you are sure the area surrounding the victim is safe. Disconnect the power source if possible. If you feel tingling in your lower body, turn around and hop to a safe place.
- Do not attempt to move wires off a victim unless you are sure the power has been disconnected.
- If it is safe to approach the victim, check ABCs (Airway, Breathing, Circulation). If necessary, begin rescue breathing and CPR. See page 68.
- Raise the victim's legs 20 to 30 cm and keep the victim warm.
- Cover burns with dry, sterile dressing.

When to Call a Health Professional

Call 911 or other emergency services immediately:

- If a person who has been electrocuted stops breathing, has no pulse, or has lost consciousness.
- If a person who has been electrocuted fell and may have other injuries.

Call your doctor for any electrical burn. Even an electrical burn that looks minor can be serious and needs to be evaluated.

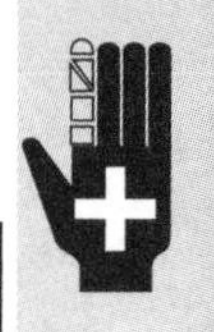

Falls

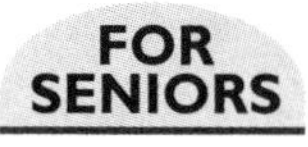

Many older adults are concerned about falling. Falls can cause serious injuries, particularly in older adults who may have weak bones. Hip fractures and other injuries caused by falling may take longer to heal or not heal as well as they would in a younger person.

Fall-related injuries can lead to permanent disability, a reduced quality of life, and for many seniors, a loss of independence.

For people of all ages, falls are often related to household and public hazards, such as loose rugs, slippery or cracked sidewalks, poorly placed electrical cords, and dark or poorly designed stairways. But older adults are at increased risk for several reasons:

- They may not see or hear as well as they used to.
- They may have weakened muscles and bones, especially if they do not have an active lifestyle.
- They may have chronic health problems that affect their strength, balance, and coordination.
- They may take medications that make them dizzy or unsteady.
- They may fear falling. This may help prevent a fall in the short term, but because it promotes inactivity, it may also make a person weaker and more likely to fall over time.

Fortunately, there are many things you can do to reduce your risk of a fall.

Prevention

1. Make your home fall-proof.

- Keep your home well lit. Install light switches at both ends of stairs and halls. Use night-lights in the bedroom, bathroom, and hallways.Turn on lights when you walk through the house at night.
- Keep pathways clear of telephone and electrical cords, shoes, and clutter. Keep the path between your bedroom and bathroom clear in case you get up during the night.
- Install handrails or banisters on both sides of the stairs. Make certain carpet is firmly attached to the stairs.
- Make sure that carpets are firmly attached to the floor without any uneven sections. Repair or replace vinyl or tiled flooring so that there are no holes or trip hazards. Remove or replace rugs that tend to slip, or attach a non-slip backing to them.
- Do not stand on a chair to reach things. Store frequently used objects where you can reach them easily. If you need to reach items on high shelves, buy a sturdy step stool with handrails.
- Use a bright colour to paint the edges of outdoor steps and any steps that are especially narrow or are higher or lower than the rest.
- Paint outside stairs with a mixture of sand and paint for better traction.
- Keep entrances and sidewalks clear and well lit, and remove snow and ice promptly.
- Add grab bars in the shower, tub, and toilet areas. Use non-slip adhesive strips or non-skid paint in the shower or tub. Consider sitting on a bench or stool in the shower. Consider using an elevated toilet seat.

2. Be careful.

- Wear low-heeled shoes or slippers that fit snugly and have non-slip soles. Do not walk around in bare feet, socks, or stockings. Have clothing hemmed if it is too long.
- Keep bags and purses light. Do not try to carry too much at once. This can upset your balance.
- Pay attention to your surroundings, especially when going through a doorway, using steps and curbs, or walking in an unfamiliar place.
- Avoid sitting in sofas and chairs that put your hips lower than your knees. When you get up from a sofa or chair, use the armrest or the edge of the chair for support, and put your feet flat on the floor, toes facing forward. Stand up slowly and hold on to the chair or sofa until you have your balance.
- Use helping devices such as canes, floor-to-ceiling poles, or chairs that raise or tilt to help you get up. If your doctor has recommended a cane or walker to help you walk, use it.
- Consider wearing a hip-protective garment, which has a hard or soft shield in a pocket over the hip area. Hip protectors may reduce your risk of breaking a hip if you fall.
- Get up slowly. Sit up first and then stand. Standing up suddenly can make you dizzy or light-headed and cause you to fall.

3. Take care of yourself.

- Have your hearing tested regularly. Inner ear problems can affect your balance.
- Have your vision checked regularly. Keep the prescription for your glasses or contact lenses up to date. Vision problems make it hard for you to see potential hazards.
- Exercise regularly to keep your muscles and bones strong and flexible. This may help prevent falls and will also help you recover faster from a fall. Inactivity can cause you to lose muscle mass and become weaker, increasing your risk of falls. Exercising with a group can help reduce fear of falling and can be a good way to socialize too.
- Limit your alcohol intake. Older adults who drink alcohol have a greater risk of falling.
- See a doctor or physical therapist about anything that makes it hard for you to walk, such as joint pain, muscle weakness, or foot problems.
- Be especially careful when you are sick (if you have the flu, for instance). Move slowly, and do not overtire yourself. You may feel weaker and less steady than usual.

4. Watch for medication side effects.

- Talk to your doctor, pharmacist, or the BC NurseLine to find out whether any of the medications

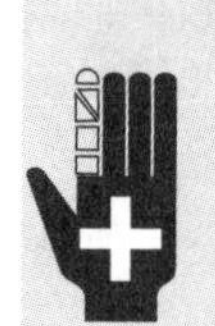

you take have side effects like drowsiness, dizziness, or confusion. Some sleeping pills, tranquilizers, and medications for depression and anxiety are associated with an increased risk of falls.

- Always take medications exactly as directed. Do not change or stop a medication without talking to your doctor first.

Home Treatment

If you fall and you are not seriously injured, you may be able to treat yourself at home. To get up from the floor safely, roll to your hands and knees and crawl to a piece of furniture that will support your weight, such as a sofa or an armchair. Use the furniture to pull yourself up gently. Sit for a minute before trying to stand up.

If you have any minor injuries, such as a bruise or sprain, see the appropriate home treatment section in this chapter.

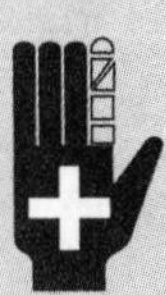

If you think you have a serious injury, do not try to stand. Crawl to the phone and call for help. (Keep your phone where you can reach it from the floor.)

When to Call a Health Professional

Call 911 or other emergency services:

- If a person remains unconscious after a fall. See Unconsciousness on page 110.
- If a fall causes a person to have a seizure.
- If you cannot get up after a fall.
- If a person appears to have a severe fracture and cannot be safely transported by car.

Call a health professional:

- If a person lost consciousness because of a fall but has now regained consciousness.
- If a person fell while having a seizure but the seizure has now stopped. (If the seizure is related to a chronic condition and a doctor has recommended treatment, begin the treatment.)
- If a fall causes severe bleeding or bruising. See Shock on page 103.
- If you think you may have a broken bone. See page 104.
- If you develop pain in your hips, lower back, or wrists after a fall. These areas are especially likely to break in older adults.
- If you think a fall was caused by a medical problem or the side effects of a medication.

Fish Hook Removal

In the excitement of fishing, sometimes fingers are hooked instead of fish. It is useful to know how to remove a fish hook, especially if you are far from medical help.

Home Treatment

Remove the hook as follows:

- Use ice, cold water, or hard pressure to provide temporary numbing.
- **Step A:** Tie a piece of fishing line to the hook near the skin's surface.
- **Step B:** Grasp the eye of the hook with one hand and press down about 3 mm to disengage the barb.
- **Step C:** While still pressing the hook down (barb disengaged), jerk the line near the skin's surface so that the hook shaft leads the barb out of the skin.

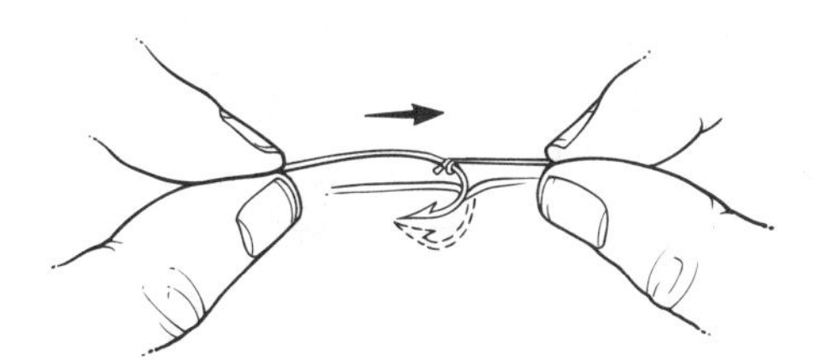

Removing a fish hook

- Another option is to push the hook the rest of the way through the skin, snip off the barb, and then pull the hook out the same way it entered the skin.
- Wash the wound thoroughly with soap if possible. Treat it as a puncture wound. See page 98.
- Do not try to remove a fish hook from an eyeball. Seek medical care immediately.

When to Call a Health Professional

- If the hook is near the eye or in the eyelid or eyeball.
- If the hook is in or near a joint, in a bone or muscle, or deep in the skin.
- If you cannot remove the hook.
- If your skin was punctured by a fish hook and your tetanus shots are not up to date. See page 17. If you need a tetanus booster, you should have it within 2 days of being injured.
- If signs of infection develop. See page 100.

Freeing Trapped Limbs

Fingers, arms, or legs sometimes get caught in objects such as bottles, jars, or pipes. Stay calm; panic will only make the situation worse.

Home Treatment

- Don't try to forcibly free the limb, because doing so will cause swelling and make the limb more difficult to remove.
- Try to relax the limb. Relaxation alone will sometimes enable you to free the limb.
- If possible, elevate the limb.
- Apply ice around the exposed part of the limb. This may reduce any swelling and allow the limb to be released.

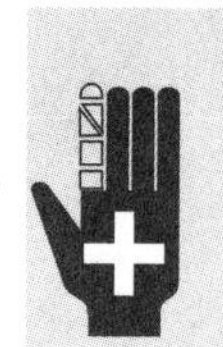

- If ice doesn't work, dribble soapy water or cooking oil on the limb. Turn the limb or the object so you "unscrew" it rather than pulling the limb out directly.

When to Call a Health Professional

Call if you are unable to free the trapped limb or if freeing the limb results in injury.

Frostbite

Frostbite is freezing of the skin or underlying tissues caused by prolonged exposure to cold.

Frostbitten skin is pale or blue, is stiff or rubbery to the touch, and feels cold and numb. Frostbite is rated by its severity:

First degree ("frostnip"): Skin is whitish or red and tingling or burning, but there is little likelihood of blistering if it is rewarmed promptly.

Second degree: Outer skin feels hard and frozen, but tissue underneath is normal. Blistering is likely.

Third degree: Skin is white or blotchy and blue. Skin and tissue underneath are hard and frozen. Blistering always occurs. Burning, throbbing, or shooting pain may follow numbness.

Fourth degree: Skin is red or blue and turns dry, black, and rubbery. Blisters may appear as small bloody spots under the skin. There is deep, aching joint pain.

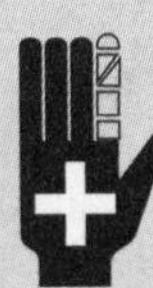

Prevention

Stay dry and out of the wind in extreme cold, and cover areas of exposed skin. Keep your body's core temperature up:

- Wear layers of clothing. Wool and polypropylene are good insulators. Wear windproof, waterproof outer layers. Wear wool socks and waterproof boots that fit well.
- Wear a hat to prevent heat loss from your head. Wear mittens rather than gloves.
- Keep protective clothing and blankets in your car in case of a breakdown in an isolated area.
- Don't drink alcoholic or caffeinated beverages or smoke when you are out in extreme cold.

Home Treatment

- Get inside or take shelter from the wind.
- Check for signs of hypothermia (see page 90). Treat it before treating frostbite.
- Protect the frozen body part from further exposure to cold.
- Warm small areas (ears, face, nose, fingers, toes) with warm breath or by tucking hands or feet inside warm clothing next to bare skin.
- Don't rub or massage the frozen area, because doing so will further damage tissues. Avoid walking on frostbitten feet if possible.
- Keep the frostbitten body part warm and elevated. Wrap it with blankets or soft material to prevent

bruising. If possible, immerse it in warm water (40° to 42°C) for 15 to 30 minutes.

- Blisters may appear as the skin warms. Do not break them. The skin may turn red, burn, tingle, or be very painful. Aspirin, ibuprofen, or acetaminophen may help relieve pain. Do not give Aspirin to anyone younger than 20.

When to Call a Health Professional

- If the skin is white or blue, and hard, rubbery, and cold, which indicates third-degree frostbite. Careful rewarming and antibiotic treatment are needed to prevent permanent tissue damage and infection.
- If blisters develop (second- or third-degree frostbite). Do not break blisters. The risk of infection is very high.
- If signs of infection develop. See page 100.

Head Injuries

Most bumps on the head are minor and heal as easily as bumps anywhere else. Minor cuts on the head often bleed heavily because the blood vessels of the scalp are close to the skin's surface. In children, blood loss from a scalp injury may be enough to cause symptoms of shock.

Head injuries that do not cause visible external bleeding may have caused life-threatening bleeding and swelling inside the skull. The more force involved in a head injury, the more likely a serious injury to the brain has occurred. Anyone who has experienced a head injury should be watched carefully for 24 hours for signs of a serious head injury. These include:

- Confusion or difficulty speaking. Ask the person his or her name, address, and age, the date, and the location.
- Numbness or weakness on one side of the body.
- Blurred or double vision that does not clear, or significant changes in pupil size or reaction.
- Lethargy, abnormally deep sleep, or difficulty waking up.
- Vomiting that continues after the first 2 hours, or violent vomiting that persists after the first 15 minutes.
- Seizures or convulsions.

Prevention

- Wear a seat belt when in a motor vehicle. Use child car seats.
- Wear a helmet while biking, motorcycling, skating, kayaking, horseback riding, skiing, or snowboarding.
- Don't dive into shallow or unfamiliar water.
- If you keep firearms in your home, store them unloaded, and lock them up. Store and lock ammunition in a separate place.

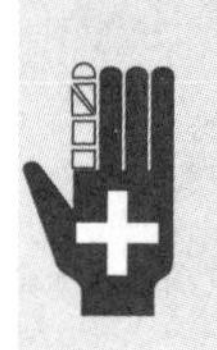

Home Treatment

- If the victim is unconscious, assume he or she has a spinal injury. Do not move the victim without first protecting the neck from movement (see page 104).
- If there is bleeding, apply firm pressure directly over the wound with a clean cloth or bandage for 15 minutes. If the blood soaks through, apply additional cloths over the first one. See Stopping Severe Bleeding on page 77.
- Check for injuries to other parts of the body, especially if the person has fallen. The alarm from seeing a head injury may cause you to overlook other injuries that need attention.
- Apply ice or cold packs to reduce the swelling. A "goose egg" may appear anyway, but ice will help ease the pain.
- A person who has a head injury should avoid contact sports until cleared by a health professional.

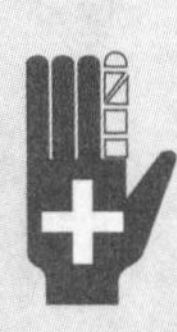

When to Call a Health Professional

Call 911 or other emergency services immediately:

- If the person loses consciousness at any time after being injured.
- If weakness or numbness occurs on one side of the body.
- If the person has seizures or convulsions.

Call your doctor now:

- If double vision or speech difficulty persists after the first minute.
- If blood or clear fluid drains from the ears or nose following a blow to the head (not due to a cut or direct blow to the nose).
- If the person is confused, does not remember being injured, or keeps repeating the same questions.
- If the person develops a severe headache.
- If vomiting occurs after the first 2 hours or violent vomiting persists after the first 15 minutes.
- If bleeding cannot be stopped (see page 77) or the wound needs stitches (see page 78).

Heart Attack

A heart attack (myocardial infarction) is caused by a complete blockage of the blood flow to a part of the heart muscle. This usually occurs when a small blood clot forms in one of the blood vessels that supply the heart muscle.

Discomfort or pain caused by a heart attack may be felt in the chest, abdomen, upper back, neck, jaw, and one or both arms.

The pain of a heart attack usually lasts longer than 10 minutes and often occurs with other symptoms such as sweating, shortness of breath, or nausea. The pain of a heart attack will not usually go away with rest.

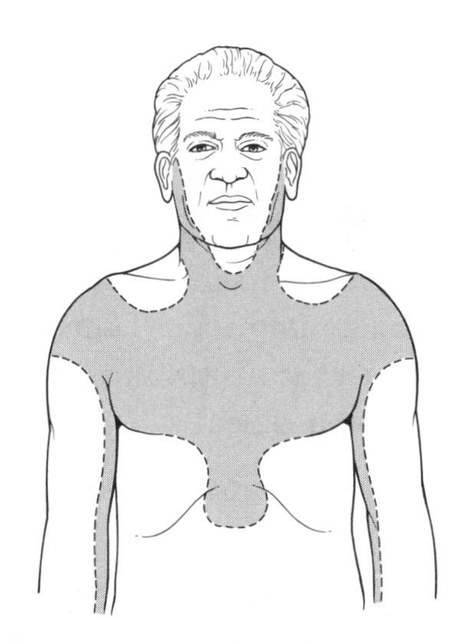

Discomfort caused by a heart attack can occur in any of the shaded areas as well as the upper back.

Many people mistake heart attack symptoms for other problems, such as indigestion, heartburn, or a pulled muscle. It is important to recognize the signals your body sends during the early stages of a heart attack and seek emergency care. Medical treatment is needed to prevent death. Sometimes medications can be given to reduce the heart muscle damage caused by a heart attack.

When to Call a Health Professional

Call 911 or other emergency services immediately if you think you may be having a heart attack. Do not try to drive yourself to the hospital. After calling 911, chew and swallow 1 adult Aspirin (unless you are allergic to or unable to take Aspirin).

Symptoms of a heart attack include chest pain or discomfort that is crushing (feels like someone is sitting on your chest), squeezing, or increasing in intensity or that occurs with any of the following symptoms:

- Sweating
- Shortness of breath
- Nausea or vomiting
- Pain in the abdomen, upper back, neck, jaw, or one or both arms
- Light-headedness
- Rapid or irregular heartbeat

Call your doctor if you have continuous chest discomfort or pain and there is no obvious cause.

Heat Exhaustion and Heatstroke

Heat exhaustion usually occurs when you are sweating a lot and do not drink enough to replace the lost fluids. It generally develops when you are working or exercising in hot weather. Symptoms include:

- Sweating a lot.
- Fatigue, weakness, headache, dizziness, or nausea.
- Skin that is cool, moist, pale, or flushed.

Heat exhaustion can sometimes lead to **heatstroke**, which requires emergency treatment. Heatstroke happens when your body fails to

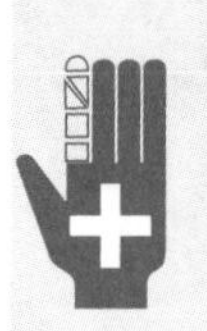

regulate its own temperature and your body temperature continues to rise, often to 40.5°C or higher. You may stop sweating entirely if you have heatstroke, or you may sweat profusely. Symptoms of heatstroke include:

- Confusion, delirium, or unconsciousness.
- Skin that is red, hot, and dry, even in the armpits.

Prevention

- Drink 8 to 10 glasses of water per day. Drink even more if you are working or exercising in hot weather.
- Avoid strenuous physical activity outdoors during the hottest part of the day (10 a.m. to 4 p.m.).
- Wear light-coloured, loose-fitting clothing and a hat with a brim to reflect the sun.
- Avoid sudden changes of temperature. Air out a hot car before getting into it. Never leave a child or an animal in a hot car.
- If you take diuretics (water pills), ask your doctor about taking a lower dose during hot weather.
- If you exercise strenuously in hot weather, drink more liquid than your thirst seems to require. Drink about 240 ml of water 10 to 15 minutes before you start exercising and another 240 ml of water every 20 to 30 minutes.

Home Treatment

- Stop your activity. Get out of the sun to a cool spot, and drink lots of cool water, a little at a time. If you are nauseated or dizzy, lie down.
- If a person's temperature exceeds 39°C, call for immediate help and try to lower the temperature as quickly as possible:
  - Remove unnecessary clothing.
  - Apply cool (not cold) water to the person's whole body; then fan the person. Apply ice packs to the groin, neck, and armpits. Do not immerse the person in ice water.
  - If you can get the person's temperature down to 39°C, take care to avoid overcooling. Stop cooling the person once his or her temperature is lowered to 37°C.
  - Do not give Aspirin or acetaminophen to reduce the temperature.
  - Watch for signs of heatstroke (confusion or unconsciousness; red, hot, dry skin).
  - If the person stops breathing, start rescue breathing (see page 68).

When to Call a Health Professional

Call 911 or other emergency services if the person's body temperature reaches 39°C and keeps rising, or if signs of heatstroke develop:

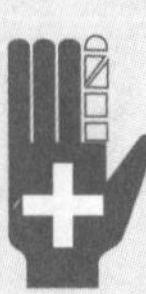

- Confusion, disorientation, unconsciousness, or seizure.
- Skin that is red, hot, and dry, even in the armpits. Sweating may be absent or excessive.

Hyperventilation

When you breathe very fast and deep (hyperventilate), the carbon dioxide (CO_2) level in your blood can drop too low. Symptoms that may occur with hyperventilation include:

- Numbness or tingling in your hands, feet, or around your mouth or tongue.
- Pounding, racing heartbeat and anxiety.
- Feeling like you can't get enough air.
- Light-headedness (feeling like you might pass out).
- Muscle cramps or spasms.
- Chest pain.
- Loss of consciousness (if hyperventilation is severe).

Prevention

If you have hyperventilated before:

- Ask people to tell you if you start to breathe too fast.
- As soon as you notice fast breathing or other symptoms, slow your breathing to 1 breath every 5 seconds, or slow enough that symptoms gradually go away.

Counting Respiration Rates

The respiration rate is the rate at which a person breathes. It increases with fever and some illnesses. The best time to count the respiration rate is when a person is resting, perhaps after you take the person's pulse while your fingers are still on the person's wrist. The person's breathing is likely to change if he or she knows you are counting it.

- Count the number of times the chest rises in 1 full minute.
- Notice whether there is any sucking in beneath the ribs or any apparent wheezing or difficulty breathing.

Normal resting respiration rate:

- Newborn to 1 year: 40–60 breaths/minute
- 1 through 6 years: 18–26 breaths/minute
- 7 years through adult: 12–24 breaths/minute

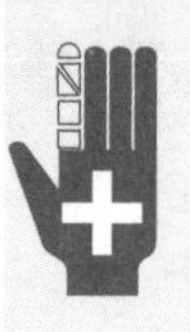

Home Treatment

- Sit down and concentrate on slowing your breathing. Try breathing through pursed lips or through your nose.
- Practise a relaxation technique. See page 386.
- Hold a paper bag over your nose and mouth and take 6 to 12 easy, natural breaths. Continue doing

this on and off for 5 to 15 minutes. Do not breathe continuously into the bag. Do not use this technique at all if you have heart or lung problems or if you are at an altitude above 1,800 metres.

When to Call a Health Professional

- If you are hyperventilating and cannot relieve the symptoms.
- If you have frequent or repeated episodes of hyperventilation and anxiety.

Hypothermia

Hypothermia is a condition of below-normal body temperature that develops when your body loses heat faster than heat can be produced by metabolism, muscle contractions, and shivering.

Early symptoms indicating mild to moderate hypothermia include:

- Shivering.
- Cold, pale skin.
- Apathy or listlessness.
- Impaired judgment.
- Clumsy movement and speech.

Later symptoms of severe hypothermia include:

- Cold abdomen.
- Rigid muscles.
- Slow pulse and breathing.
- Weakness or drowsiness.
- Confusion.

Shivering may stop if your body temperature drops below 32.2°C.

Hypothermia is an emergency and can quickly lead to unconsciousness and death. Hypothermia can happen at temperatures of 10°C or even higher in wet and windy weather or in 15.5°C to 21°C water. Frail and inactive people can develop hypothermia indoors if they are not dressed warmly.

Early recognition is very important in the treatment of hypothermia. Often a hiker or skier will lose heat to a critical degree before others notice anything is wrong. If someone starts to shiver violently, stumble, or respond incoherently to questions, suspect hypothermia and warm the person quickly.

Prevention

Whenever you plan to be outdoors for several hours in cold weather, take the following precautions:

- Dress warmly and wear windproof, waterproof clothing. Wear fabrics that remain warm even when they are wet, such as wool or polypropylene.
- Wear a warm hat. An unprotected head loses a great deal of the body's total heat.
- Keep your hands and feet dry.
- Head for shelter if you get wet or cold.
- Eat well before going out and carry extra food.

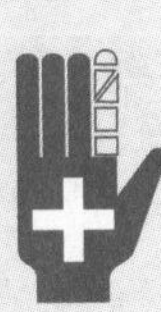

- Don't drink beverages containing alcohol while in the cold. They make your body lose heat faster.
- Older or less active people can prevent indoor hypothermia by dressing warmly and keeping room temperatures above 18°C.

Home Treatment

The goal of home or "in-the-field" treatment is to stop additional heat loss and slowly rewarm the person.

- For a mild case of hypothermia, get the person out of the cold and wind. Remove cold, wet clothes first, and give the person dry or wool clothing to wear.
- For a moderate case of hypothermia, remove cold, wet clothes first. Then warm the person with your own body heat by wrapping a blanket or sleeping bag around both of you.
- Give warm liquids to drink and high-energy foods, such as candy, to eat. Do not give food or drink if the person is disoriented or unconscious. Do not give alcoholic or caffeinated beverages.
- Rewarming the person in warm water can cause shock or heart attack. However, in emergency situations when help is not available and other home treatments are not working, you can use a warm-water bath (38° to 40.5°C) as a last resort.

When to Call a Health Professional

Call 911 or other emergency services if the person seems confused, stumbles repeatedly, or loses consciousness and remains unconscious.

Call your doctor:

- If the victim is a child or an older adult. It's a good idea to call regardless of the severity of the symptoms.
- If the person's body temperature remains below 35.5°C after 2 hours of warming.

Insect and Spider Bites and Stings

Insect and spider bites and bee, yellow jacket, and wasp stings usually cause a localized reaction with pain, swelling, redness, and itching. In some people, especially children, the redness and swelling may be worse, and the local reaction may last up to a few days. In most cases, bites and stings do not cause reactions all over the body.

Some people have severe skin reactions to insect or spider bites or stings, and a few have severe allergic reactions that affect the whole body (anaphylactic shock). Symptoms may include hives all over the body, shortness of breath and tightness in the throat or chest, dizziness, wheezing, or swelling of the tongue

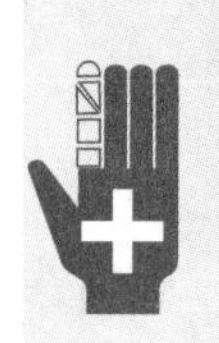

and face. If these symptoms develop, immediate medical attention is needed.

Spider bites are rarely serious, although any bite may be serious if it causes a person to have an allergic reaction. A single bite from a poisonous spider, such as a black widow, brown recluse, or hobo spider, may cause a severe reaction and requires immediate medical attention.

Black widow spiders can be up to 5 cm across (although they are generally much smaller) and are shiny black with a red or yellow hourglass mark on their undersides. Bites from female black widows may cause chills, fever, nausea, and severe abdominal cramps.

Brown recluse (fiddler) spiders are smaller than black widows and have long legs. They are brown with a violin-shaped mark on their heads. **Hobo** spiders are light brown with a yellowish green tint on their abdomens. They are about 1.25 cm across. A bite from a brown recluse or hobo spider results in intense pain, and a blister may develop that turns into a large, open sore. Their bites may also cause nausea, vomiting, headaches, and chills.

Also see Tick Bites on page 109.

Prevention

- To avoid bee stings, wear white or light-coloured solid fabrics. Bees are attracted to dark colours and flowered prints.
- Avoid wearing perfumes and colognes when you are outside.
- Apply an insect repellent containing DEET according to the product directions when in insect- and spider-infested areas. See page 209 for more information about using DEET.
- Wash DEET off when you go inside. Citronella and other products also seem to repel insects, but DEET works the best.
- Wear gloves and tuck pants into socks when working in woodpiles, sheds, and basements where spiders are found.

Home Treatment

- Remove a bee stinger by scraping or flicking it out. Don't squeeze the stinger; you may release more venom into the skin. If the stinger isn't visible, assume there isn't one.
- If you are bitten by a black widow, brown recluse, or hobo spider, apply ice to the bite and call your doctor immediately. Do not apply a tourniquet.
- Apply a cold pack or ice cube to the bite or sting. For some people, applying a paste of baking soda or unseasoned meat tenderizer mixed with a little water helps relieve pain and decrease the reaction.
- Take an oral antihistamine (such as Benadryl or Chlor-Tripolon) to relieve pain, swelling, and itching. Calamine lotion or hydrocortisone cream may also help.

- Carry an emergency kit containing an epinephrine syringe (such as EpiPen) if you have had a severe allergic reaction to insect venom in the past. Ask your doctor or pharmacist how and when to use the kit.

To prevent skin infection:

- Wash the area with soap and water.
- Trim your fingernails to prevent scratching, because scratching can lead to infection.
- Avoid breaking any blisters that develop.

When to Call a Health Professional

Call 911 or other emergency services if you develop the following signs of a severe allergic reaction soon after you are bitten or stung by an insect or spider:

- Wheezing or difficulty breathing.
- Swelling around the lips, tongue, or face, or significant swelling around the site of the bite or sting (for example, your entire arm or leg is swollen).
- Signs of shock. See page 103.

Call your doctor:

- If you develop a spreading skin rash, itching, feeling of warmth, or hives.
- If you have been bitten by a type of spider or insect that caused you to have a serious reaction in the past.
- If a blister appears at the site of a spider bite, or if the surrounding skin becomes discoloured.
- If symptoms are not improving in 2 to 3 days or if signs of infection develop. See page 100.
- To talk about adrenaline kits or allergy shots (immunotherapy) for insect venom if you have had a serious allergic reaction.

Nosebleeds

Most nosebleeds are not serious and can usually be stopped with home treatment. Some common causes of nosebleeds are low humidity, colds and allergies, injuries to the nose, medications (especially Aspirin), and high altitude. Blowing or picking your nose can also cause a nosebleed.

Prevention

- Low humidity is a common cause of nosebleeds. Humidify your home, especially the bedrooms, and keep the temperature cooler (15° to 18°C) in sleeping areas.
- If your nose becomes very dry, breathe moist air for a while (such as in the shower) and then put a little petroleum jelly on the inside of your nose to help prevent bleeding. A saline nasal spray may also help. See page 406.
- Limit your use of Aspirin, which can contribute to nosebleeds.

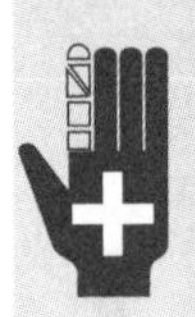

Home Treatment

- Sit up straight and tip your head slightly forward. Tilting your head back may cause blood to run down your throat.

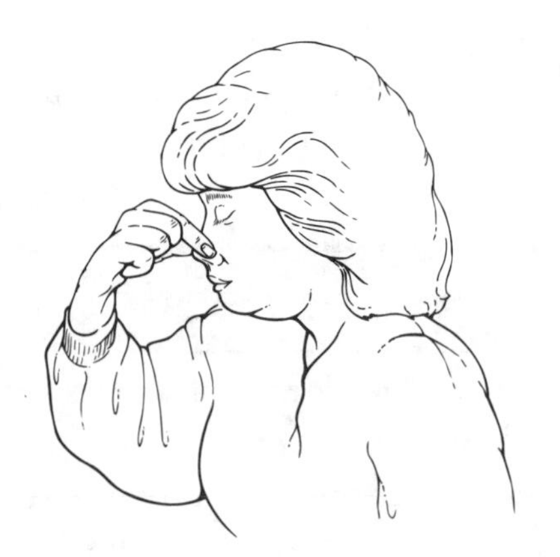

Stopping a nosebleed

- Blow all the clots out of your nose. Pinch your nostrils shut between your thumb and forefinger or apply firm pressure against the bleeding nostril for 10 full minutes. Resist the urge to peek after a few minutes to see if your nose has stopped bleeding.
- After 10 minutes, check to see if your nose is still bleeding. If it is, hold it for 10 more minutes. Most nosebleeds will stop after you apply direct pressure for 10 to 30 minutes.
- Stay quiet for a few hours and do not blow your nose for at least 12 hours after the bleeding has stopped.

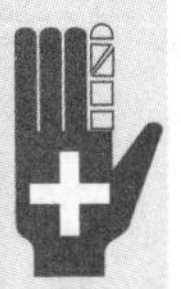

When to Call a Health Professional

- If the bleeding hasn't stopped after you have applied direct pressure for 30 minutes.
- If blood runs down the back of your throat even when you pinch your nose.
- If your nose is deformed after an injury and may be broken.
- If nosebleeds recur often (more than four in a week).
- If you take blood thinners (anti-coagulants) or high doses of Aspirin and have had more than one nosebleed in a single day.

Objects in the Ear

Children sometimes place food items or other small objects in their ears. A piece of cotton from a swab or cotton ball may become lodged in the ear canal. An insect may crawl into the ear. These objects usually cause only mild symptoms, such as minor discomfort or unusual noises in the ear. However, if an object stays in the ear too long, it can lead to infection.

Home Treatment

- Don't try to kill an insect inside a person's ear. Pull the ear up and back and let the sun or a bright light shine into the ear. Insects are attracted to light, so the insect may crawl out.

- If the insect doesn't crawl out, fill the ear canal with warm mineral, olive, or baby oil. The insect may float out.
- To remove an object other than an insect from the ear, tilt the person's head to the side and shake it gently. (Never shake a baby.) Gently pulling the ear up and back may straighten the ear canal and help dislodge the object.
- If you can see the object, try carefully to remove it with tweezers. Do not try this if the person will not hold very still or if the object is in the ear so far that you can't see the tips of the tweezers. Use care not to push the object in farther.

When to Call a Health Professional

- If you cannot remove the insect or object or it does not fall out on its own within 24 hours.
- If pain, fever, swelling, bleeding, or drainage develops.
- If hearing loss or dizziness develops.

Objects in the Eye

A speck of dirt or small object in the eye will often wash out with your tears. If the object is not removed, it may scratch the eye (corneal abrasion). Most corneal abrasions are minor and will heal on their own in 1 to 2 days.

When an object is thrown forcefully into the eye (from a machine, for example), it is possible that the eyeball will be punctured and emergency care will be needed.

Prevention

Wear safety glasses or other protective eyewear when working with machines or tools, mowing the lawn, or cycling.

Home Treatment

- Wash your hands before touching the eye.
- Don't rub the eye; you could scratch the cornea.
- Do not try to remove an object that is over the coloured part of the eye or stuck in the white of the eye. Try flushing it out with water or saline solution. If that doesn't work, call a health professional.
- If the object is at the side of the eye or on the lower lid, moisten a cotton swab or the tip of a twisted piece of tissue and touch the end to the object. The object should cling to the swab or tissue. Some minor irritation is common after you have removed the object.

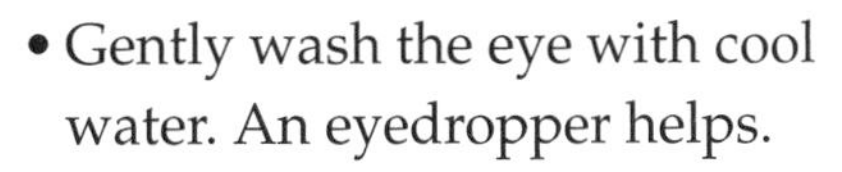

- Gently wash the eye with cool water. An eyedropper helps.
- Never use tweezers, toothpicks, or other hard items to remove an object from the eye.

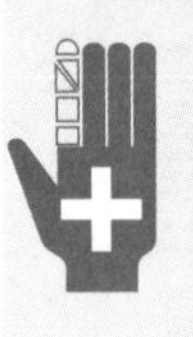

When to Call a Health Professional

Call 911 or other emergency services if the eyeball seems to be punctured.

Call your doctor:

- If the object is over the coloured part of the eye or is embedded in the eye. Do not pull out an object that is stuck in the eye.
- If you cannot remove the object.
- If there is blood over or in front of the coloured part of the eye.
- If pain is severe or persists; if it feels like there is still something in your eye; if your eye is sensitive to light; or if your vision is blurred after the object has been removed. Your cornea may be scratched. Keep your eye closed.

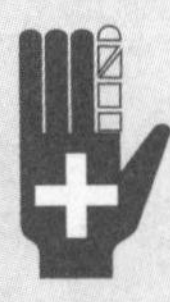

Objects in the Nose

Children sometimes put small objects, like beads, popcorn, or small batteries, up their noses. If the child doesn't tell you about it, your first clue may be a foul-smelling, green or yellow discharge from just one nostril. The nose may also be tender and swollen.

Home Treatment

- Have the child pinch the other nostril closed and try to blow the object out.
- If you can see the object, try to remove it with blunt-nosed tweezers. Hold the child's head still and use care not to push the object in farther. If the child resists, do not try tweezers. Minor bleeding from the nostril is not serious.
- Spray a nasal decongestant (see page 406) in the affected nostril to reduce the swelling, unless you suspect the object is a disc battery.

When to Call a Health Professional

- If a disc battery is stuck in the nose. The moist tissue in the nose can cause the battery to release harmful chemicals, often in less than an hour.
- If you are unable to remove the object after several tries.
- If removing the object causes a severe nosebleed. See page 93.

Poisoning

FOR ANY POISONING: Call 911 or Poison Control immediately.

Children will swallow just about anything, including poisons. When in doubt, assume the worst.

Always believe a child who indicates that he or she has swallowed poison, no matter how unappetizing the substance is.

If you suspect food poisoning, see page 133.

Carbon Monoxide Poisoning

Carbon monoxide is a colourless, odourless, tasteless gas produced from burning fuels such as natural gas, gasoline, fuel oil, charcoal, or wood. If fuel-burning appliances are not used properly, dangerous levels of carbon monoxide can build up in enclosed areas.

When a person inhales carbon monoxide, the carbon monoxide begins to replace the oxygen in the blood. This condition is called carbon monoxide poisoning. Symptoms include headache, dizziness, and nausea. If the exposure to carbon monoxide continues, the person may lose consciousness and even die. Infants, small children, older adults, and people with chronic health problems are more easily affected by high amounts of carbon monoxide in the blood, and their symptoms may be more severe.

To protect yourself and your family from carbon monoxide poisoning, install a carbon monoxide detector in your home. Also, have your heating appliances, chimneys, and vents inspected each year. Do not leave your car's engine running when the car is in an enclosed area such as a garage, even if the garage door is open.

If you know or suspect that someone has carbon monoxide poisoning, seek medical care immediately.

Prevention

More than half of all poisonings occur in children under age 6. Develop poison prevention habits before your child is born or certainly before he or she is crawling. Infants grow so fast that sometimes they are crawling and walking before you have time to protect them.

- Never leave a poisonous product unattended, even for a moment.
- Lock all drugs and vitamins away from children. Aspirin is a common source of childhood poisoning, especially flavoured baby Aspirin. Lock up drugs between doses.
- Do not keep poisons, such as drain opener, dishwasher detergent, oven cleaner, or plant food, under your kitchen sink. Keep them completely out of the reach of children. Dishwasher detergent is especially dangerous.
- Keep products in their original containers. Never store poisonous products in food containers.
- Use childproof latches on your cupboards.
- Keep the number for Poison Control near your phone.
- Talk with your health professional about including activated charcoal in your first aid supplies at home. Activated charcoal reduces the toxic effect of some poisons.

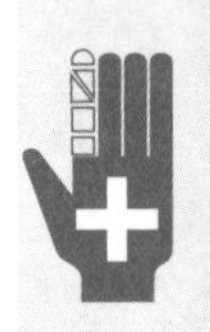

Lead Poisoning

Infants and young children who inhale or eat dust, food, or other things that contain lead are at risk for developing learning disabilities and growth problems. Lead poisoning can cause serious problems in adults as well.

Lead is present in old paint, water pipes, and other substances. Lead-based paint may be a hazard in older homes, especially if the paint is flaking or peeling and a child eats the paint flakes.

To reduce the risk of lead poisoning:

- Keep painted surfaces in good repair. Clean paint flakes and chips from older painted surfaces (such as floors and windowsills) carefully.
- Keep young children away from home remodelling and refinishing projects.
- If your home has lead or lead-soldered water pipes, use cold water and let the water run for a few minutes before using it for drinking, cooking, or making baby formula.
- Have your child's blood tested for lead at about 1 year of age.
- Call your local public health unit for more information about preventing lead poisoning.

When to Call a Health Professional

For poisoning of any kind, call 911, Poison Control, a hospital, or a health professional immediately for instructions. Have the poison container with you so you can describe the poison.

Puncture Wounds

Puncture wounds are caused by sharp, pointed objects that penetrate the skin. Nails, tacks, ice picks, knives, needles, and teeth can all cause puncture wounds. Puncture wounds become infected easily because they are difficult to clean and provide a warm, moist place for bacteria to grow.

Home Treatment

- If the object that caused the wound is small, such as a tack or sewing needle, remove it, checking to make sure it is intact. If the object is large or caused a deep wound, leave it in place and call a health professional immediately.
- Allow the wound to bleed freely for up to 5 minutes to clean itself out, unless there has been a large loss of blood or the blood is squirting out. If bleeding is heavy, see Stopping Severe Bleeding on page 77.

- Clean the wound thoroughly with soap and water. Do not use alcohol, hydrogen peroxide, iodine, or Mercurochrome.
- Watch for signs of infection (see page 100). If the wound closes, an infection under the skin may not be detected for several days.

Removing Splinters

Try using Scotch tape first. Simply put the tape over the splinter, and then pull it up.

If that doesn't work, grasp the end of the splinter with tweezers and try to gently pull it out. If the splinter is embedded in the skin, clean a needle with alcohol and make a small hole in the skin over the end of the splinter. Then lift the splinter with the tip of the needle until it can be grasped with the tweezers and pulled out.

After the splinter has been removed, wash the area with soap and water. Apply a bandage if needed to keep the wound clean; otherwise, leave the wound open to the air. Watch for signs of infection (see page 100).

Call a health professional if the splinter is very large or deeply embedded and cannot be easily removed, or if the splinter is in the eye.

When to Call a Health Professional

- If severe bleeding cannot be controlled. See page 77.
- If the wound is in your head, neck, chest, or abdomen, unless it is minor.
- If the skin near the wound is blue, white, or cold; if there is numbness, tingling, or loss of feeling; or if you are unable to move a limb below the wound.
- If an animal bite is severe and may need stitches, or if it is on your face, hand, or foot. Stitches usually need to be done within 8 hours.
- If the wound was caused by a cat or human bite.
- If you are unable to remove an object from the wound or if you think part of the object may still be in the wound.
- If the wound was caused by an injection of a substance under high pressure (such as from a paint sprayer).
- If you have a puncture wound and your tetanus shots are not up to date (see page 17).
- If a deep wound to the foot occurred through a shoe.
- If signs of infection develop. See page 100.

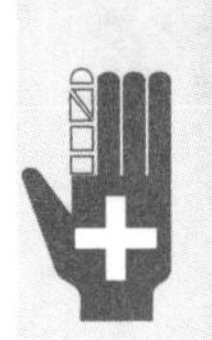

Scrapes

Scrapes or abrasions happen so often that they seem unimportant. Good home treatment will reduce scarring and prevent infection.

Home Treatment

- Scrapes are usually very dirty. Remove large pieces of debris with tweezers. Then scrub well with soap and water and a face cloth. The injured person will probably complain loudly, but thorough cleaning is necessary to prevent infection and scarring. Scrubbing may cause some minor bleeding. Using a water sprayer from the kitchen sink is a good way to wash a scrape.
- Apply steady pressure with a clean bandage or cloth to stop bleeding.
- Apply ice to reduce swelling and bruising.
- If the scrape is large or in an area that may be rubbed by clothing, apply an antibiotic ointment (such as Bacitracin or Polysporin) to the scrape and cover it with a non-stick bandage.

When to Call a Health Professional

- If bleeding continues after 30 minutes of pressure.
- If your tetanus shots are not up to date. See page 17.
- If you cannot clean the scrape well because it is too large, deep, or painful or because dirt and debris are embedded under the skin.
- If signs of infection develop. See page 100.

Signs of Infection

Infection can develop after a wound to the skin or mucous membranes, especially if the wound is not cleaned well. Cuts, scrapes, puncture wounds, burns, blisters, stings, bites, and rashes can all become infected. Bruises, sprains, broken bones, and other conditions can lead to infection under the skin.

Signs of infection include:

- Increased pain, swelling, redness, warmth, or tenderness.
- Red streaks extending from the affected area.
- Discharge of pus.
- Swollen lymph nodes in the neck, armpits, or groin.
- Fever of 38°C or higher with no other cause.

Call a health professional if signs of infection develop after a wound or injury. You may need to be treated with antibiotics.

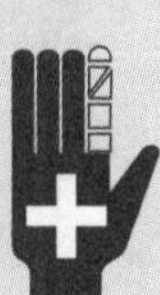

Seizures and Convulsions

The brain controls how the body moves by sending out small electrical signals through the nerves to the muscles. Seizures, or convulsions, may occur if the normal signals from the brain change.

Seizures are different from person to person. Some people have only slight shaking of a hand and do not pass out. Other people may pass out and have violent shaking of the whole body. Some people briefly lose touch with their surroundings and appear to stare into space. Although awake, they cannot respond normally, and afterwards may not remember what happened. A single seizure usually lasts less than 3 minutes and is not followed by a second seizure.

Any normally healthy person can have a single seizure under certain conditions. For instance, a sharp blow to the head may cause a seizure. However, a seizure may also be caused by a more serious medical problem, so it is important to follow up with your doctor to find the cause. Seizures have many possible causes, including extremely low blood sugar, alcohol or drug withdrawal, stroke, and other problems.

One common cause of recurring seizures is epilepsy. Epilepsy is a nervous system problem that can develop at any age. Usually a cause cannot be found, although sometimes epilepsy is the result of another condition, such as head injury, stroke, birth injury, or brain tumour.

A rapidly rising fever is a common cause of seizures in children. Fever seizures are scary but usually harmless. For information about fever seizures in children, see page 280.

Prevention

If you are being treated for seizures:

- Take your medications exactly as directed. Taking too little or too much medication, abruptly stopping your medication, or changing your medication schedule can cause seizures.
- Avoid activities that might trigger a seizure, such as games that have flashing or flickering lights. In rare cases, the flashing lights and geometric patterns of video games can trigger seizures in children.
- If your seizures are not well controlled, avoid potentially dangerous activities, such as operating heavy machinery, swimming, climbing ladders, and driving. In British Columbia, the law requires that you be seizure-free for a full year before driving.

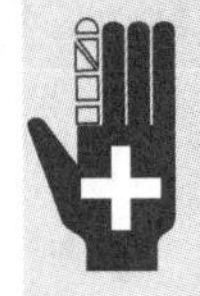

Home Treatment

No matter what the cause of the seizure, you can take steps to protect a person during a seizure and to get help after the seizure.

During a seizure:

- Protect the person from injury. If possible, keep the person from falling. Try to move furniture or other objects that might cause injury during the seizure.
- Do not force anything, including your fingers, into the person's mouth. This may cause injuries such as chipped teeth or a fractured jaw. You could also get bitten.
- Do not try to hold down or move the person.
- Try to stay calm.
- Pay close attention to what the person is doing so you can describe the seizure to rescue or health professionals.
- Time the length of the seizure, if possible.

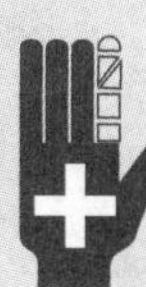

After a seizure:

- Check the person for injuries.
- Turn the person onto his or her side when the seizure ends and he or she is more relaxed.
- If the person has trouble breathing, use your finger to gently clear the mouth of any vomit or saliva.
- Loosen tight clothing around the person's neck and waist.
- Provide a safe area where the person can rest.
- Do not give the person anything to eat or drink until he or she is fully awake and alert.
- Stay with the person until he or she is awake and familiar with the surroundings. Most people will be sleepy or confused after a seizure.

When to Call a Health Professional

For information about fever seizures in children, see page 280.

Call 911 or other emergency services if:

- A seizure lasts longer than 3 minutes, or more than one seizure occurs within 1 hour.
- A seizure occurs with any signs of stroke (see page 108).
- A seizure occurs with signs of serious illness, such as severe headache, fever, stiff neck, trouble breathing, or an unexplained rash.
- A seizure follows a head injury.
- A seizure occurs after using street drugs or drinking a lot of alcohol.
- A pregnant woman has a seizure.
- A person with diabetes has a seizure.

Call a health professional if:

- You have a seizure and you have not been diagnosed with epilepsy.
- You have been diagnosed with epilepsy and notice a change in your seizures.

Taking a Pulse

The pulse is the rate at which a person's heart beats. As the heart pumps blood through the body, you can feel a throbbing in the arteries wherever they come close to the skin's surface. Most of the time, the pulse is taken at the wrist, neck, or groin.

- Count the pulse after a person has been sitting or resting quietly for 10 minutes or more.
- Place two fingers gently against the wrist as shown (don't use your thumb).
- If it is hard to feel the pulse in the wrist, locate the carotid artery in the neck, just to either side of the windpipe. Press gently.
- Count the beats for 30 seconds; then double the result to calculate beats per minute.

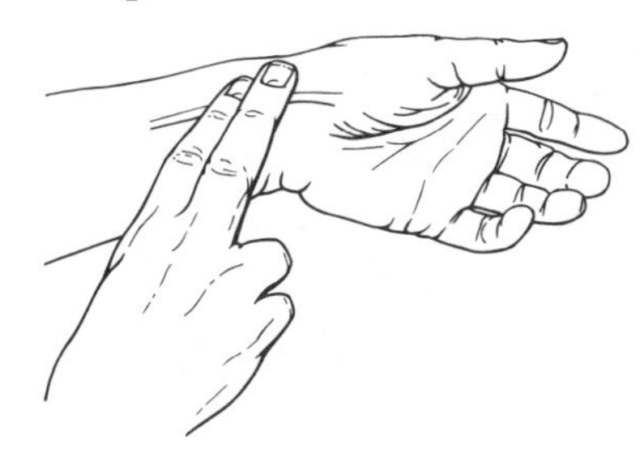

Normal resting pulse:

- Newborn to 12 months: 100–160 beats/minute
- 1 through 6 years: 65–140 beats/minute
- 7 through 10 years: 60–110 beats/minute
- 11 years through adult: 50–100 beats/minute

Certain illnesses can cause the pulse to increase, so it is helpful to know what your resting pulse rate is when you are well. The pulse rate rises about 10 beats per minute for every degree of fever.

Shock

Shock may develop as a result of sudden illness or injury. When the circulatory system is unable to get enough blood to the vital organs, the body goes into shock. Sometimes even a mild injury will lead to shock.

The signs of shock include:

- Cool, pale, clammy skin.
- Weak, rapid pulse.
- Shallow, rapid breathing.
- Low blood pressure.
- Thirst, nausea, or vomiting.
- Confusion or anxiety.
- Faintness, weakness, dizziness, or loss of consciousness.

Shock is a life-threatening condition. Prompt home treatment can save the person's life.

Home Treatment

- After calling for emergency care, have the person lie down and elevate his or her legs 30 cm or more. If the injury is to the head, neck, or chest, keep the legs flat. If the person vomits, roll the person to one side to let fluids drain from the mouth. Use care if there could be a spinal injury (see page 104).
- Control any bleeding (see page 77) and splint any fractures (see page 106).
- Keep the person warm, but not hot. Place a blanket underneath the person, and cover the person with

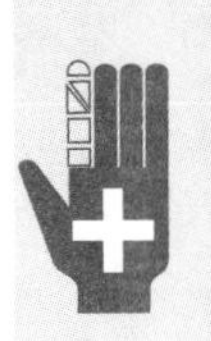

a sheet or blanket, depending on the weather. If the person is in a hot place, try to keep the person cool.

- Take and record the person's pulse every 5 minutes. See page 103.
- Comfort and reassure the person to relieve anxiety.

When to Call a Health Professional

Call 911 or other emergency services if a person develops signs of shock.

Spinal Injuries

Injury to the spine must be considered anytime there has been an accident involving the neck or back. Permanent paralysis may be avoided if the injured person is immobilized and transported correctly.

Signs of a spinal injury include:

- Severe pain in the neck or back.
- Bruises on the head, neck, shoulders, or back.
- Weakness, tingling, or numbness in the arms or legs.
- Loss of bowel or bladder control.
- Loss of consciousness.

Home Treatment

- If you suspect a spinal injury, do not move the person unless there is an immediate threat to life, such as fire. Don't drag victims from automobile accidents.
- If the person is in immediate danger and must be moved, do whatever you can to move the person's head, neck, and shoulders together as a unit while you move him or her to safety.
- If the person was injured in a diving accident, don't pull the injured person from the water, because you may cause permanent damage. Float the person face up in the water until help arrives. The water will act as a splint and keep the person's spine immobile.

When to Call a Health Professional

Call 911 or other emergency services to transport the injured person if you suspect a spinal injury.

Strains, Sprains, Fractures, and Dislocations

A **strain** is an injury caused by overstretching or tearing a muscle or tendon. A **sprain** is an injury to the ligaments or soft tissues around a joint. A **fracture** is a broken bone. A **dislocation** occurs when one end of a bone is pulled or pushed out of its normal position.

All four injuries cause pain and swelling. Unless a broken bone is obvious, it may be difficult to tell if an injury is a strain, sprain, fracture, or dislocation. An injury may involve all four. Rapid swelling often

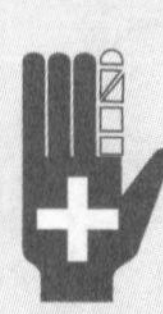

indicates a more serious injury. If a bone is poking through the skin, or if a limb turns white, cold, or clammy below the injured area, immediate medical care is needed.

Most minor strains and sprains can be treated at home, but severe sprains, fractures, and dislocations need professional care. Apply home treatment while you wait to see your health professional.

A **stress fracture** is a weak spot or small crack in a bone caused by repeated overuse. Stress fractures in the small bones of the foot may occur during intensive training for basketball, running, and other sports. The most common symptom is persistent pain at the site of the fracture. The pain may improve during exercise but will be worse before and after activity. There may not be any visible swelling.

Prevention

It may not always be possible to prevent accidents that cause strains, sprains, fractures, or dislocations. However, if you train properly for activities, try not to push too hard during activities, wear protective gear, and use equipment that is in good condition, you will improve your chances of avoiding serious injury.

Other tips for preventing accidents include the following:

- Make sure you can always see where you are going.
- Don't carry objects that are too heavy.
- Use a step stool to reach objects that are above your head. Don't stand on chairs, countertops, or unstable objects.
- Keep toddlers away from objects that may cause injuries if the child falls on them (coffee tables, stairs, and fireplaces).
- See the prevention tips in Sports Injuries on page 174.

Home Treatment

Generally speaking, whether the injury affects soft tissue or bone, the basic treatment is the same: **RICE**, which stands for rest, ice, compression, and elevation. Begin the RICE process immediately for most injuries.

R. Rest. Do not put weight on the injured joint for at least 24 to 48 hours.

- Use crutches to support a badly sprained knee or ankle.
- Support a sprained wrist, elbow, or shoulder with a sling, which will help the injury heal faster.
- Rest a sprained finger by taping it to the healthy finger next to it (this works for toes too). Always put padding between the two fingers or toes you are taping together.

Injured muscle, ligament, or tendon tissue needs time and rest to heal. Stress fractures need rest for 2 to 4 months.

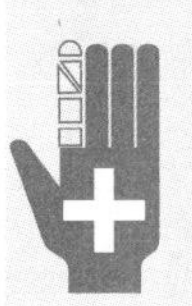

Splinting

Splinting immobilizes a limb that you suspect is fractured to prevent further injury until you can see a health professional. Splinting may also be helpful after a snakebite while you wait for help to arrive. There are two ways to immobilize a limb: tie the injured limb to a stiff object, or fasten it to some other part of the body.

For the first method, tie rolled-up newspapers or magazines, a stick, a cane, or anything that is stiff to the injured limb, using a rope, a belt, or anything else that will work. Do not tie too tightly.

Position the splint so the injured limb cannot bend. A general rule is to splint from a joint above the suspected fracture to a joint below it. For example, splint a broken forearm from above the elbow to below the wrist.

For the second method, tape a broken toe to the next toe, or immobilize an injured arm by tying it across the chest.

Note: These splinting methods are for short-term, emergency use only. Your doctor will provide you with a splint or cast that is appropriate for the type of injury you have.

I. Ice. Cold will reduce pain and swelling and promote healing. Heat feels nice, but it does more harm than good if it is applied too soon (less than 48 hours) after an injury.

Apply ice or cold packs immediately to prevent or minimize swelling. For difficult-to-reach injuries, a cold pack works best. See Ice and Cold Packs on page 167.

C. Compression. Wrap the injured area with an elastic bandage (such as an Ace wrap) or compression sleeve to immobilize and protect the area. Don't wrap it too tightly, because doing so can cause more swelling. Loosen the bandage if the area below the wrap feels numb, tingles, or feels cool. A tightly wrapped sprain may fool you into thinking you can keep using the joint. With or without a wrap, the joint needs total rest for 1 to 2 days.

E. Elevation. Elevate the injured area on pillows while you apply ice and anytime you are sitting or lying down. Try to keep the injury at or above the level of your heart to help minimize swelling and bruising.

Heat (hot water bottle, warm towel, heating pad) may be used after 48 to 72 hours of cold treatments if the swelling is gone. Some experts recommend going back and forth between heat and cold treatments.

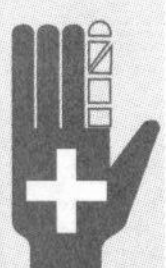

Removing a Ring

If you did not remove a ring before an injured finger started to swell, try the following method to remove the ring:

- Stick one end of a slick piece of string, such as dental floss, under the ring toward your hand.
- Starting at the side of the ring closest to the middle knuckle, wrap the string snugly around your finger, wrapping beyond the middle knuckle. Each wrap should be right next to the one before it.
- Grasp the end of the string that is stretched under the ring and pull the string toward the ring. As the string unwraps, push the ring ahead of it, until the ring passes the middle knuckle.

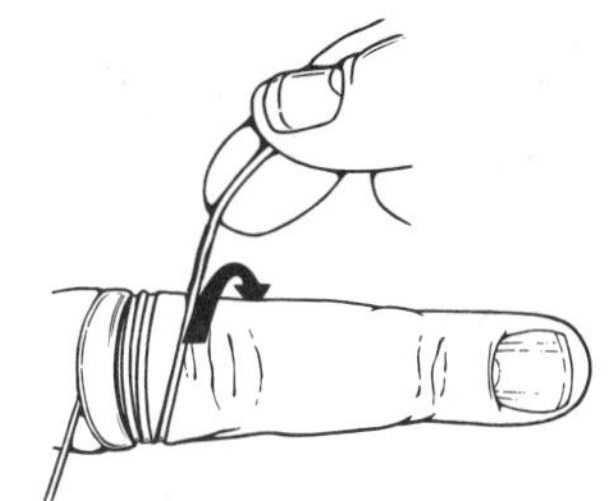

Wrap toward the end of the finger.

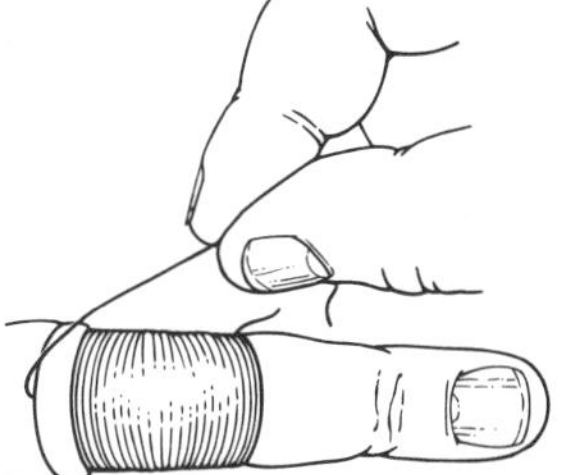

Pull the ring over the wrapped joint.

You may be able to prevent further damage by following these tips:

- Splint an arm, leg, finger, or toe that you suspect is broken. Use a splint or a sling for a short period of time (a few hours) while waiting to see your health professional. See page 106.
- Apply a sling to support an injured arm. Do not put an arm sling on a baby.
- Remove all rings, watches, and bracelets immediately from a sprained finger or hand. Swelling is likely to occur, making removal of these items more difficult later. See Removing a Ring on page 107.
- Use Aspirin, ibuprofen, naproxen sodium, or ketoprofen to help ease inflammation and pain. Do not give Aspirin to anyone younger than 20.
- Start gentle exercise as soon as the initial pain and swelling have gone away. If you have a broken bone or a severe sprain, your doctor may put the limb in a cast.

When to Call a Health Professional

- If the injured limb or joint is deformed or out of its normal position.
- If the skin over the site of an injury is broken.
- If there are signs of nerve or blood vessel damage:
  - Numbness, tingling, or a pins-and-needles sensation.

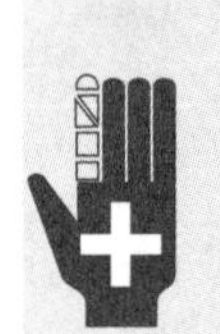

- Skin that is pale, white, or blue, or feels colder than the skin on the limb that is not hurt.
- Inability to move the limb normally because of weakness, not just pain.

- If you cannot bear weight on or straighten an injured limb, or if an injured joint wobbles or feels unstable.
- If pain is severe or lasts longer than 24 hours.
- If a lot of swelling develops within 30 minutes of the injury or if swelling does not improve after 48 hours of home treatment.
- If signs of infection develop following an injury. See page 100.

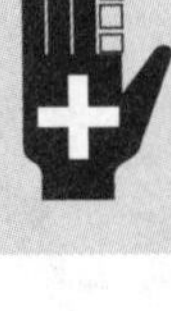

Stroke

A stroke occurs when a blood vessel (artery) supplying blood to the brain bursts or becomes blocked by a blood clot. Within minutes, the nerve cells in that area of the brain are damaged and die. As a result, the part of the body controlled by those cells cannot function properly.

Call 911 or other emergency services immediately if you think you may be having a stroke. Do not try to drive yourself to the hospital. If medical treatment is sought as soon as stroke symptoms are noticed, fewer brain cells may be permanently damaged by the stroke.

The effects of a stroke may range from mild to severe and may be temporary or permanent. A stroke can affect vision, speech, behaviour, thought processes, and the ability to move parts of the body. Sometimes it can cause a coma or death. The effects of a stroke depend on:

- Which brain cells are damaged.
- How much of the brain is affected.
- How quickly blood supply is restored to the affected area.

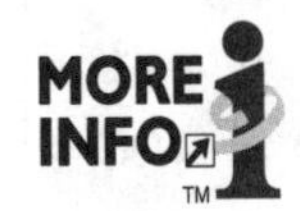

A person may have one or more transient ischemic attacks (TIAs) before having a stroke. TIAs are often called mini strokes because their symptoms are similar to those of a stroke. The difference between a TIA and a stroke is that TIA symptoms usually disappear within 10 to 20 minutes; however, TIA symptoms may last up to 24 hours. A TIA can occur months before a stroke occurs. It is a warning signal that a stroke may soon follow. The first TIA should always be treated as an emergency, even if the symptoms go away after just a few minutes.

When to Call a Health Professional

Call 911 or other emergency services immediately if you have any of the following symptoms of stroke:

- Any new weakness, numbness, or paralysis in your face, arm, or leg, especially on only one side of your body.

- Blurred or decreased vision in one or both eyes that does not clear with blinking.
- New difficulty speaking or understanding simple statements.
- Sudden, unexplainable, and intense headache that is different from any headache you have had before.
- Severe dizziness, loss of balance, or loss of coordination, especially if another warning sign is present at the same time.

If a symptom was definitely there and then went away after a few minutes, call your doctor immediately. Symptoms that go away in a few minutes may be caused by a TIA. A TIA is a strong sign that a major stroke may soon occur and should be treated as an emergency.

Tick Bites

Ticks are small, spider-like insects that bite into the skin and feed on blood. Ticks live in the feathers of birds and in the fur of other animals. Tick bites occur more often from early spring to late summer.

Most ticks do not carry diseases, and most tick bites do not cause serious health problems. However, it is important to remove a tick as soon as you find one.

You can get Lyme disease from ticks in BC. If not diagnosed and treated, Lyme disease can cause chronic illness, including serious joint and heart problems.

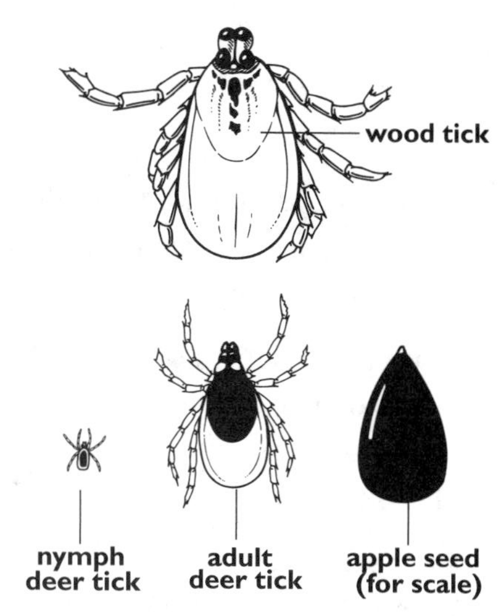

Lyme disease is usually spread by nymph deer ticks, which are difficult to see. Adult deer ticks are about the size of an apple seed. All ticks grow larger as they fill up with blood.

Many of the diseases ticks may pass to humans (including Rocky Mountain spotted fever, relapsing fever, Colorado tick fever, and Lyme disease) have the same flu-like symptoms: fever, headache, muscle aches, and a general feeling of illness. Sometimes a rash or crater-like sore (ulcer) may accompany the flu-like symptoms. An expanding red rash is an early symptom of Lyme disease. It may appear 1 day to 1 month after you have been bitten by a deer tick. If you develop flu-like symptoms or a rash after being bitten by a tick, be sure to tell your health professional.

Prevention

Before going outdoors in a tick-infested area:

- Put on light-coloured clothing and tuck pant legs into socks.

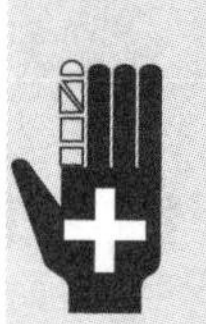

- Apply an insect repellent containing DEET to exposed areas of skin or to clothing. Apply carefully around eyes and mouth.
  - Children and pregnant women should use a lower concentration of DEET. See page 209.
  - Don't put repellent on small children's hands, because children often put their hands in their mouths.
  - After returning indoors, wash the repellent off with soap and water.

Home Treatment

- Regularly check your body for ticks when you are out in the woods, and thoroughly examine your clothes, skin, and scalp when you return home. Check your pets too. The sooner ticks are removed, the less likely they are to spread infection.
- Remove a tick by gently pulling on it with tweezers, as close to the skin as possible. Fine-tipped tweezers may work best. Pull straight out and try not to crush the body. Save the tick in a jar for tests in case you develop flu-like symptoms after you have been bitten.
- Wash the area and apply an antiseptic.

When to Call a Health Professional

- If you are unable to remove the entire tick.
- If you develop a red rash that expands over several days, especially if you know you were recently exposed to ticks. The rash may or may not be in the area where you were bitten and may be accompanied by flu-like symptoms, such as fatigue, headache, stiff neck, fever, chills, or body aches.

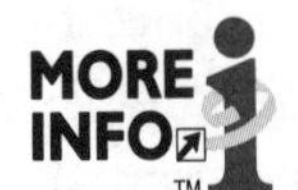

Your doctor will probably be able to tell if you have Lyme disease based on your symptoms and whether you may have been exposed to deer ticks. In most cases, blood tests to diagnose Lyme disease are not necessary.

Unconsciousness

An unconscious person is completely unaware of what is going on and is unable to make purposeful movements. Fainting is a brief form of unconsciousness; a coma is a deep, prolonged state of unconsciousness.

Causes of unconsciousness include stroke, epilepsy, heatstroke, diabetic coma, insulin shock, head injury, suffocation, alcohol or drug overdose, shock, bleeding, irregular heartbeat, and heart attack.

Fainting is a short-term loss of consciousness, usually lasting only a few seconds. It is most often caused by a momentary drop in blood flow to the brain. When you fall or lie down, blood flow is improved and

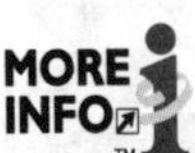

you regain consciousness. Fainting is a mild form of shock and is usually not serious. If it happens often, there may be a more serious problem. Dizziness and fainting can also be brought on by sudden emotional stress or injury. See page 222.

Home Treatment

- Make sure the unconscious person can breathe. Check for breathing, and if necessary, begin rescue breathing. See page 68.
- Check for signs of circulation, such as coughing, normal breathing, or movement in response to rescue breaths. If there are none, call for help and start cardiopulmonary resuscitation (CPR). See page 68.
- Keep the person lying down on his or her side.
- Look for a medical alert bracelet, necklace, or card that identifies a medical problem such as epilepsy, diabetes, or drug allergy.
- Treat any injuries.
- Do not give the person anything to eat or drink.

When to Call a Health Professional

Call 911 or other emergency services if a person remains unconscious for longer than a few seconds.

Call your doctor:

- If a person completely loses consciousness, even if the person is now awake.
- If unconsciousness follows a head injury and the person is now awake. A person with a head injury needs to be carefully observed. See page 85.
- Whenever a person with diabetes loses consciousness, even if he or she is now awake. He or she may have insulin shock (low blood sugar) or be in a diabetic coma (too much sugar in the blood).
- If fainting has occurred more than once.

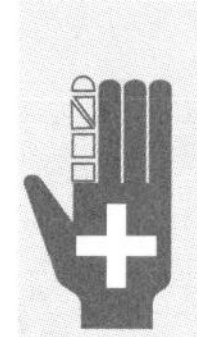

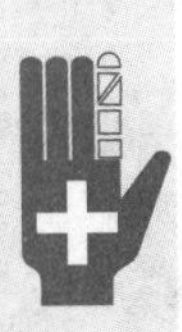

A great step towards independence is a good-humoured stomach.
Seneca

6

Digestive and Urinary Problems

The cause of a digestive or urinary problem can be hard to pinpoint. Sometimes both serious and minor problems start with the same symptoms. Fortunately, most digestive and urinary problems are minor and home treatment is all that is needed.

Use the chart on page 114 to find the symptoms that most closely match the ones you are having. Some illnesses that can cause digestive and urinary problems are covered more thoroughly in other chapters. Use the chart or the index to find those topics.

Abdominal Pain

You can get clues about the cause of abdominal pain and how serious the problem may be by noting the following:

- The severity of the pain. A visit to a health professional is usually needed when severe abdominal pain comes on suddenly and continues, or when new or different pain becomes more severe over several hours or days.
- The location of the pain. See illustration on page 113.

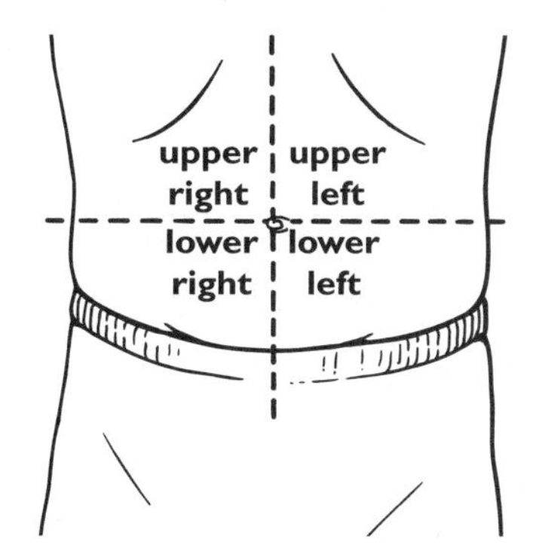

If you have abdominal pain, it helps to tell your doctor exactly where the pain is.

Digestive and Urinary Problems	
Symptoms	**Possible Causes**
Nausea or vomiting	Nausea and Vomiting, p. 129; Hepatitis, p. 122; Medication reaction—call your doctor or pharmacist; Adverse Drug Reactions, p. 411.
Bowel Movements	
Frequent, watery stools	Diarrhea, p. 120; Stomach Flu and Food Poisoning, p. 133; Antibiotics, p. 410.
Stools are dry and difficult to pass	Constipation, p. 116.
Bloody or black, tarry stools	Ulcers, p. 134; Diarrhea, p. 120.
Pain during bowel movements; bright red blood on surface of stool or on toilet paper	Hemorrhoids, p. 130; Anal fissure, p. 132; Constipation, p. 116.
Abdominal Pain	
Pain and tenderness localized to one place with possible nausea, vomiting, and fever	Appendicitis, p. 115; Urinary Tract Infections, p. 138; Ovarian cyst, p. 115; Gallstones, p. 126; Kidney Stones, p. 141; also see p. 113.
Bloating and gas with diarrhea, constipation, or both	Irritable Bowel Syndrome, p. 125.
Burning or discomfort behind or below breastbone	Heartburn, p. 121; Ulcers, p. 134; Chest Pain, p. 190.
Pain in lower abdomen and lower back just before menstrual period	Menstrual Cramps, p. 313; Ovarian cyst, p. 115.
Pain on one side of lower abdomen with possible pregnancy	Ectopic pregnancy, p. 309.
Urination	
Pain or burning while urinating	Urinary Tract Infections, p. 138; Kidney Stones, p. 141; Prostate Infection, p. 323; Sexually Transmitted Diseases, p. 332.
Difficulty urinating or weak urine stream (males)	Prostate problems, pp. 323 to 326.
Leaking urine or loss of bladder control	Urinary Incontinence, p. 137.
Blood in urine	Urinary Tract Infections, p. 138; Kidney Stones, p. 141; also see p. 136.
Abdominal Lumps or Swelling	
Painless lump or swelling in groin that comes and goes	Hernia, p. 124.
Very rigid or distended abdomen	Blunt Abdominal Wounds, p. 65; Appendicitis, p. 115; Watch for shock, p. 103.

Generalized pain is pain that occurs in more than half of the abdomen. Generalized pain can occur with many different illnesses, most of which will go away without medical treatment. Heartburn (indigestion) and stomach flu are common problems that can cause generalized abdominal pain. **Cramping**, which can be very painful, is rarely serious if passing gas or a stool relieves it. Many women have cramping pain with their periods. Unless it is significantly different than usual, or it localizes to one area of the abdomen, generalized pain is usually not a cause for concern.

Localized pain is pain that is most intense in one part of the abdomen. Localized pain that comes on suddenly and persists, that gradually becomes more severe, or that gets worse when you move or cough may indicate a problem in an abdominal organ, such as appendicitis, pancreatitis, diverticulitis, an ovarian cyst, or gallbladder disease.

Any new abdominal pain that lasts more than a few days needs to be evaluated by a health professional.

Home Treatment

Most of the time, abdominal pain improves with home treatment and does not require a visit to a health professional.

Specific home treatment for abdominal pain often depends on the symptoms that accompany the pain, such as diarrhea or nausea and vomiting. Be sure to review the home treatment guidelines for any other symptoms you have that are covered in this or other chapters.

Appendicitis

The appendix is a small sac attached to the large intestine. (See illustration on page 121.) Sometimes the appendix becomes inflamed or infected (appendicitis). If not treated, appendicitis can cause the appendix to burst and spread infection throughout the abdomen (peritonitis). This can cause a rigid or distended abdomen.

Typical symptoms of appendicitis include:

- Pain in the abdomen that begins around the navel or a little higher. The pain becomes more intense and then moves (localizes) to the lower right part of the abdomen below the navel. The pain is steady and gets worse when you walk or cough.
- Loss of appetite, nausea, vomiting, and constipation.
- Fever and chills.

Call your health professional:

- If you think you have appendicitis.
- If continuous pain in the lower right abdomen lasts longer than 4 hours.

Also see When to Call a Health Professional on page 116.

If you have mild abdominal pain without other symptoms, try the following:

- Rest until you are feeling better.
- Drink plenty of fluids to avoid dehydration. You may find that taking small, frequent sips of a beverage is easier on your stomach than trying to drink a whole glass at once.
- Try eating several small meals instead of two or three large ones. Eat mild foods, such as rice, dry toast or crackers, bananas, and applesauce. Avoid spicy foods, other fruits, alcohol, and drinks that contain caffeine until 48 hours after all symptoms have gone away.

When to Call a Health Professional

Call 911 or other emergency services if you have any of the following:

- Signs of shock (see page 103).
- Pain in the upper abdomen with chest pain that is crushing or squeezing, feels like a heavy weight on your chest, or occurs with any other symptoms of a heart attack (see page 191).
- Signs of severe dehydration (see When to Call a Health Professional on pages 119 to 120).
- Severe abdominal pain following an injury to the abdomen.
- Severe abdominal pain and fainting.

Call your doctor if you have:

- Ongoing severe abdominal pain.
- Localized pain that lasts longer than 4 hours.
- Generalized abdominal pain or cramping pain that has lasted longer than 24 hours and is not improving.
- Inability to keep down fluids.
- Pain that gets worse when you move or cough and does not feel like a pulled muscle.
- Any abdominal pain that has lasted longer than 3 days.

Constipation

Constipation occurs when stools are difficult to pass. Some people are overly concerned with stool frequency because they have been taught that a healthy person has a bowel movement every day. This is not true. Most people pass stools anywhere from 3 times a day to 3 times a week. If your stools are soft and pass easily, you are not constipated.

Constipation may occur with cramping and pain in the rectum caused by straining to pass hard, dry stools. There may be some bloating and nausea. There may also be small amounts of bright red blood on the stools or toilet paper; the blood comes from slight tears in the anus, which occur when hard stools are pushed through it. The bleeding should stop when the constipation is relieved.

If a stool becomes lodged in the rectum (impacted), mucus and fluid may leak out around the stool, which sometimes leads to leakage of fecal material (fecal incontinence). You may experience this as constipation alternating with diarrhea.

Lack of fibre and too little water in the diet are common causes of constipation. Other causes include inactivity, delaying bowel movements, medications, pain caused by a tear (fissure) in the lining of the rectum, and laxative overuse. Irritable bowel syndrome (see page 125) may also cause constipation.

Toilet training may contribute to constipation in young children. Children who are involved in play or other activities and ignore the urge to pass stools may become constipated. Children and adults who are reluctant to use toilets away from home may become constipated.

Prevention

- Eat plenty of high-fibre foods such as fruits, vegetables, and whole grains. You can also add fibre to your diet in the following ways (also see page 354):
  - Eat a bowl of bran cereal with 10 g of bran per serving.
  - Add 30 g of wheat bran to cereal or soup.
  - Try a product that contains a bulk-forming agent, such as Citrucel, FiberCon, or Metamucil. Start with 15 g or less and drink extra water to avoid bloating.
- Avoid foods that are high in fat and sugar.
- Drink plenty of water and other fluids every day. Drink extra fluids in the morning.
- Be more physically active. A walking program is a good start. See Fitness starting on page 343.
- Set aside relaxed times for having bowel movements. Urges usually occur sometime after meals. Establishing a daily routine (after breakfast, for example) may help.
- Go when you feel the urge and encourage your children to do the same. Your bowels send signals when a stool needs to pass. If you ignore the signal, the urge will go away and the stool will eventually become dry and difficult to pass.

Home Treatment

- Follow the diet outlined in Prevention to help relieve and prevent constipation.
- If necessary, use a stool softener or a very mild laxative such as Milk of Magnesia. Do not use mineral oil or any other laxative for more than 2 weeks without consulting your doctor.
- If an infant or child up to age 10 is having rectal pain because he or she is unable to have a bowel movement, put the child in a warm bath and add a little baking soda to the tub. This may help relax the muscles that normally keep stool inside the rectum, allowing the child to pass the stool.

- If your child is 6 months old or older and the warm bath does not work, use 1 or 2 glycerine suppositories to make the stool easier to pass. Use glycerine suppositories only once or twice. If constipation is not relieved or develops again, discuss the problem with your doctor.
- Do not give laxatives or enemas to a child without talking to your child's doctor first.

When to Call a Health Professional

- If constipation persists after home treatment has been followed for several days for an adult or according to a doctor's recommendation for an infant.
- If rectal bleeding is heavy (more than a few bright red streaks) or if the blood is reddish brown or black.
- If rectal bleeding lasts longer than 2 to 3 days after constipation has improved, or if bleeding occurs more than once.
- If you have sharp or severe abdominal pain.
- If you have rectal pain that either continues after you pass a stool or keeps you from passing stools at all.
- If you experience stool leakage (fecal incontinence).
- If your stools have become consistently more narrow (they may be no wider than a pencil).
- If you are unable to have bowel movements without using laxatives.

Dehydration

Dehydration occurs when your body loses too much water. When you stop drinking water or lose large amounts of fluids because of diarrhea, vomiting, or sweating, your body's cells reabsorb fluid from the blood and other tissues. Severe dehydration can lead to shock, which can be life-threatening.

Dehydration is very dangerous for everyone, but especially for infants, small children, and older adults. Watch closely for its early signs anytime there is an illness that causes high fever, vomiting, or diarrhea. The early symptoms are:

- Dry mouth and sticky saliva.
- Urinating smaller amounts than usual.
- Dark yellow urine.

Prevention

- Prompt home treatment for illnesses that cause diarrhea, vomiting, or fever will help prevent dehydration. See the chart on page 114.
- To prevent dehydration during hot weather or exercise, drink 8 to 10 glasses of fluid (water and sports drinks) each day. Drink extra water before, during, and after exercise.

Rehydration Drinks

Diarrhea and vomiting can cause your body to lose large amounts of water and essential minerals called electrolytes. If you are unable to eat for a few days, you are also losing nutrients. This happens faster and is more serious in infants, young children, and older adults.

A rehydration drink (Pedialyte, Gastrolyte, Rehydralyte) will replace fluids and electrolytes in amounts that are best used by your body. Sports drinks and other sugared drinks will replace fluid, but most contain too much sugar (which can make the diarrhea worse) and not enough of the other essential ingredients. Plain water won't provide any necessary nutrients or electrolytes.

Rehydration drinks won't make diarrhea or vomiting go away faster, but they will prevent serious dehydration from developing.

Home Treatment

Treatment of mild dehydration is simple: stop the fluid loss and restore lost fluids as soon as possible.

- To stop vomiting or diarrhea, do not eat any solid foods for several hours or until you are feeling better. During the first 24 hours, take frequent, small sips of water or a rehydration drink.
- Once the vomiting or diarrhea is controlled, drink water, diluted broth, or sports drinks a sip at a time until your stomach can handle larger amounts. Drinking too much fluid too soon can cause vomiting to recur.
- If vomiting or diarrhea lasts longer than 24 hours, sip a rehydration drink to replace lost minerals. See Rehydration Drinks on page 119.
- Watch for signs of more severe dehydration (see When to Call a Health Professional below).

For home treatment of vomiting or diarrhea in infants and children, see page 275.

When to Call a Health Professional

Call 911 or other emergency services if the following signs of severe dehydration develop:

- Sunken eyes, no tears, dry mouth and tongue.
- Sunken soft spot on an infant's head.
- Little or no urine for 8 hours.
- Extreme dizziness or lightheadedness when moving from lying down to sitting upright.
- Rapid breathing and heartbeat.
- Sleepiness, difficulty awakening, listlessness, and extreme irritability.

Call a health professional:

- If vomiting lasts longer than 24 hours in an adult.
- If a person is unable to hold down even small sips of fluid and therefore cannot drink enough to replace lost fluids.
- If severe diarrhea (large, loose stools every 1 to 2 hours) lasts longer than 2 days in an adult.

Diarrhea

Diarrhea occurs when the intestines push stools through before the water in the stools can be reabsorbed by the body. This causes bowel movements to occur more frequently and stools to become watery and loose. A person who has diarrhea may also have abdominal cramps and nausea.

The exact cause of diarrhea is often difficult to pinpoint. Viral stomach flu (gastroenteritis) or food poisoning often causes diarrhea. Many medications, especially antibiotics, can cause diarrhea; so can laxatives, if they are overused. Sorbitol (a sugar substitute) and olestra (a fat substitute used in some processed foods) may cause diarrhea. For some people, emotional stress, anxiety, or food intolerance may bring on this problem. Irritable bowel syndrome (see page 125) may also cause diarrhea.

Drinking untreated water that contains parasites, viruses, or bacteria is another cause of diarrhea. Symptoms may develop a few days to a few weeks after you drink the contaminated water.

Home Treatment

To treat diarrhea in infants and children 11 years and younger, see Home Treatment starting on page 275.

- Don't eat any food for several hours or until you are feeling better. Take frequent, small sips of water or a rehydration drink.
- Avoid antidiarrheal drugs for the first 6 hours. After that, use them only if there are no other signs of illness, such as fever, cramping or discomfort, or bloody stools. Stop taking antidiarrheal medications as soon as stools thicken. See Antidiarrheals on page 405.
- After the first 24 hours (or sooner, depending on how you feel), begin eating mild foods, such as rice, dry toast or crackers, bananas, and applesauce. Avoid spicy foods, other fruits, alcohol, and drinks that contain caffeine until 48 hours after all symptoms have disappeared. Avoid dairy products for 3 days after symptoms disappear.
- Take care to avoid dehydration. See page 118.

When to Call a Health Professional

- If you develop signs of dehydration (see page 118).
- If you have severe diarrhea (large, loose bowel movements every 1 to 2 hours) that lasts more than 1 or 2 days.
- If diarrhea lasts longer than 2 weeks.
- If stools are bloody or black.
- If abdominal pain increases or localizes, especially to the lower right or lower left part of the abdomen.
- If diarrhea occurs with a fever.
- If your symptoms become more severe or frequent.
- If diarrhea occurs after drinking untreated water.

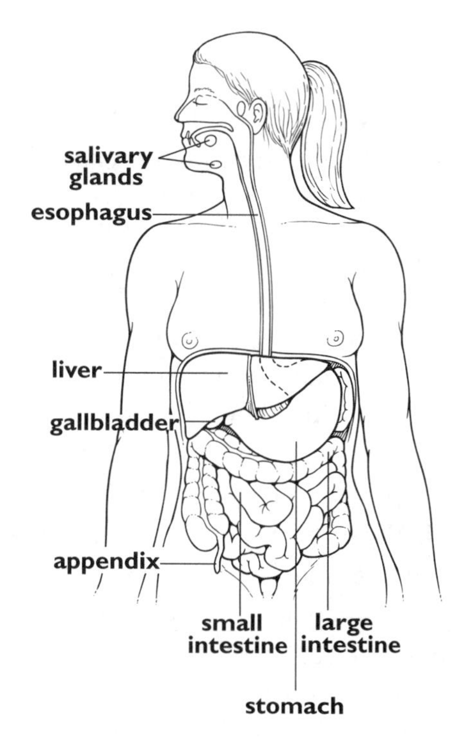

Organs of the digestive tract

Heartburn

Heartburn occurs when there is an abnormal backflow of stomach juices into the esophagus, the tube that leads from the mouth to the stomach. The backflow (reflux) causes a feeling of burning, warmth, or heat beneath the breastbone. The discomfort may spread in waves upward into your neck, and you may get a sour taste in your mouth. Heartburn can last up to 2 hours or longer. Symptoms often start after you eat. They grow worse when you lie down or bend over and improve when you sit or stand up.

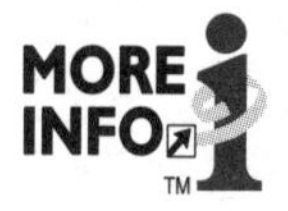

Don't be concerned if you have heartburn now and then; nearly everyone does. Following the home treatment tips can prevent most cases of heartburn. However, if backflow of stomach acid into your esophagus happens regularly, you may have gastroesophageal reflux disease (GERD). GERD can cause continuous irritation of the lining of the esophagus, which can lead to other health problems. It is important to visit a health professional if you have frequent heartburn and home treatment does not relieve the discomfort.

Hepatitis

Hepatitis means "liver inflammation." Viruses cause hepatitis A, B, and C, the most common types of hepatitis.

The hepatitis A virus (HAV) is spread mainly by oral contact with stool containing the virus. Most people become infected through contact with a household member who is infected. Large groups of people can become infected with HAV if someone who has hepatitis A prepares food for them. HAV infection usually goes away without medical treatment, causing no long-term problems.

The hepatitis B virus (HBV) lives in blood and other body fluids. It is commonly spread during sexual contact and when people share needles to inject drugs, but it can also be spread when an infected person shares items like razors or toothbrushes with others. A pregnant woman who is infected with HBV can pass the virus to her baby. Young people who become infected with HBV are more likely to develop chronic HBV infection and long-term liver problems than are people who become infected later in life.

The hepatitis C virus (HCV) is spread when HCV-infected blood enters a person's body. Blood transfusions were once a common means of spreading HCV, but this is now rare. The virus is commonly spread among people who share needles to inject drugs. Many people develop chronic HCV infection, which can lead to severe liver damage after many years.

Hepatitis symptoms are similar to flu symptoms. They include nausea, headache, sore muscles, and fatigue. Some people have pain in the upper right side of the abdomen. Jaundice may develop, causing the skin and whites of the eyes to turn yellow and making the urine dark. Call a health professional if you develop hepatitis symptoms or if you may have been exposed to hepatitis. Because all three types of viral hepatitis have similar symptoms, blood tests are needed to determine which hepatitis virus is causing the infection.

Vaccines can prevent hepatitis A and B (see page 19), but there is no vaccine for hepatitis C. If you are exposed to HAV or HBV before you have been vaccinated, getting a shot of immune globulin is likely to keep you from becoming infected.

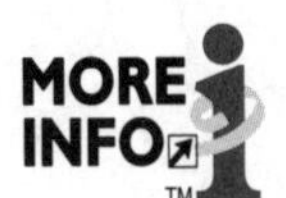

Drug treatment may be available for people with chronic hepatitis infection (HBV or HCV) who are likely to develop liver problems.

Home Treatment

Try other home treatment measures before taking antacids or stomach acid reducers to relieve heartburn. If you take medications to relieve your heartburn without doing other home treatment, your heartburn is likely to keep coming back. If symptoms are not relieved by home treatment, or if symptoms last longer than 2 weeks, call your doctor.

- Eat smaller meals, and avoid late-night snacks. After eating, wait 2 to 3 hours before lying down.
- Avoid foods that bring on heartburn. These may include chocolate, fatty or fried foods, peppermint- or spearmint-flavoured foods, coffee and other caffeinated drinks, alcohol, and carbonated drinks.
- Limit acidic foods that can irritate your esophagus. These include citrus fruits and juices such as orange juice and tomato juice. Limit spicy foods.
- Avoid clothes with tight belts or waistbands.
- Stop smoking. Smoking promotes heartburn.
- Lose weight if you are overweight. Being overweight can worsen heartburn, and the loss of even a few kilograms can help prevent heartburn.
- If you get heartburn at night, raise the head of your bed 15 to 20 cm by putting blocks underneath your bed frame or placing a foam wedge under the head of your mattress. (Adding extra pillows does not work well.)
- Avoid Aspirin, ibuprofen, naproxen sodium, and other anti-inflammatory drugs. These can cause heartburn. Try acetaminophen instead.
- Take a non-prescription product for heartburn. Antacids, such as Maalox, Mylanta, Tums, and Gelusil, neutralize stomach acid. Stomach acid reducers, such as Pepcid AC, Tagamet HB, and Zantac 75, reduce the production of stomach acid. Ask your pharmacist to help you choose one of these medications, and follow the package instructions and your doctor's advice for its use.

When to Call a Health Professional

Call 911 or other emergency services if you have any of the following:

- Pain in the upper abdomen with chest pain that is crushing or squeezing, feels like a heavy weight on your chest, or occurs with any other symptoms of a heart attack (see page 191).
- Signs of shock (see page 103).

Call your doctor:

- If there is blood in your vomit.
- If you suspect that a medication is causing heartburn. Antihistamines, antianxiety medications, and anti-inflammatory drugs,

including Aspirin, ibuprofen, and naproxen sodium, can sometimes cause heartburn.

- If you are routinely having pain or difficulty when swallowing solid foods.
- If you are losing weight and you don't know why.
- If heartburn persists for more than 2 weeks despite home treatment. Call sooner if symptoms are severe or are not relieved at all by antacids or stomach acid reducers. See Ulcers on page 134.

Hernia

A hiatal hernia is a common problem that occurs when a portion of the stomach bulges into the chest cavity. Hiatal hernias often do not cause symptoms. However, sometimes a hiatal hernia will cause a backflow of stomach acid into the esophagus (the tube leading from the mouth to the stomach), which can cause heartburn and a sour taste in the mouth. See Heartburn on page 121.

An inguinal hernia occurs when abdominal tissue bulges through a weak spot in the abdominal wall in the groin area. Inguinal hernias are more common in men than in women. In a man, an inguinal hernia may bulge into the scrotum.

A person with an inguinal hernia may sense that something has "given way." Other symptoms may include:

- A tender bulge in the groin or scrotum. The bulge may appear gradually, or it may form suddenly after heavy lifting, coughing, or straining. The bulge may disappear when the person lies down.
- Groin discomfort or pain that may extend into the scrotum. Discomfort may increase with bending or lifting.
- Nausea and abdominal swelling.

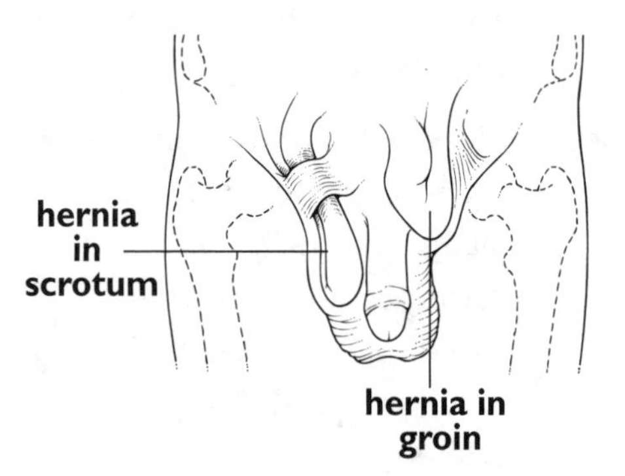

A hernia can cause a bulge or lump in the groin or scrotum.

Inguinal hernias can be caused by increased abdominal pressure resulting from lifting heavy weights, coughing, or straining to pass stools or urine. Sometimes a weak spot in the abdominal wall is present at birth. An inguinal hernia is called reducible if the bulging tissue can be pushed back into place in the abdomen. If the tissue cannot be pushed back into place, the hernia is called irreducible.

If an inguinal hernia is irreducible, the tissue may become trapped outside the abdominal wall. If the blood supply to the tissue is cut off (strangulated hernia), the tissue will swell and die. The dead tissue will quickly become infected, requiring immediate medical attention. Rapidly increasing pain in the groin or scrotum is a sign that a hernia has become strangulated.

A hernia can develop anywhere there is a weakness in the abdominal wall. Common places for hernias to develop are the belly button (umbilical hernia) and at the site of an incision from abdominal surgery (incisional hernia).

Prevention

- Use proper lifting techniques (see page 146), and avoid lifting weights that are too heavy for you.
- Lose weight if you are overweight.
- Avoid constipation and do not strain during bowel movements and urination.
- Stop smoking, especially if you have a chronic cough.

When to Call a Health Professional

Call a health professional immediately:

- If a testicle swells and is painful, particularly in a child or adolescent.
- If you have sudden, severe pain in the groin area, along with nausea, vomiting, and fever.

Also call a health professional:

- If mild groin pain or an unexplained bump or swelling in the groin continues for more than 1 week.
- If the skin over a hernia or bulge in the groin or abdomen becomes red.

If you have been diagnosed with a hernia, call a health professional if the hernia cannot be pushed back into place with gentle pressure when you are lying down.

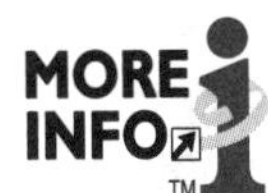

If you suspect that you have a hernia, see your doctor to confirm the diagnosis and discuss your treatment options.

Irritable Bowel Syndrome

Irritable bowel syndrome (IBS) is one of the most common disorders of the digestive tract. Symptoms of IBS often increase with stress or after eating and include:

- Abdominal bloating, pain, and gas.
- Mucus in the stool.
- Feeling as if a bowel movement hasn't been completed.
- Irregular bowel habits, with constipation, diarrhea, or both.

The cause of IBS is unknown. Symptoms are thought to be related to abnormal muscle contractions in the intestines. However, when tests are done, they find no changes (such as inflammation or tumours) in the physical structure of the intestines.

Gallstones

Gallstones are small stones (usually made of cholesterol) that form in the gallbladder. Most people who have gallstones do not have any symptoms.

Sometimes gallstones cause the gallbladder to become inflamed. The main symptom is a dull aching or cramping pain that starts in the upper right abdomen and may radiate to the centre of the upper abdomen or to the right upper back or shoulder blade. The pain may be severe and usually lasts several hours. Fever and vomiting also may be present.

Symptoms often occur at night, usually at about the same time every night. Pain may or may not be related to a meal.

Risk factors for gallstones include a high-fat, high-sugar diet; obesity; lack of exercise; rapid weight loss; estrogen replacement therapy; and diabetes. Gallstones are more common in women than in men.

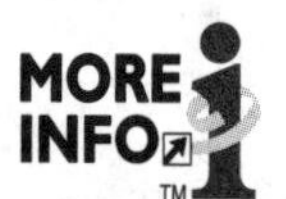

Gallstones that don't cause symptoms don't require treatment. If you have gallstones that cause pain or infection, you may want to consider having gallbladder surgery.

If you have mild symptoms, it is safe to wait until symptoms recur several times before seeking treatment. See When to Call a Health Professional on page 116 to decide what to do if your symptoms become more severe.

IBS can persist for many years. An episode may be more severe than the one before it, but the disorder itself does not worsen over time or lead to more serious diseases such as cancer. Symptoms tend to get better over time.

If you have not yet been diagnosed with IBS, try to rule out other causes of stomach problems, such as eating a new food, nervousness, or stomach flu. Try home treatment for 1 to 2 weeks. If there is no improvement, or if your symptoms worsen, call your doctor for an appointment.

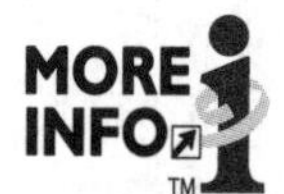

Your doctor may prescribe medication for you to take in addition to doing home treatment. There are no tests that can diagnose irritable bowel syndrome, but your doctor may recommend testing to rule out other possible causes of your symptoms. The amount of testing your doctor will do depends on your age, the pattern and severity of your symptoms, and your response to initial treatment.

Prevention

There is no way to prevent IBS. However, symptoms often worsen or improve because of changes in your diet, your stress level, your medications, the amount of exercise you are getting, or for other reasons. Identifying the things that trigger your symptoms may help you avoid or minimize attacks.

Home Treatment

If constipation is your main symptom:

- Eat more fruits, vegetables, legumes, and whole grains. Add these fibre-rich foods to your diet slowly so they do not worsen gas or cramps. See page 354.
- Add unprocessed wheat bran to your diet. Start by using 15 g per day, and gradually increase to 60 g per day. Sprinkle bran on cereal, soup, and casseroles. Drink extra water to avoid becoming bloated.
- Try a product that contains a bulk-forming agent, such as Citrucel, FiberCon, or Metamucil. Start with 15 g or less per day, and drink extra water to prevent bloating.
- Use laxatives only if your doctor recommends them.
- Be more physically active. Exercise helps the digestive system work better.

If diarrhea is your main symptom:

- Try the dietary suggestions for relieving constipation. Fibre-rich foods and wheat bran can sometimes help relieve diarrhea by absorbing liquid in the large intestine.
- Avoid foods that make diarrhea worse. Try eliminating one food at a time; then add it back gradually. If a food doesn't seem to be related to symptoms, there is no need to avoid it. Many people find that the following foods or ingredients make their symptoms worse:
  - Alcohol, caffeine, nicotine
  - Beans, broccoli, cabbage, apples
  - Spicy foods
  - Foods high in acid, such as citrus fruit
  - Fatty foods, including bacon, sausage, butter, oils, and anything deep-fried
- Avoid dairy products that contain lactose (milk sugar) if they seem to worsen symptoms. However, be sure to get enough calcium in your diet from other sources. See Lactose Intolerance on page 360.
- Avoid sorbitol (an artificial sweetener found in some sugarless candies and gum) and olestra (a fat substitute used in some processed foods, such as potato chips).
- Add more starchy food (bread, rice, potatoes, pasta) to your diet.
- If diarrhea persists, a non-prescription medication such as loperamide (the active ingredient in products such as Imodium) may help. Check with your doctor if you are using loperamide twice a month or more.

To reduce stress:

- Keep a record of the life events that occur with your symptoms. This may help you see any connection between your symptoms and stressful occasions.
- Get regular, vigorous exercise such as swimming, jogging, or brisk walking to help reduce tension.
- See page 386 for more tips on managing stress.

Crohn's Disease

Crohn's disease is a chronic inflammatory bowel disease that causes parts of the digestive tract to swell and develop sores. Crohn's disease usually occurs in the last part of the small intestine and the first part of the large intestine. But it can develop anywhere from the mouth to the anus.

The main symptoms of Crohn's disease are abdominal pain, rectal bleeding, and diarrhea. Constipation, fever, and loss of appetite may also occur.

Antidiarrheal medications can sometimes control mild cases of Crohn's. Some people need prescription medications to help reduce inflammation. These self-care tips may also help:

- Cut down on sugar and processed foods, and avoid foods that make your symptoms worse. These might include milk, alcohol, or spicy foods.
- Eat a healthy diet. Make sure to get enough iron. Rectal bleeding may make you lose iron. Good sources of iron include lean beef, lentils, spinach, raisins, and enriched breads and cereals.
- Do not take anti-inflammatory medicines, such as Aspirin, ibuprofen, or naproxen. They may make your symptoms worse. If you need pain relief, try acetaminophen.
- Do not smoke. Smoking makes Crohn's disease worse.

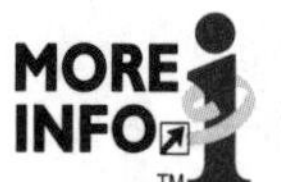

If your symptoms are severe and do not respond to medications, or if you develop complications, you may need surgery to remove the damaged part of the colon. However, most people with Crohn's disease do not need surgery.

When to Call a Health Professional

- If you have been diagnosed with irritable bowel syndrome and your symptoms get worse, begin to disrupt your usual activities, or do not respond as usual to home treatment.
- If you are becoming increasingly fatigued.
- If your symptoms frequently wake you.
- If your pain gets worse with movement or coughing.
- If you have abdominal pain and a fever.
- If you have abdominal pain that does not get better when you pass gas or stools.

- If you are losing weight and you don't know why.
- If your appetite has decreased.
- If there is blood in your stools.

Nausea and Vomiting

Nausea is a very unpleasant feeling in the pit of the stomach. A person who is nauseated may feel weak and sweaty and produce lots of saliva.

Intense nausea often leads to vomiting, which forces stomach contents up the esophagus and out of the mouth. Home treatment will help ease the discomfort.

Nausea and vomiting may be caused by:

- Viral stomach flu or food poisoning (see page 133).
- Stress or nervousness.
- Medications, especially antibiotics and anti-inflammatory drugs, such as Aspirin, ibuprofen, and naproxen sodium.
- Pregnancy (see Morning Sickness on page 305).
- Diabetes.
- Migraine headache (see page 238).
- Head injury (see page 85).

Nausea and vomiting can also be signs of other serious illnesses involving abdominal organs such as the liver (hepatitis, see page 122), pancreas, gallbladder (gallstones, see page 126), stomach (ulcers, see page 134), or appendix (appendicitis, see page 115).

Home Treatment

Home treatment may be all that is needed to treat occasional vomiting. For home treatment of vomiting in children under age 4, see page 276. For older children and adults:

- Watch for and treat early signs of dehydration. See page 118. Older adults and young children can quickly become dehydrated from vomiting.
- After vomiting has stopped for 1 hour, drink 30 ml of a clear liquid every 20 minutes for 1 hour. Clear liquids include apple or grape juice mixed to half strength with water; rehydration drinks; weak tea with sugar; clear broth; and gelatin dessert. Avoid citrus juices.
- If vomiting lasts longer than 24 hours, sip a rehydration drink to restore lost fluids and nutrients. See page 119.
- When you are feeling better, begin eating clear soups, mild foods, and liquids until all symptoms have been gone for 12 to 48 hours. Gelatin dessert, dry toast, crackers, and cooked cereal are good choices.
- Rest in bed until you are feeling better.

When to Call a Health Professional

- If signs of severe dehydration develop (see When to Call a Health Professional on pages 119 to 120).
- If vomiting occurs with:
  - Severe headache, sleepiness, lethargy, or stiff neck. See Encephalitis and Meningitis on page 201.
  - Chest pain. See Heart Attack on page 86.
  - Fever and increasing pain in the lower right abdomen.
  - Fever and shaking chills.
  - Abdominal swelling.
  - Pain in the upper right or upper left abdomen. See illustration on page 113.
- If vomit contains blood or material that looks like coffee grounds. See Shock on page 103.
- If vomiting and fever last longer than 48 hours.
- If you suspect that a medication is causing the problem. Antibiotics and anti-inflammatory medications (Aspirin, ibuprofen, naproxen sodium) may cause nausea or vomiting. Learn which of your medications can cause these symptoms.
- If vomiting occurs after a head injury. See page 85.
- If any vomiting lasts longer than 1 week.

Rectal Problems

The rectum is the lower part of the large intestine. At the end of the rectum is the anus, where stools pass out of the body.

Rectal problems are common. Most people experience itching, pain, or bleeding in the rectal or anal area at some time. These problems are often minor and will go away on their own or with home treatment.

Anal itching can have many causes. Skin around the anus may become irritated because of stool leakage. Anal itching can also be a sign of pinworms (see page 282), especially in households with children. Caffeine and spicy foods can irritate the lining of the rectum, causing anal itching and discomfort. If the anus is not kept clean, itching may result. However, trying to keep the area too clean by rubbing it with dry toilet paper or using harsh soap may injure the skin.

Hemorrhoids are enlarged and inflamed veins that may develop inside or outside the anus. Straining to pass hard stools, being overweight or pregnant, and prolonged sitting or standing can all cause hemorrhoids.

Hemorrhoids generally last several days and often come back (recur). The symptoms of hemorrhoids include bright red streaks of blood on stools or toilet paper or blood dripping from the anus; leakage of mucus from the anus; irritation or itching around the anus; and feeling as if a bowel movement hasn't been completed. Sometimes an internal hemorrhoid will actually stick out of the anus and may have to be pushed back into place with a finger.

Colorectal Cancer

Cancer of the colon and rectum is one of the leading causes of cancer deaths. Treatment is very successful in the early stages of the disease, but because colorectal cancer usually has no symptoms in its early stages, it is often not detected until much later. Regular screening tests are therefore the best prevention for colorectal cancer. Routine screening can detect pre-cancerous changes that may lead to cancer or detect the cancer early enough that it can be successfully treated.

Screening for colorectal cancer may include one or more of the following tests:

- **Colonoscopy**. During this test, the doctor uses a flexible lighted tube to view the rectum and the entire length of the colon. Polyps found during the colonoscopy or a previous test can be removed during the procedure. The test usually takes 30 to 60 minutes. Colonoscopy is the most thorough screening method for colorectal cancer, but it is also the most invasive and the most expensive.
- **Flexible sigmoidoscopy**. Like colonoscopy, this test uses a flexible lighted tube to look for pre-cancerous growths and cancers of the colon and rectum. However, in flexible sigmoidoscopy, the doctor is only able to view the rectum and the lower third of the colon. The examination takes about 15 minutes, is only mildly uncomfortable, and is very safe.
- **Fecal occult blood test**. This test can detect hidden blood in your stool. It is inexpensive and easy to do at home, but it does not detect colon cancer nearly as well as flexible sigmoidoscopy or colonoscopy.
- **Barium enema**. This is an X-ray examination of the colon and rectum. To make the intestine visible on the X-ray, the colon is filled with a contrast material containing barium. Barium enema is now used infrequently to screen for colorectal cancer.

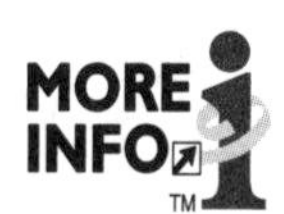

Screening tests are recommended for all adults older than 50 and for adults older than 40 who are at increased risk. You are at increased risk if you have a family history of colorectal cancer or if you have a personal history of colon polyps, ulcerative colitis, or Crohn's disease. Talk with your doctor about which tests and screening schedules are most appropriate for you.

Pain is not usually a symptom, unless a blood clot forms in a hemorrhoid or the blood supply to a hemorrhoid is cut off (strangulated). A clotted hemorrhoid may be extremely painful but is not dangerous. However, a strangulated hemorrhoid may need emergency treatment.

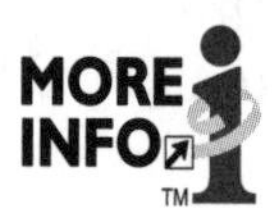

You may want to consider surgery if you have hemorrhoids that bleed persistently, are very uncomfortable, or make it difficult to keep your anal area clean. Talk to your doctor about your options for surgery.

An **anal fissure** may cause pain during bowel movements and streaks of blood on stools. Anal fissures are long, narrow sores that usually develop when the tissue in the anal area is torn during a bowel movement.

Rectal bleeding, recent changes in bowel habits, and rectal pain are also symptoms of colorectal cancer (see page 131). People who have these symptoms, especially people age 50 or older who have a family history of cancer, should talk to their health professional.

Prevention

- Keep your stools soft. Include plenty of water, fresh fruits and vegetables, and whole grains in your diet. Include up to 30 g of bran or a commercial stool softener, such as Metamucil, in your diet each day. Regular exercise promotes smooth bowel movements. Also see Constipation on page 116.
- Try not to strain during bowel movements, and never hold your breath. Take your time, but don't sit on the toilet too long.
- Avoid sitting or standing too much. Take short walks to increase blood flow in your pelvic region.
- Keep the anal area clean, but be gentle when cleansing it. Use water and a fragrance-free soap, or use baby wipes or Tucks pads.

Home Treatment

- Take warm baths. They are soothing and cleansing, especially after you have a bowel movement. Sitz baths (warm baths with just enough water to cover the anal area) are also helpful for hemorrhoids but may worsen anal itching.
- Wear cotton underwear and loose clothing to decrease moisture in the anal area.
- Apply a cold compress on the anus for 10 minutes, 4 times a day.
- Ease itching and irritation with zinc oxide, petroleum jelly, or hydrocortisone (1%) cream. Use medicated suppositories (such as Preparation H) to relieve pain and lubricate the anal canal during bowel movements. Ask your doctor before using any product that contains a local anaesthetic (these products have the suffix

"-caine" in the name or ingredients). Such products cause allergic reactions in some people.

When to Call a Health Professional

- If rectal bleeding occurs for no apparent reason and is not associated with trying to pass stools.
- If rectal bleeding continues for more than 1 week or occurs more than once.
- If stools become more narrow than usual (they may be no wider than a pencil).
- If pain caused by hemorrhoids is severe, or if moderate anal pain continues after a full week of home treatment.
- If any unusual material or tissue seeps or sticks out of the anus.
- If a lump near the anus gets bigger or becomes more painful and you develop a fever.
- If fever accompanies bloody stools.

Stomach Flu and Food Poisoning

Stomach flu and food poisoning are different ailments with different causes. However, many people confuse the two because the symptoms are so similar.

Stomach flu is usually caused by a viral infection in the digestive system. To prevent stomach flu, you must avoid contact with the virus, which is not always easy to do.

Food poisoning is usually caused by a toxin produced by bacteria in food that is not handled or stored properly. Bacteria can grow rapidly when certain foods, especially meats, dairy products, and sauces, are not handled properly during preparation or are kept at temperatures between 4° and 60°C.

Suspect food poisoning when symptoms are shared by others who ate the same food, or when symptoms develop after eating unrefrigerated foods. Symptoms of food poisoning may begin as soon as 1 or 2 hours or as late as 48 hours after eating. Nausea, vomiting, and diarrhea may last from 12 to 48 hours.

Botulism is a rare but often fatal type of food poisoning. It is generally caused by improper home canning methods for low-acid foods like beans and corn. Bacteria that survive the canning process may grow and produce toxins in the jar. Symptoms include blurred or double vision and difficulty swallowing or breathing.

Prevention

To prevent food poisoning:

- Keep hot foods hot and cold foods cold.
- Don't eat meat, dressings, salads, or other foods that have been kept for more than 2 hours between 4° and 60°C.
- Use a thermometer to check your refrigerator. It should be between 0° and 4°C.

- Defrost meats in the refrigerator or microwave, not on the kitchen counter.
- Keep your hands and your kitchen clean. Wash your hands, cutting boards, and countertops frequently. After handling raw meats, especially chicken, wash your hands and utensils with hot, soapy water before preparing other foods.
- Cook meat until it is well done, chicken until the juices run clear, fish until it flakes with a fork, and shellfish until it is opaque.
- Do not eat raw eggs or uncooked sauces made with raw eggs.
- Discard any cans or jars with bulging lids or leaks.
- Follow home canning and freezing instructions carefully. Look in the BC HealthFiles at www.bchealthguide.org.

Home Treatment

- Viral stomach flu and food poisoning will usually go away within 24 to 48 hours. Good home care can speed recovery. For adults and older children, see Nausea and Vomiting on page 129 and Diarrhea on page 120. For infants and young children, see page 275.
- Watch for and treat early signs of dehydration (see page 118). Older adults and young children can quickly become dehydrated from diarrhea and vomiting.

When to Call a Health Professional

- If vomiting lasts longer than 1 day in an adult.
- If severe diarrhea (large, loose stools every 1 to 2 hours) lasts longer than 2 days in an adult.
- If signs of severe dehydration develop. See When to Call a Health Professional on pages 119 to 120.
- If you suspect food poisoning from a canned food or have symptoms of botulism (blurred or double vision, difficulty swallowing or breathing). If you still have a sample of the food you suspect caused your symptoms, take it to the doctor for testing.

Ulcers

A peptic ulcer is a sore or crater in the lining of the digestive tract. Most ulcers develop in the stomach (gastric ulcers) or in the upper part of the small intestine (duodenal ulcers).

Until recently, the cause of ulcers was not well understood. It is now believed that most people who develop ulcers are infected with *Helicobacter pylori (H. pylori)* bacteria. Most people who are infected with *H. pylori* do not develop ulcers unless other factors are also present. Such factors may include:

- Use of certain medications.
- Excessive alcohol use.

- Smoking.
- Physical stress, such as surgery or trauma.
- Other illnesses.

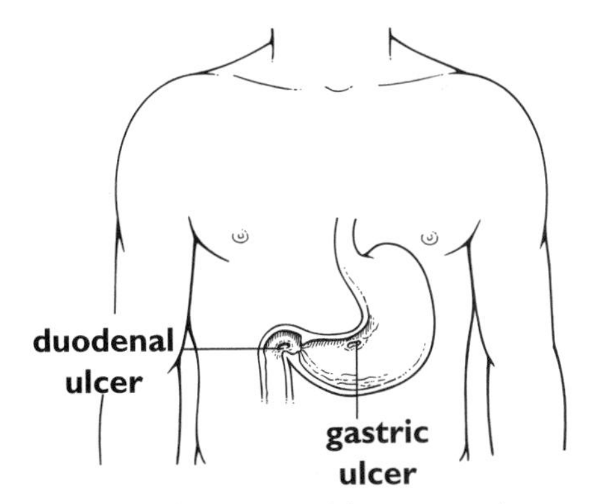

Most ulcers occur in the stomach (gastric ulcer) or in the opening to the small intestine (duodenal ulcer).

Most ulcers that are not caused by *H. pylori* infection are caused by frequent use of Aspirin or other nonsteroidal anti-inflammatory drugs (such as ibuprofen, indomethacin, and naproxen sodium), which can damage the digestive tract's lining.

The symptoms of an ulcer are often similar to symptoms of other common stomach problems like heartburn or inflammation of the stomach lining (gastritis). Symptoms may include a burning or gnawing pain between the navel and the breastbone. The pain often occurs between meals and may wake you during the night. Eating something or taking an antacid usually relieves the pain. Ulcers may also cause bloating, nausea, or vomiting after meals.

Ulcers can cause bleeding in the stomach and small intestine, which may cause stools to appear dark red, black, or tarry. Without treatment, ulcers may sometimes cause a blockage between the stomach and the small intestine. An ulcer may occasionally break through (perforate) the stomach wall, causing severe abdominal pain and a rigid abdomen. Ulcers that bleed or perforate the stomach wall require immediate medical treatment.

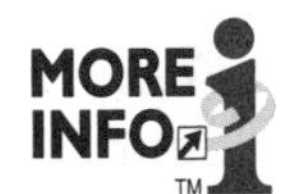

If you think you have an ulcer and your symptoms do not improve after 10 to 14 days of home treatment, make an appointment with your doctor. He or she can evaluate your symptoms and prescribe a treatment plan that may include antacids or other medications.

Home Treatment

- Avoid foods, especially spicy or greasy foods, that seem to bring on symptoms. It isn't necessary to eliminate any particular food from your diet if it doesn't cause you problems.
- Avoid coffee, tea, cola, and other products that contain caffeine. Many people find that caffeine makes their pain worse.
- Try eating smaller, more frequent meals. If it doesn't help, return to a regular diet.
- Stop smoking. Smoking slows healing of ulcers and increases the likelihood that they will come back.

- Limit your alcohol intake. Excessive amounts of alcohol may make an ulcer heal more slowly and may make symptoms worse.
- Do not take Aspirin, ibuprofen, or naproxen sodium. Try acetaminophen instead. Review any prescription medications with your doctor or pharmacist.
- Antacids (such as Tums, Maalox, and Mylanta) reduce the amount of acid in your stomach. Stomach acid reducers (such as Pepcid AC, Tagamet HB, Zantac 75, and Axid AR) decrease the amount of acid your stomach produces. Proton pump inhibitors, including Prevacid, Prilosec, and Nexium, reduce the production of stomach acid even more. Reducing the amount of acid in your stomach helps your ulcer heal. Talk with your doctor about the best medication and best dose for you. Also see page 403.
- Learn to relax and manage stress. Too much stress may slow ulcer healing. Practise the relaxation techniques on page 386.

When to Call a Health Professional

- If you have pain in the upper abdomen with chest pain that is crushing or squeezing, feels like a heavy weight on your chest, or occurs with any other symptoms of a heart attack (see page 191).
- If you have been diagnosed with an ulcer and you have severe, continuous abdominal pain, severe vomiting, blood in vomit or stools, dizziness or light-headedness, or signs of shock (see page 103).
- If your symptoms continue or get worse after 10 to 14 days of treatment with antacids or stomach acid reducers.
- If you are losing weight and you don't know why.
- If nausea or vomiting often occurs right after meals.
- If abdominal pain awakens you from sleep.
- If you have pain or difficulty when swallowing.

Blood in the Urine

A blow to the kidneys, kidney stones, excessive running, a urinary tract infection or, rarely, cancer can cause blood in the urine. Blood in the urine can be a sign of a serious illness and should always be discussed with a health professional.

Eating foods such as beets, blackberries, and foods containing red artificial food colourings can temporarily colour the urine pink or red. Certain medications can also discolour the urine.

Urinary Incontinence

If you suffer from loss of bladder control (urinary incontinence), you are not alone. Many people are coping with this problem.

Many cases of incontinence can be controlled or cured if the underlying problem is corrected. Water pills (diuretics) and many other common medications can cause temporary incontinence. Constipation, urinary tract infections, stones in the urinary tract, multiple pregnancies, and being overweight are other causes of incontinence.

The two most common types of persistent or chronic loss of bladder control are described here.

Stress incontinence occurs when small amounts of urine leak out during exercise or when you cough, laugh, or sneeze. It is more common in women than in men, but it may affect some men after prostate surgery. Kegel exercises often help relieve stress incontinence. See page 137. Ask your doctor about devices that can be used to prevent urine from leaking.

Urge incontinence happens when the need to urinate comes on so quickly that there is not enough time to get to the toilet. Causes include bladder infection, prostate enlargement, tumours that press on the bladder, Parkinson's disease, and nerve-related disorders such as multiple sclerosis or stroke.

Kegel Exercises

Kegel exercises can help cure or improve stress incontinence by strengthening the pelvic muscles that control the flow of urine. No one will know you are doing them except you.

- Locate the muscles by repeatedly stopping your urine in midstream and starting again.
- Practise squeezing these muscles while you are not urinating. If your stomach or buttocks move, you are not using the right muscles.
- Hold the squeeze for 3 seconds; then relax for 3 seconds.
- Repeat the exercise 10 to 15 times per session. Do at least three Kegel exercise sessions per day.

Home Treatment

- Don't let incontinence keep you from doing the things you like to do. Absorbent pads or briefs, such as Depend or Poise, are available in pharmacies and supermarkets. No one will know you are wearing an absorbent pad.
- Avoid beverages that contain caffeine, which overstimulates the bladder. Do not cut down on fluids overall; you need fluids to keep the rest of your body healthy.

- Stop smoking. This may reduce your coughing, which may in turn reduce your problem with incontinence.
- Lose weight if you are overweight.
- Practise "double-voiding." Empty your bladder as much as possible, relax for a minute, and then try to empty it again.
- If you have stress incontinence, practise Kegel exercises daily. See Kegel Exercises on page 137.
- Urinate on a schedule, perhaps every 3 to 4 hours during the day, whether the urge is there or not. This may help you restore control.
- Wear clothing that can be removed quickly, such as pants with elastic waistbands.
- Clear a path from your bed to the bathroom, or consider placing a portable commode by your bed.
- Keep skin in the genital area dry to prevent rashes. Vaseline or Desitin ointment or zinc oxide will help protect the skin from irritation caused by urine.
- Incontinence is sometimes caused by a urinary tract infection. If you feel pain or burning when you urinate, see Urinary Tract Infections on page 138.
- Ask your doctor or pharmacist whether any medications you are taking, including non-prescription drugs, can affect bladder control. Do not stop taking any medication without first discussing it with your doctor.

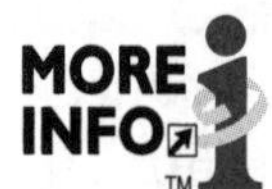

Try not to let incontinence embarrass you. Take charge and work with your doctor to treat any underlying condition that may be causing the problem.

When to Call a Health Professional

- If you suddenly become incontinent.
- If you are urinating frequently, but only passing small amounts of urine.
- If your bladder feels full even after you urinate.
- If you have difficulty urinating when your bladder feels full.
- If you feel burning or pain while urinating. See Urinary Tract Infections on page 138.
- If your urine looks bloody. See Blood in the Urine on page 136.
- If your urine has an unusual odour.
- If urinary incontinence interferes with your life in any way.

Urinary Tract Infections

The urinary tract includes the kidneys, ureters, bladder, and urethra. The kidneys filter the blood, and the waste products from the blood

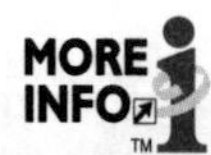

become urine. The ureters carry urine from the kidneys to the bladder. The bladder holds the urine until the urine is expelled from the body through the urethra.

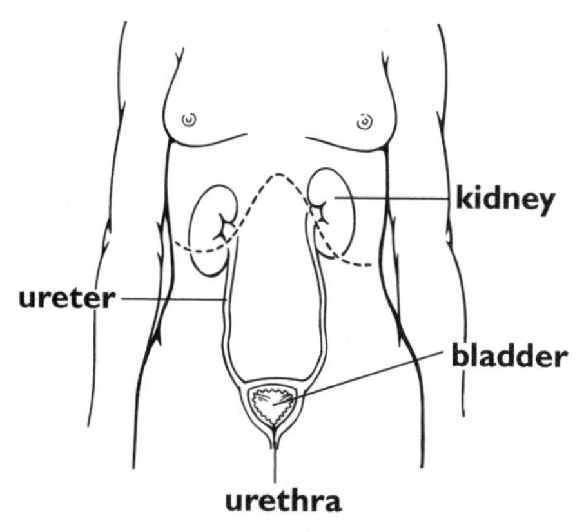

Infections can occur in any of the structures of the urinary tract.

Urinary tract infections (UTIs), including bladder infections (cystitis) and kidney infections (pyelonephritis), are generally caused by bacteria that are normally present in the digestive system. Females get UTIs more often than males do.

Early symptoms of a UTI may include burning or pain during urination as well as itching or pain in the urethra. The urine may be cloudy or reddish in colour and may have an unusual odour. You may feel some discomfort in the lower abdomen or back and have a frequent urge to urinate without being able to pass much urine. Chills and fever may be present if the infection is severe, especially if it has spread to the kidneys.

Men with symptoms similar to those caused by a UTI may have an infection of the prostate gland or the epididymis (the tube that transports sperm from the testicle). See Prostate Infection on page 323 and Testicular Problems on page 326.

Men who have enlarged prostates, women who have had multiple pregnancies, people with kidney stones or diabetes, and those who are paralyzed may be at higher risk for chronic urinary tract infections.

Other causes of irritation to the genital area that may be associated with UTIs include having sexual intercourse, using a diaphragm or spermicide for birth control, wearing tight pants, riding a bike, using perfumed soaps and powders, or even eating spicy foods.

If urinary pain or vaginal burning and redness occur in a young girl, consider the possibility of an allergy to bubble bath or soap. Urinary pain or vaginal burning may also be a symptom of a sexually transmitted disease (STD) or a sign of sexual abuse. If you are concerned about possible sexual abuse of a child, call a health professional.

Prevention

- Drink plenty of fluids; water is best. Aim for at least 2 litres per day.
- Urinate frequently.
- Females should wipe from front to back after going to the toilet. This will reduce the spread of bacteria

from the anus to the urethra. Teach young girls this habit during toilet training.

- Avoid douching and bubble baths, and don't use vaginal deodorants or perfumed feminine hygiene products.
- Wash the genital area once a day with plain water or mild soap and water. Rinse well and dry the area thoroughly.
- Drink extra water before sexual intercourse and urinate promptly afterwards. This is especially important if you tend to get UTIs.
- Wear cotton underwear, cotton-lined panty hose, and loose clothing.
- Avoid alcohol, caffeine, and carbonated beverages, which can irritate the bladder.
- Include cranberry and blueberry juice in your diet. These may protect against UTIs, especially in females.

Home Treatment

Start home treatment at the first sign of genital irritation or painful urination. A day or so of self-care may clear up a minor infection. However, if your symptoms last longer than 1 or 2 days or worsen despite home treatment, call your doctor. Because the organs of the urinary tract are connected, untreated UTIs can spread, which may lead to kidney infections and other serious problems.

- Drink extra fluids (think in terms of litres) as soon as you notice symptoms and for the next 24 hours. This will help dilute the urine, flush bacteria out of the bladder, and decrease irritation.
- Urinate frequently and follow the other tips outlined in Prevention.
- Check your temperature twice daily. Fever may indicate a more serious infection.
- A hot bath may help relieve pain. Avoid using bubble bath and harsh soaps. Apply a heating pad over your genital area to help relieve the pain. Never go to sleep with a heating pad in place.
- Avoid sexual intercourse until symptoms improve. Do not use a diaphragm. It may put pressure on your urethra and slow down or prevent complete emptying of the bladder.

When to Call a Health Professional

- If painful urination occurs with any of the following symptoms:
  - Fever of 38°C or higher and chills.
  - Inability to urinate when you feel the urge.
  - Pain in the back, side, groin, or genital area.
  - Blood or pus in the urine.
  - Unusual vaginal or penile discharge.
  - Nausea and vomiting.

- If symptoms get worse despite home treatment.
- If symptoms do not improve after 1 to 2 days of home treatment.
- If you are pregnant or have diabetes and you have symptoms of a urinary tract infection.
- If you suspect that your child has a urinary tract infection or has been sexually abused.

Kidney Stones

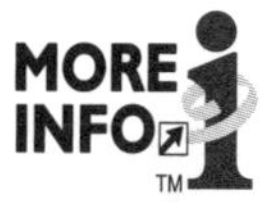

Kidney stones can form from the minerals in urine. The most common cause of kidney stones is not drinking enough water.

If a stone blocks the urine flow in the kidney or the tube that leads to the bladder (ureter), you may have severe pain.

Symptoms that may develop when a kidney stone moves through a ureter include:

- Pain in the side, groin, or genital area that begins suddenly and gets worse over 15 to 60 minutes until it is steady and nearly unbearable. The pain may stop for a while when the stone is not moving, and pain often vanishes suddenly when the stone moves into the bladder.
- Nausea and vomiting.
- Blood in the urine.
- Feeling like you need to urinate often or pain when urinating.
- Diarrhea, constipation, or loss of appetite.
- Inability to find a comfortable body position.

Call your doctor immediately if you suspect that you are passing a kidney stone. Most small kidney stones pass without the need for any treatment other than pain medication. If a stone is too large to pass on its own or gets stuck, you may need a procedure or surgery to help you pass it.

Stand up straight!
Mom

7

Back and Neck Pain

Although back and neck pain are usually preventable, most of us will suffer from one or both at some time in our lives. Fortunately, most acute back injuries will heal on their own within 6 to 12 weeks.

By following the prevention and home treatment guidelines in this chapter, you can recover from most back and neck pain and prevent it from recurring.

Back Pain

Your back includes the area from below your head to your tailbone. It is composed of the bones of the spine (vertebrae); the joints that guide the direction of movement of the spine; the discs that separate the bones of the spine and absorb shock as you move; and the muscles and ligaments that hold them all together. One or more of these structures can be stressed or injured, causing back pain.

Most back pain is the result of repeated forceful movements or prolonged postures that strain the back. A sudden or awkward movement that twists the back can result in a strain or sprain of the spinal ligaments, the muscles in the back, or the sacroiliac joints (the joints between the spine and the pelvic bones).

You can damage your discs the same way, causing them to tear or rupture. If a tear in a disc is large enough, the jelly-like material inside the disc may leak out and press against a nerve. The nerve may also become irritated by swelling or inflammation in other parts of the spine.

First Aid for Back Pain

When you first feel a catch or strain in your back, try these steps to avoid or reduce pain. These are the most important home treatments for the first few days of back pain. Also see Home Treatment on page 151.

First Aid No. 1: Relax

Lie down in a comfortable position. This will allow your spinal muscles to relax.

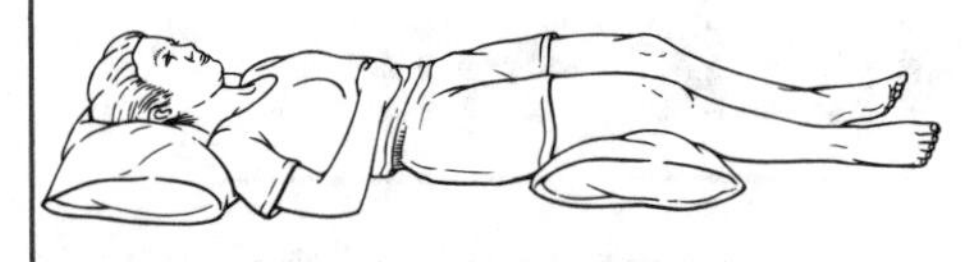

First Aid No. 2: Ice

As soon as possible, apply ice or a cold pack to your injured back (10 to 15 minutes every hour). Cold applied for the first 3 days reduces pain and speeds healing.

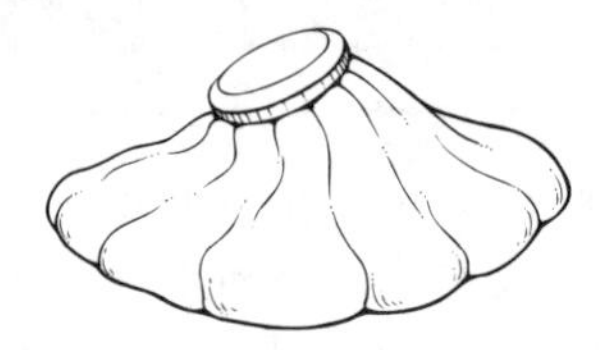

First Aid No. 3: Pelvic tilts

This exercise gently moves the spine and stretches the lower back.

- Lie on your back with knees bent and feet flat on the floor.
- Slowly tighten your stomach muscles and press your lower back against the floor. Hold for 10 seconds (do not hold your breath). Slowly relax.

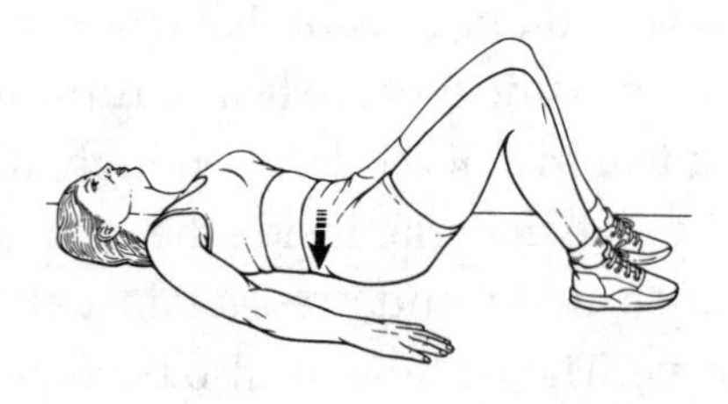

First Aid No. 4: Walk

Take a short walk (3 to 5 minutes) on a level surface (no slopes) every 3 hours. Walk only distances you can manage without pain, especially leg pain.

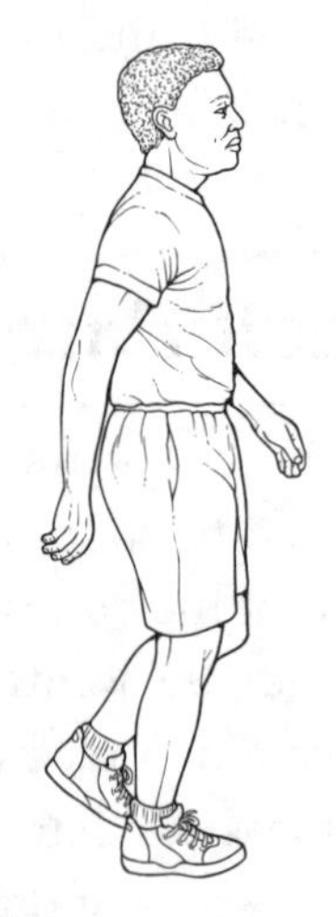

If you have an undiagnosed medical problem with your back or have a recurring back injury that does not respond to first aid, call your doctor for advice.

Any of these injuries can result in 2 to 3 days of pain and swelling in the injured tissue, followed by slow healing and a gradual reduction in pain. The pain may be felt in the low back, in the buttock, or down the leg. The goals of self-care are to relieve pain, promote healing, and avoid reinjury. Fortunately, most acute back injuries heal on their own in 6 to 12 weeks.

Back pain can also be caused by conditions that affect the bones and joints of the spine. Arthritis pain may be a steady ache, unlike the sharp, acute pain of strains, sprains, and disc injuries. If you think arthritis may be causing your back pain, combine the self-care guidelines for back pain with those for arthritis on page 158.

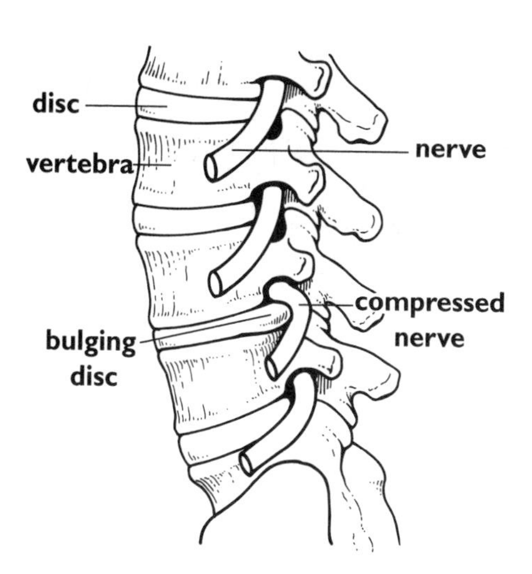

A bulging or ruptured (herniated) disc can put pressure on a nerve, causing pain.

Osteoporosis weakens all bones, including those of the spine, which can lead to broken bones and compression fractures. Compression fractures cause vertebrae to collapse. This can cause misalignment of the spine, which may lead to varying degrees of pain. See page 172 for more information about osteoporosis.

Sciatica

Sciatica is an irritation of the sciatic nerve, which is formed by the nerve roots coming out of the spinal cord into the lower back. The sciatic nerve extends down through the buttocks to the feet. Sciatica can occur when an injured disc presses against a spinal nerve root. Its main symptom is radiating pain, numbness, or weakness that is usually worse in the leg than in the back. For relief, see Home Treatment on page 151, and follow these tips:

- Avoid sitting if possible, unless it is more comfortable than standing.
- Alternate lying down with short walks. Increase your walking distance as you are able to do so without pain.
- Apply ice or a cold pack to the middle of your lower back. See page 144.

Prevention

The keys to preventing back pain are to use good body mechanics and to practise good health habits, such as getting regular exercise, maintaining a healthy body weight, and avoiding tobacco (nicotine weakens the discs in your back). Some of the tips presented here are things you will want to do every day, not only because they are good for your back, but because they are good for your overall health. The rest will come in handy if you are ever suffering from acute back pain.

Body Mechanics

Good body mechanics will reduce the stress on your back. Use good body mechanics all the time, not just when you have back pain.

Sitting

- Avoid sitting in one position for more than an hour at a time. Get up or change positions often.
- If you must sit a lot, the extension exercises on page 148 are particularly important.
- If your chair doesn't give enough support, use a small pillow or rolled towel to support your lower back.
- When driving, pull your seat forward so that the pedals and steering wheel are within comfortable reach. Stop often to stretch and walk around. Consider placing a small pillow or towel roll behind your lower back.

Lifting

- Keep your upper back straight. Do not bend forward from the waist to lift.
- Bend your knees and let your arms and legs do the work. Tighten your buttocks and abdomen to further support your back.
- Keep the load as close to your body as possible, even if the load is light.
- While holding a heavy object, turn your feet, not your back. Try not to turn or twist your body.
- If possible, don't lift heavy objects above shoulder level.
- Use a hand truck or ask someone to help you carry heavy or awkward objects.

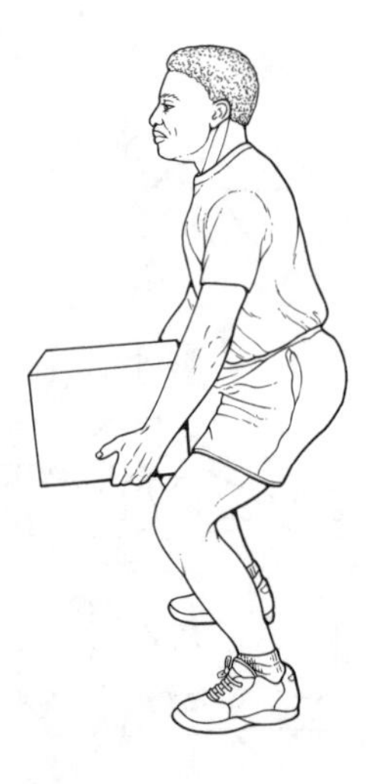

Avoid back strain when lifting heavy objects by keeping your upper back straight, bending your knees, and keeping the load close to your body.

Lying Down

If you have back pain at night, your mattress may be the problem. Try sleeping on a firmer mattress. Or, if you think your mattress is too firm, try one that's a little softer. Try these additional tips for more comfortable sleep:

- If you sleep on your back, you may want to use a towel roll to support your lower back or put a pillow under your knees.
- If you sleep on your side, try placing a pillow between your knees.
- Sleeping on your stomach is fine if it doesn't increase your back or neck pain.

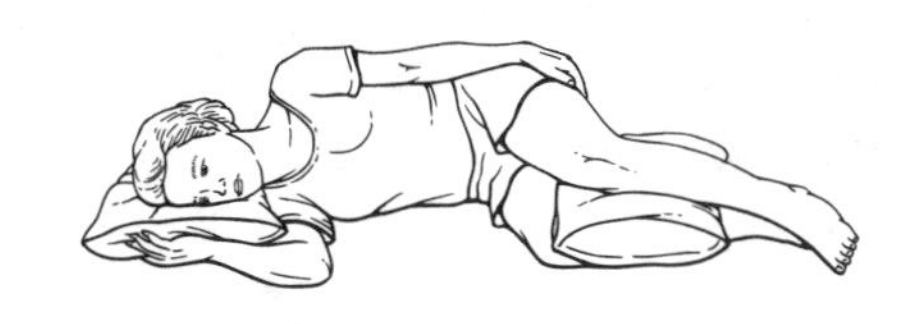

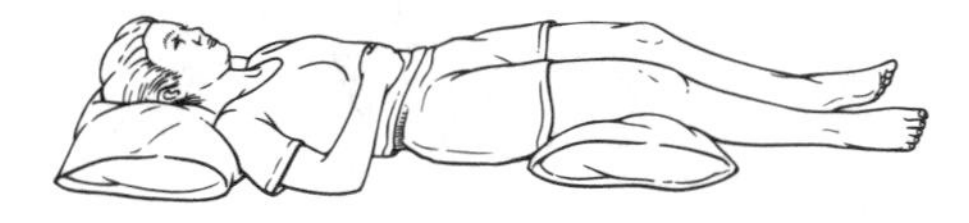

Try placing pillows between or under your knees to relieve back pain while lying in bed.

Exercise

Regular exercise (stretching, strengthening, and aerobic exercise) helps you maintain your overall fitness and flexibility and strengthens the muscles that support your spine. Exercising also helps you maintain a healthy body weight, which reduces the load on your lower back. If you are interested in creating a personalized fitness plan, see Fitness starting on page 343.

Although there is no clear evidence that specific exercises can help prevent back pain, the exercises presented here are a common, practical approach to helping you maintain strength and flexibility. You may choose to make the exercises a part of your regular fitness routine.

Do not do these exercises if you have just injured your back. Instead, see First Aid for Back Pain on page 144.

Extension exercises strengthen your lower back muscles and stretch the stomach muscles and ligaments. Flexion exercises stretch the lower back muscles and strengthen the stomach muscles.

- You do not need to do every exercise. Do the ones that help you the most.
- If any exercise makes your back pain worse, stop the exercise and try something else. Stop any exercise that causes the pain to radiate away from your spine into your buttocks or legs, either during or after the exercise.
- Start with 5 repetitions, 3 to 4 times a day, and gradually increase to 10 repetitions. Do all exercises slowly.

Extension Exercises

Press-Ups

Begin and end every set of exercises with a few press-ups.

- Lie face down with your arms bent, palms flat on the floor.
- Lift yourself up on your elbows, keeping the lower half of your body relaxed. If it's comfortable, press your chest forward.

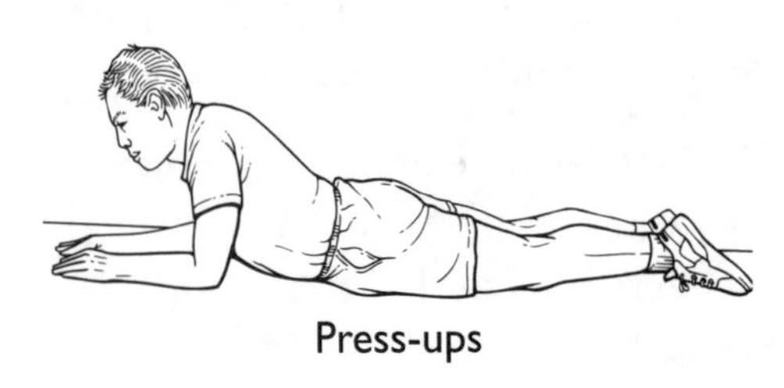

Press-ups

- Keep your hips pressed to the floor. Feel the stretch in your lower back.
- Lower your upper body to the floor. Repeat this exercise slowly.

Shoulder Lifts

Shoulder lifts will strengthen the back muscles that support the spine.

- Lie face down with your arms beside your body.
- Lift your shoulders straight up from the floor as high as you can without pain. Keep your chin down and your eyes facing the floor. Keep your torso and hips pressed to the floor.

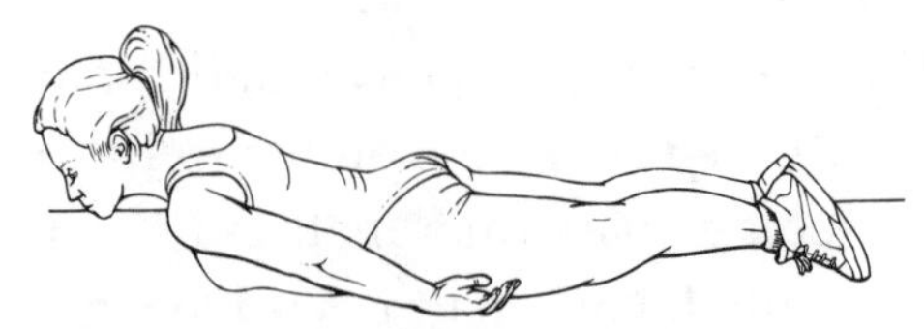

Shoulder lifts
(keep neck straight and chin down)

Backward Bend

Practise the backward bend at least once a day and whenever you work in a bent-forward position.

- Stand upright with your feet slightly apart. Back up to a countertop for greater support and stability.
- Place your hands in the small of your back and gently bend backward. Keep your knees straight (not locked) and bend only at the waist. See illustration. Hold the backward stretch for 1 to 2 seconds.

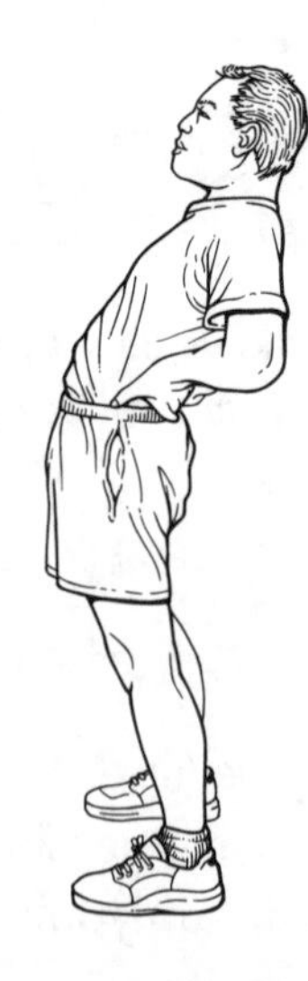

Backward bend
(keep neck straight and chin down)

Flexion Exercises

Curl-Ups

Curl-ups strengthen your abdominal muscles, which work with your back muscles to support your spine.

- Lie on your back with knees bent (60° angle), feet flat on the floor, and arms crossed on your chest. Do not hook your feet under anything.
- Slowly curl your head and shoulders up until your shoulder blades barely rise from the floor. Keep your lower back pressed to the floor. To avoid neck problems, remember to lift your shoulders, and do not force your head up or forward. Hold for 5 to 10 seconds (do not hold your breath), and then curl down very slowly.

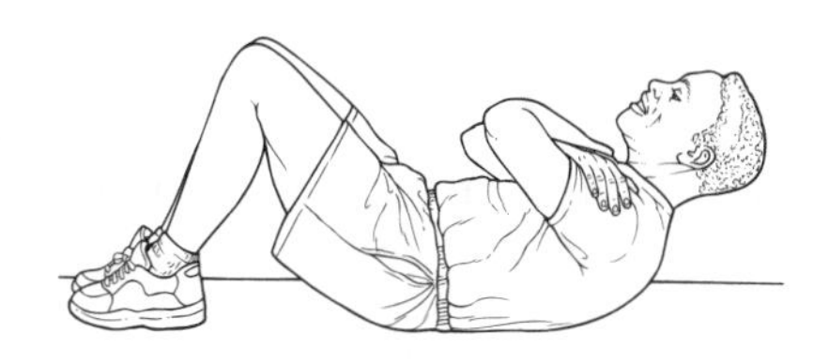

Curl-ups
(keep neck straight and chin tucked in)

Knee-to-Chest Stretch

The knee-to-chest exercise stretches the lower back muscles and relieves pressure on the joints where the vertebrae come together.

- Lie on your back with knees bent and feet close to your buttocks.
- Bring one knee to your chest, keeping the other foot flat on the floor (or the other leg straight, if that is more comfortable for your lower back). Keep your lower back pressed to the floor. Hold for 5 to 10 seconds.
- Relax and lower your knee to the starting position. Repeat with the other leg.

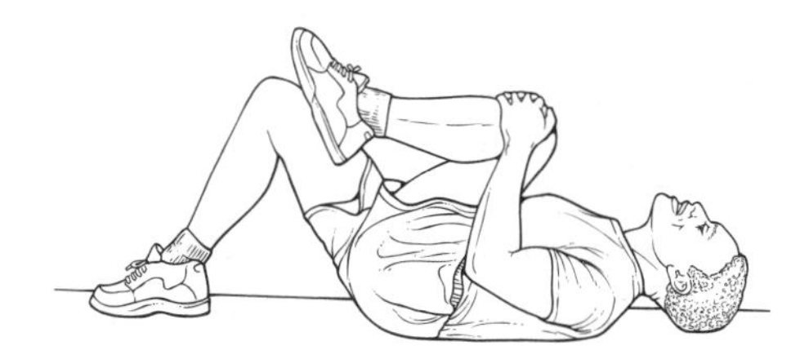

Knee-to-chest stretch

Additional Strengthening and Stretching Exercises

Prone Buttocks Squeeze

This exercise strengthens the buttocks muscles, which support the back and help you lift with your legs. You may need to place a small pillow under your stomach for comfort.

- Lie flat on your stomach with your arms at your sides.
- Slowly tighten your buttocks muscles and hold for 5 to 10 seconds (don't hold your breath). Relax slowly.

Pelvic Tilts

See instructions on page 144.

Hamstring Stretch

This exercise stretches the muscles in the back of your thigh, which will allow you to bend your legs without putting stress on your back.

- Lie on your back in a doorway. Keep one leg resting on the floor of the doorway, and extend the leg you want to stretch straight up, resting the heel on the wall next to the doorway.
- Keep the leg straight and slowly move your heel up the wall until you feel a gentle pull in the back of your thigh. Do not overstretch.
- Relax in this position for 30 seconds; then bend the knee to relieve the stretch. Repeat with the other leg.

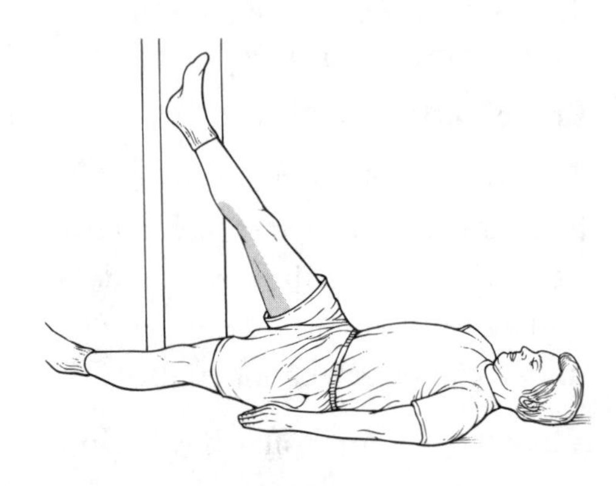

Hamstring stretch
(shading shows where stretch is felt)

Hip Flexor Stretch

This exercise stretches the muscles in the front of your hip.

- Kneel on one knee with your other leg bent in front of you.
- Slowly sink your hips so your weight shifts onto your front foot. The knee of your forward leg should be aligned over the ankle. Hold for 10 seconds. You should feel a stretch in the groin of the leg you are kneeling on. Repeat with the other leg.

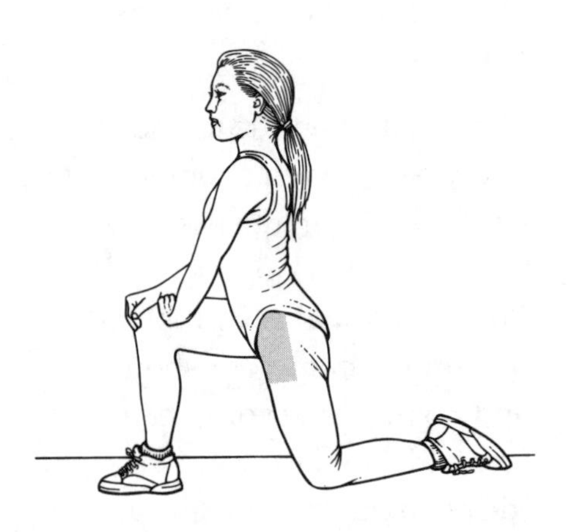

Hip flexor stretch
(shading shows where stretch is felt)

Exercises to Avoid

Many common exercises actually increase the risk of low back pain. Avoid the following:

- Straight-leg sit-ups.
- Bent-leg sit-ups when you have acute back pain.
- Leg lifts (lifting both legs while lying on your back).
- Lifting heavy weights above the waist (military press, biceps curls while standing).
- Any stretching done while sitting with the legs in a V.
- Toe touches while standing.

Home Treatment

Immediately after an injury and for the next few days, the most important home treatment includes the following:

- Follow the First Aid for Back Pain guidelines on page 144.
- Sit or lie in positions that are most comfortable and reduce your pain, especially any leg pain.
- Do not sit up in bed, and avoid soft couches and twisted positions. Avoid sitting for long periods of time. Follow the body mechanics guidelines on pages 146 to 147.
- Bed rest can help relieve back pain but may not speed healing. Unless you have severe leg pain, 1 to 2 days of bed rest should relieve pain. More than 3 days of bed rest is not recommended and can actually delay healing in some cases.
- For bed rest, try one of the following positions (see illustrations on page 147):
    - Lie on your back with your knees bent and supported by large pillows, or lie on the floor with your legs on the seat of a sofa or chair.
    - Lie on your side with your knees and hips bent and a pillow between your legs.
    - If it doesn't increase your pain, lie on your stomach.
- Take Aspirin or ibuprofen regularly as directed. Do not give Aspirin to anyone younger than 20. Call your doctor if you've been told to avoid anti-inflammatory medications. Acetaminophen may also be used. Take these medications sensibly; the maximum recommended dose will reduce the pain. Masking the pain completely might allow movement that could lead to reinjury.
- Relax your muscles. See page 387 for progressive muscle relaxation.

You can try the following home treatment 2 to 3 days after the injury occurs:

- Apply heat to your sore back for 20-minute periods. Moist heat (hot packs, baths, showers) works better than dry heat. Some people find comfort in alternating between heat and ice packs, or using ice only.
- Continue daily walks (increase to 5 to 10 minutes, 3 to 4 times a day).
- Try swimming, which is good for your back. It may be painful immediately after a back injury, but lap swimming or kicking with swim fins often helps prevent back pain from recurring.
- When your pain has improved, begin easy exercises that do not increase your pain. One or two of the exercises described on pages 147 to 150 may be helpful. Start with 5 repetitions, 3 to 4 times a day, and increase to 10 repetitions as you are able.

When to Call a Health Professional

- If back pain occurs with chest pain or other symptoms of a heart attack (see page 191). **Call 911 or other emergency services immediately.**
- If you lose bowel or bladder control.
- If you cannot walk or stand.
- If you have new numbness in the buttocks, genital or rectal area, or legs.
- If you have leg weakness that is not solely due to pain. Many people with low back pain say their legs feel weak. If leg weakness is so severe that you are unable to bend your foot upward, get up out of a chair, or climb stairs, you should see a doctor.
- If you have new or increased back pain with unexplained fever, painful urination, or other signs of a urinary tract infection. See page 138.
- If you have a dramatic increase in your chronic back pain, especially if it is unrelated to a new or changed physical activity.
- If you have a history of cancer or HIV infection and you develop new or increased back pain.
- If you have severe back pain that does not improve after a few days of home treatment.
- If you develop a new, severe pain in your lower back that does not change with movement and is not related to stress, muscle tension, or a known injury.
- If back pain does not improve after 2 weeks of home treatment.

Back Surgery

Rest, pain relievers, and exercise can relieve almost all back problems, including most disc problems.

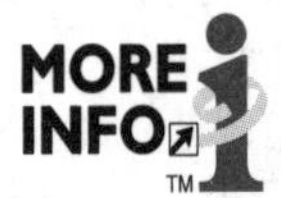

Most back surgeries are done to treat disc problems that have not improved with time and exercise. Surgery may also be appropriate in cases of spinal fracture, spinal infection, and other conditions. If you are considering surgery to treat your back pain, getting all the facts and thinking about your own needs and values will help you make a wise decision about treatment.

If you do plan to have surgery, the body mechanics guidelines and exercises in this chapter are still important. A strong, flexible back will help you recover more quickly after surgery.

Who Can Help?

When you have back or neck pain or an injury to these areas, it is important to take care of yourself early to prevent symptoms from getting worse. In BC, the following health professionals can help you with back and neck problems:

- Acupuncturists
- Chiropractors
- Massage therapists
- Medical doctors
- Occupational therapists
- Physical therapists

Remember, it is important to get a diagnosis from a medical doctor for new symptoms, especially if the pain is severe and has not improved after a few days of home treatment.

For more information about the approaches, services, and treatments available from each of the professionals above, or to learn about possible costs per visit, see Health Care in British Columbia starting on page 417, visit BC HealthGuide OnLine at www.bchealthguide.org, or call the health professional's office directly.

Neck Pain

Most people occasionally feel pain, stiffness, or a kink in the neck. Neck pain may spread to the shoulders, upper back, or upper arms, and it may also cause headache. Pain may limit neck movement. This usually affects one side of the neck more than the other.

Neck pain is most often caused by tension, strain, or spasm in the neck muscles or inflammation of the ligaments, tendons, or joints in the neck. These problems typically result from prolonged or repeated activities or movements that stress the neck. Postures that put your neck in awkward positions—cradling the telephone between your ear and shoulder, sleeping on your stomach or with your neck twisted, or using a workstation that strains your neck—are also common causes.

Other causes of neck pain include:

- Injury resulting from a sudden movement of the head and neck (whiplash), a direct blow to the neck, or a fall.
- Arthritis or damage to the discs in the neck that results in a "pinched nerve." When this is the cause of neck pain, the pain usually spreads down the arm. Numbness, tingling, or weakness in the arm or hand may occur. When you have symptoms of a pinched nerve, you need to see your doctor.
- Meningitis, a serious illness that requires emergency care. Meningitis causes a severe stiff neck with headache and fever (see page 201).

Neck Exercises

You do not need to do every exercise. Stick with the ones that help you the most. Do each exercise slowly. Stop any exercise that increases pain. Start by doing the exercises twice a day.

Dorsal glide: Sit or stand tall, looking straight ahead (a "palace guard" posture). Slowly tuck your chin as you glide your head backward over your body. Hold for a count of 5; then relax. Repeat 6 to 10 times. This stretches the back of the neck. If you feel pain, do not glide so far back. You may find this exercise easier to do while lying on your back with ice on your neck.

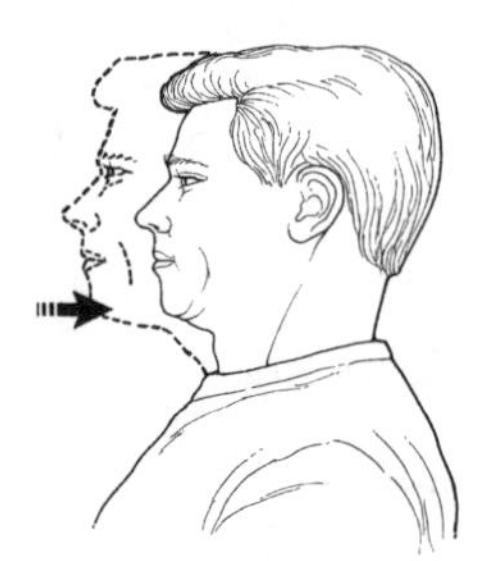

Dorsal glide

Chest and shoulder stretch: Sit or stand tall and glide your head backward as in the dorsal glide exercise. Raise both arms so that your hands are next to your ears. As you exhale, lower your elbows down and back. Feel your shoulder blades slide down and together. Hold for a few seconds and then relax. Repeat 6 to 10 times.

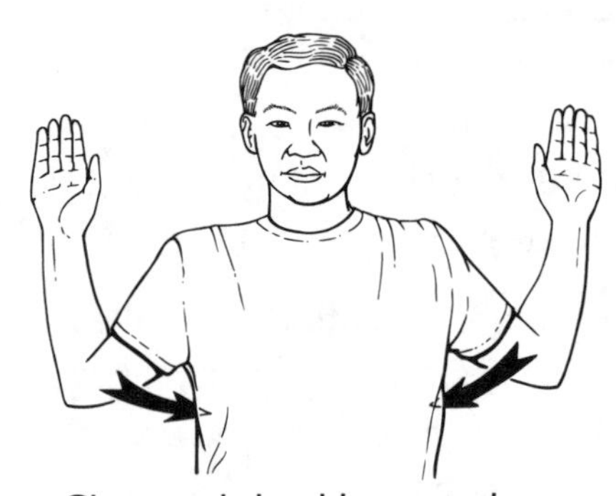

Chest and shoulder stretch

Shoulder lifts: Lie face down with your arms beside your body. Lift your shoulders straight up from the floor as high as you can without pain. Keep your chin down and your eyes facing the floor. Keep your torso and hips pressed to the floor. Repeat 6 to 10 times.

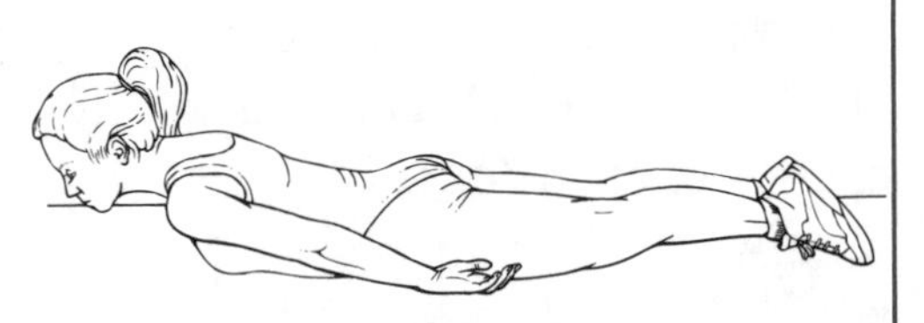

Shoulder lifts

Hands on head: Move your head backward, forward, and side to side against gentle pressure from your hands, holding each position for several seconds. Repeat 6 to 10 times.

Prevention

Most neck pain can be prevented by using good posture, getting regular exercise, and avoiding prolonged periods in positions that stress the neck. You can also strengthen and protect your neck by doing neck exercises once a day. See page 154. If stress may be the cause of your neck pain, practise the progressive muscle relaxation exercises on page 387.

If your pain is **worse at the end of the day**, evaluate your posture and body mechanics during the day.

- Sit straight in your chair with your lower back supported. Avoid sitting for long periods without getting up or changing positions. Take short breaks several times each hour to stretch your neck muscles.
- If you work at a computer, adjust the monitor so that the top of the screen is at eye level. Use a document holder that puts the copy at the same level as the screen.
- If you use the telephone a lot, consider using a headset or speakerphone.

If your neck stiffness is **worse in the morning**, you may need better neck support when you sleep.

- Try folding a towel lengthwise into a 10-cm-wide pad and wrapping it around your neck. Pin it for good support.
- You may need a special neck support pillow. Look for a pillow that supports your neck comfortably when you lie on your back and on your side (try before buying). Avoid pillows that force your head forward when you are on your back.
- Avoid sleeping on your stomach with your neck twisted or bent.
- Morning neck pain may also be the result of activities done the day before.

Home Treatment

Much of the home treatment for back pain is also helpful for neck pain. See page 151.

- If you have just been in an accident involving your neck, see Spinal Injuries on page 104.
- See the icing guidelines on page 144. If the problem is near your shoulder or upper back, it will usually help more to ice the back of your neck.
- After the first 72 hours (or if you have chronic pain), you may apply heat to the sore area for 20-minute periods.
- Use Aspirin, ibuprofen, or acetaminophen to help relieve pain. Do not give Aspirin to anyone younger than 20.
- Walking also helps relieve and prevent neck pain. The gentle swinging motion of your arms often relieves pain. Start with short walks of 5 to 10 minutes, 3 to 4 times a day.

- If neck pain occurs with headache, see Tension Headaches on page 240.
- Once the pain starts to get better, do the exercises on page 154.

When to Call a Health Professional

- If neck pain occurs with chest pain or other symptoms of a heart attack (see page 191). **Call 911 or other emergency services immediately**.
- If a stiff neck occurs with headache and fever. See Encephalitis and Meningitis on page 201.
- If you have severe neck pain after an injury or fall. See Spinal Injuries on page 104.
- If you develop new weakness or continuous numbness in your arms or legs.
- If pain extends or shoots down one arm, or if you have numbness or tingling in your hands.
- If a blow or injury to your neck (whiplash) is causing new pain.
- If you are unable to manage your pain with home treatment.
- If the pain has lasted 2 weeks or longer without improvement despite home treatment.

I don't deserve this award, but then I have arthritis and I don't deserve that either.
Jack Benny

8

Bone, Muscle, and Joint Problems

Our aches and pains remind us that life isn't always easy. But pain can be managed. This chapter covers pain from arthritis to plantar fasciitis. As with most chapters in this book, we hope you rarely have to refer to these pages. But when you do, we hope these guidelines will make your life more comfortable.

In many cases, you can determine the cause of bone, muscle, or joint problems by thinking back to how or when the pain started.

- A single episode of overuse or repeated heavy use of a joint can cause bursitis or tendinosis. See page 161.
- Joint pain that comes on gradually and seems unrelated to any specific injury may be due to arthritis.
- Traumatic injuries (turning an ankle or twisting a knee) usually cause strains, sprains, fractures, or dislocations. See page 104.

Arthritis

Arthritis refers to a variety of joint problems that cause pain, swelling, and stiffness. Simply put, arthritis means inflammation of a joint. Arthritis can occur at any age, but it affects older people the most.

There are more than 100 different types of arthritis. The chart on page 158 describes three common kinds of arthritis. Osteoarthritis is the most common type and can usually be managed at home. Rheumatoid arthritis and gout can improve with a combination of self-care and professional care.

Little is known about what causes most types of arthritis. Some seem to run in families; others seem to be related to imbalances in body chemistry or immune system problems. Many arthritis problems are the result of injury or long-term wear and tear on the joints.

Common Types of Arthritis			
Type	**Cause**	**Symptoms**	**Comments**
Osteoarthritis	Breakdown of joint cartilage.	Pain and stiffness; common in knees, fingers, hips, feet, and back.	Most common after age 50.
Rheumatoid Arthritis	Inflammation of the membrane (synovium) lining the joint.	Pain, stiffness, warmth, and swelling in joints on both sides of the body; common in hands, wrists, elbows, feet, knees, and neck.	Onset most often around age 40; more common in women.
Gout	Buildup of uric acid crystals in the joint fluid.	Sudden onset of burning pain, stiffness, and swelling; common in big toe, ankle, knee, wrist, and elbow.	Most common in men ages 30 to 50; may be aggravated by alcohol and exposure to cold.

Prevention

It may not be possible to prevent arthritis, but you can prevent a lot of pain by being kind to your joints. This is especially important if you already have arthritis.

- If activities that jar your body (such as running) cause pain, try activities that involve less impact (such as swimming).
- Control your weight.
- Exercise regularly. Exercise nourishes joint cartilage and removes waste products from the joints. It also strengthens the muscles around the joints, providing support and reducing injuries caused by fatigue. Stretching maintains your range of pain-free motion.

Home Treatment

- Take a warm shower or bath to help relieve morning stiffness. Try to avoid sitting still afterwards.
- If the joint is not swollen, apply moist heat for 20 to 30 minutes, 2 to 3 times a day. Do not apply heat to a swollen, inflamed joint.
- If the joint is swollen, apply cold packs for 10 minutes, once an hour. Cold will help relieve pain and reduce swelling and inflammation.
- Rest sore joints. Avoid activities that put weight or strain on the joints for a few days. Take short rest breaks from your regular activities throughout the day.

- Put each of your joints gently through its full range of motion once or twice each day.
- Exercise regularly to help maintain strength and flexibility in your muscles and joints. Try low-impact activities, such as swimming, water aerobics, biking, or walking.
- Take acetaminophen to relieve pain caused by osteoarthritis. Anti-inflammatory medications, such as Aspirin, ibuprofen, or naproxen sodium, may help ease pain but can cause stomach upset.
- Enroll in an arthritis self-management program. Participants in these programs usually have less pain and fewer limitations on their activities.

Joint Replacement Surgery

FOR SENIORS

When severe arthritis pain and loss of function interfere with your quality of life and do not respond to medications, physical therapy, and other treatments, you may want to think about joint replacement surgery. Hip and knee joints are the most commonly replaced joints.

Joint replacement relieves pain and may improve your ability to use the joint. It does not restore the joint to how it was before arthritis developed, but it may let you get back to activities and hobbies that you had to give up because of pain and stiffness. Basic activities like getting up from a chair and climbing stairs may also be easier.

Here are a few other points to keep in mind as you think about surgery:

- Surgery helps most when a single joint is causing most of your problems.
- To make the most of a new joint after surgery, you will need to do regular exercises and work with a physical therapist for several weeks or months.
- The chance of success is better if you are in good shape. Regular exercise and weight control are important both before and after the surgery.
- Artificial joints do not last forever. You may need to replace the joint again in 10 to 20 years.

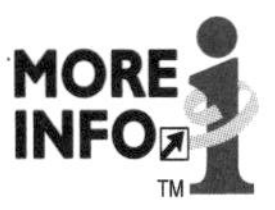

Work with your doctor to decide whether joint replacement is a good choice for you.

When to Call a Health Professional

- If you have fever or a skin rash along with severe joint pain.
- If the joint is so painful that you cannot use it.
- If there is sudden, unexplained swelling, redness, warmth, or pain in one or more joints.
- If sudden back pain occurs with weakness in the legs or loss of bowel or bladder control.
- If joint pain continues for more than 6 weeks and home treatment is not helping.
- If you experience side effects (stomach pain, nausea, persistent heartburn, or dark, tarry stools) from Aspirin or other arthritis medications. Do not exceed recommended doses of these medications without your doctor's advice.

Bunions and Hammer Toes

A bunion is an enlargement of the joint at the base of the big toe. A bunion develops when the big toe bends toward and sometimes overlaps the second toe. A hammer toe is a toe that bends up permanently at the middle joint. These foot problems sometimes run in families. Tight or high-heeled shoes increase the risk of both conditions and may make an existing problem worse.

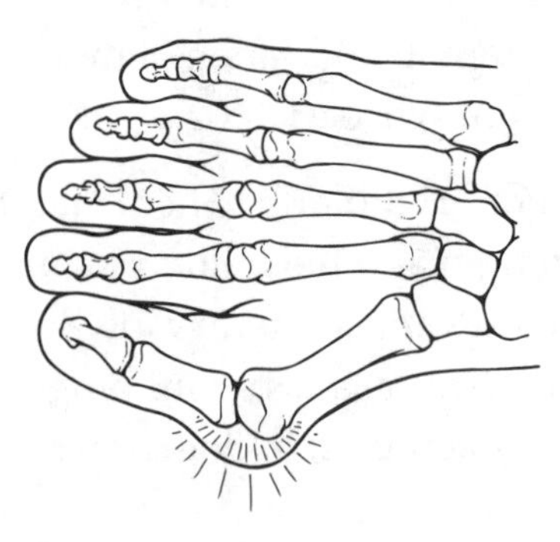

A bunion is an enlargement of the joint at the base of the big toe.

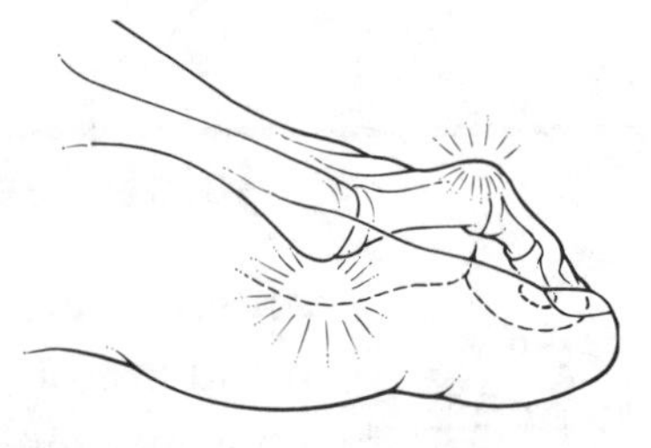

A hammer toe is a toe that bends up permanently at the middle joint.

Prevention

Wear shoes with low or flat heels and roomy toe areas. Tennis or basketball court shoes are often best. Make sure your shoes fit properly.

Home Treatment

Once you have a bunion or hammer toe, there is usually no way to completely get rid of it. Home treatment will help relieve discomfort and keep the problem from getting worse.

- Wear low-heeled shoes that have roomy toe areas.
- Cushion the joint with moleskin or doughnut-shaped pads to prevent rubbing and irritation.

- Modify an old pair of shoes by cutting out the area over the bunion or hammer toe; then wear them around the house. You could also wear comfortable sandals that don't press on the area.
- Try ibuprofen or acetaminophen to relieve pain. Ice or cold packs may also help.

When to Call a Health Professional

- If severe pain in the big toe comes on suddenly and you have not been diagnosed with gout.
- If your big toe starts to overlap your second toe.
- If you have diabetes, poor circulation, or peripheral vascular disease. In people with these conditions, irritated skin over a bunion or hammer toe can easily become infected.
- If you develop a sore over the bunion or hammer toe.
- If pain does not respond to home treatment in 2 to 3 weeks.

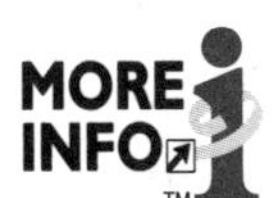

If severe pain or joint deformity interferes with walking or daily activities, you may want to consider surgical treatment. Surgery may not cure the problem completely. The more information you gather about the risks and benefits of surgery for bunions and hammer toes, the easier it will be for you to make a wise health decision.

Bursitis and Tendinosis

A bursa is a small sac of fluid that helps the tissues surrounding a joint slide over one another easily. Injury or overuse of a joint can result in pain, redness, heat, and inflammation of the bursa, a condition known as bursitis. Bursitis often develops quickly, over just a few days, usually after a specific injury, overuse, or prolonged direct pressure on a joint.

Tendons are tough, rope-like fibres that connect muscles to bones. Tendinosis develops when general wear and tear or overuse of a tendon causes tiny tears in the tissue, eventually leading to tenderness, inflammation, and breakdown in the tendons or the tissues surrounding them.

Both bursitis and tendinosis can be related to job, sports, or household activities that require repeated twisting or rapid joint movements. The same home treatment is good for both problems.

Prevention

Stretch and warm up well before exercising, and increase the intensity of the activity gradually. Cool down afterward by doing gentle stretches. See pages 162 to 164 for additional, joint-specific prevention tips.

Home Treatment

Bursitis or tendinosis will usually improve in a few days or weeks if you avoid the activity that caused it.

The most common mistake in recovery is thinking that the problem is gone when the pain is gone. Chances are, the problem will recur if you do not take steps to strengthen and stretch the muscles around the joint and change the way you do some activities.

- Rest the affected area. Change the way you do the activity that causes pain so that you can do it without pain. See pages 162 to 164 for joint-specific guidelines. To maintain fitness, substitute activities that don't stress the affected area.
- As soon as you notice pain, apply ice or cold packs for 10-minute periods, once an hour or as often as you can for 48 hours. Continue applying ice (10 minutes, 3 times a day) as long as it relieves pain. See page 167. Although heating pads or hot baths may feel good, ice or cold packs will reduce inflammation and promote healing.
- Aspirin, ibuprofen, or naproxen sodium may help ease pain and inflammation, but don't use medication to relieve pain while you continue overusing a joint. Do not give Aspirin to anyone younger than 20.
- To prevent stiffness, gently move the joint through as full a range of motion as you can without pain. As the pain subsides, continue range-of-motion exercises, and add exercises that strengthen the affected muscles.
- Gradually resume the activity at a lower intensity. Increase the intensity slowly and only if pain does not recur.
- Warm up before and stretch after the activity. Apply ice to the injured area after exercise to prevent pain and swelling.

In addition to the general prevention and home treatment information for bursitis and tendinosis above, the following tips will be useful if you have a specific joint problem.

Wrist pain may be caused by tendinosis. Though this is not the same as carpal tunnel syndrome, the same home care may help. See page 166.

Elbow pain is often caused by one of the following common types of tendinosis in the forearm tendons. (The inside or outside of the elbow is defined by holding your arm at your side with the palm of your hand facing forward. The inside is the side closest to your body.)

- **Tennis elbow** causes pain on the outside of the elbow where the muscles that bend the wrist back are attached.
- **Golfer's elbow** causes pain on the inside of the elbow where the muscles that bend the wrist down are attached.

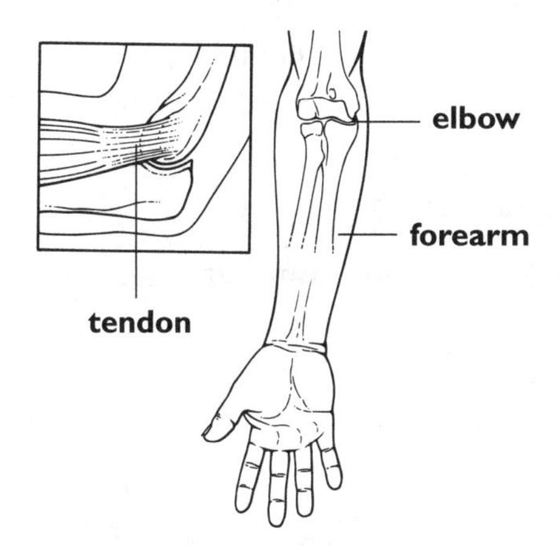

Elbow pain is often caused by tendinosis in the forearm.

To relieve elbow pain and prevent further injury:

- Rest the elbow and give it time to heal.
- Wear a brace or elbow sleeve.
- Support a sore elbow with a sling for 1 to 2 days. Do range-of-motion exercises daily.
- Strengthen the wrist, arm, shoulder, and back muscles to help protect the elbow.
- Avoid activities that require repetitive use of the wrist.
- Make changes in your activities to avoid irritating the tendon:
  - Use tools with larger handles.
  - Use a two-handed tennis backhand stroke and a more flexible, midsize racket.
  - Try to avoid hitting divots when playing golf.
  - Try to avoid sidearm pitching and throwing curveballs.

Shoulder pain that occurs on the outside of the upper arm is often caused by bursitis or tendinosis in the shoulder joint. Pain on the top of the shoulder or in the neck may be caused by tension in the trapezius muscles, which run from the back of the head across the back of the shoulders. See Neck Pain on page 153.

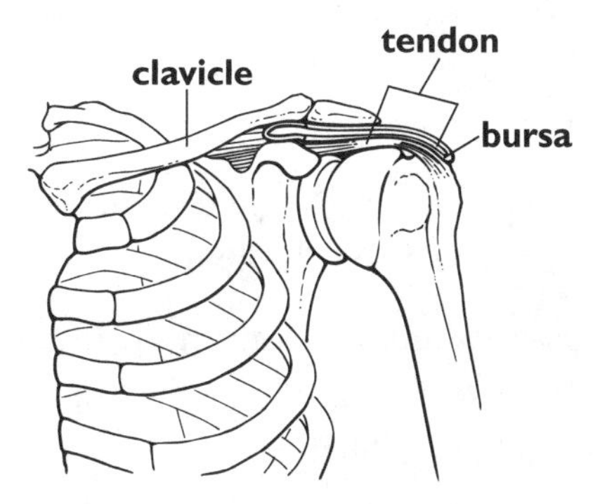

Bursitis, tendinosis, and muscle tension are common causes of shoulder pain.

Common symptoms of bursitis or tendinosis in the shoulder are pain, pinching, and stiffness when you raise your arm. The symptoms are often brought on by doing repeated overhead movements. Problems develop when you continue to use your shoulder without giving it time to rest. This leads to further swelling and pain.

For home treatment of shoulder pain, see page 162. Also consider the following suggestions:

- Avoid activities that involve overhead reaching, but continue to use your shoulder.

- Practise the pendulum exercise to prevent stiffness: Bend forward and grasp the back of a chair with the hand of your "good" arm. Let the other arm dangle straight down from the shoulder. Move the dangling arm in clockwise circles; start with small circles and gradually make them bigger. Then make counterclockwise circles (small to large). Next, swing the arm forward and backward, then from side to side. Do this exercise 10 times a day.
- Use proper throwing techniques for baseball and football.
- Use a different swim stroke: breaststroke or sidestroke instead of the crawl or butterfly.
- Put your shoulder through its full range of motion every day to prevent stiffness.

Hip pain caused by tendinosis or bursitis may be felt at the side of the hip when you rise from a chair and take the first few steps, while you climb stairs, or while you drive. If pain is severe, sleeping on your side may also be painful. Pain in the front of the hip may also be caused by arthritis. See page 157. Hip pain can also cause knee or thigh pain. This is known as referred pain.

To relieve hip pain and avoid further hip problems:

- Wear well-cushioned shoes and avoid high heels.
- Avoid activities that force one side of your pelvis higher than the other, such as running in only one direction on a track or working sideways on a slope.
- Sleep on your uninjured side with a pillow between your knees, or on your back with pillows beneath your knees.
- See the hip stretches on pages 150 and 348. Stretch after activity, when your muscles are warm.

Knee pain may be caused by bursitis or tendinosis. See Knee Problems on page 169.

Heel or foot pain may be caused by plantar fasciitis or Achilles tendinosis. See page 167. Pain in the front of the lower leg may be due to shin splints. See page 171.

When to Call a Health Professional

- If there is fever, rapid swelling, or redness, or if you are unable to use a joint.
- If severe pain continues when the joint is at rest and you have applied ice.
- If the pain persists for 2 weeks or longer despite home treatment. Your doctor or a physical therapist can help you develop a specific exercise and home treatment plan.

Carpal Tunnel Syndrome

The carpal tunnel is a narrow passageway between the bones and ligaments in your wrist. The median nerve, which controls sensation in the fingers and some muscles in the hand, passes through this tunnel along with some of the finger tendons. Carpal tunnel syndrome (CTS) develops when there is pressure on the median nerve where it goes through the carpal tunnel.

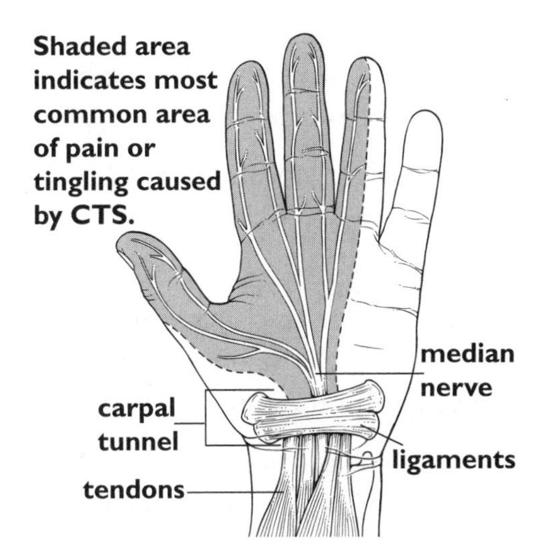

Pain and tingling in the hand may be caused by pressure on a nerve in the wrist.

Doing activities that use the same finger or hand movements over and over can cause CTS. We do these activities in every part of our lives, including work, home, hobbies, and sports. Other causes of CTS include being overweight, having a cyst (ganglion) on the tendon sheath in the wrist, or having rheumatoid arthritis. Previous wrist injuries, pregnancy, diabetes, thyroid disease, and taking birth control pills also may increase your risk for CTS.

Pressure on the median nerve causes the following symptoms of CTS:

- Numbness or pain in your hand or wrist that wakes you up at night.
- Numbness or tingling in the fingers of one or both hands, except for the little finger.
- Numbness or pain that gets worse when you use your hand or wrist, especially when you grip an object or flex your wrist.
- Occasional aching pain in your arm from your hand to your elbow.
- A weak grip.

Prevention

- Stop any activity that you think may be causing finger, hand, or wrist numbness or pain. If your symptoms improve when you stop an activity, resume that activity gradually and with greater efforts to keep your wrist straight or only slightly bent.
- Use your whole hand (not just your fingers and thumb) to grasp objects.
- Reduce the speed and force of repetitive hand movements such as those used for typing.
- Switch hands and change positions often when you are doing repetitive motions.

- Take frequent breaks and rest your hands.
- If you are not able to change positions or equipment at work often enough to prevent numbness or pain, ask your health professional about wearing a wrist splint that will reduce the stress on your fingers, hand, or wrist.
- Pay attention to your posture. When you are typing, make sure your fingers are lower than your wrists (using a keyboard wrist support may help). When your forearms are hanging by your sides, keep your shoulders relaxed.
- Keep your arm, hand, and finger muscles strong and flexible and maintain good overall fitness.
- Avoid using too much salt if you tend to retain fluid.

Home Treatment

- Follow the prevention tips above.
- Use ibuprofen or naproxen sodium to relieve pain and reduce swelling. (Vitamin B_6 has not been shown to be an effective treatment for CTS.)
- Apply ice or a cold pack to the palm side of the wrist. See Ice and Cold Packs on page 167.
- Avoid sleeping on your hands.
- Ask your health professional about using a wrist splint to relieve pressure on your wrist.
- Do simple range-of-motion exercises with your fingers and wrist to prevent stiffening. Stop if it hurts.
- Other lifestyle changes such as losing weight, quitting smoking, reducing the amount of alcohol you drink, and controlling diabetes may help relieve symptoms of CTS that are related to swelling.

When to Call a Health Professional

- If tingling, numbness, weakness, or pain in your fingers and hand has not gone away after 2 weeks of home treatment.
- If you have little or no feeling in your fingers or hand.
- If you cannot do simple hand movements, or if you accidentally drop things.
- If you cannot pinch your thumb and first finger together or you have no thumb strength.
- If you have problems at work because of pain in your fingers or hand.

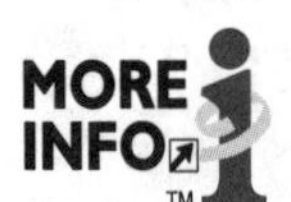

Most cases of carpal tunnel syndrome are treated without surgery. If you are considering surgery, gather as much information as possible about its risks and benefits. Getting all the facts and thinking about your own needs and values will help you work with your doctor to make a wise health decision.

Ice and Cold Packs

Ice can relieve pain, swelling, and inflammation from injuries and other conditions such as arthritis. Apply ice consistently as long as you have symptoms. Use either a commercial cold pack or one of the following:

- Ice towel: Wet a towel with cold water and squeeze it until it is just damp. Fold the towel, place it in a plastic bag, and freeze it for 15 minutes. Remove the towel from the bag and place it on the affected area.
- Ice pack: Put about 0.5 kg of ice in a plastic bag. Add water to barely cover the ice. Squeeze the air out of the bag and seal it. Wrap the bag in a wet towel and apply it to the affected area.
- Homemade cold pack: See instructions on page 399.

Ice the area at least 3 times a day. For the first 48 hours, ice for 10 minutes once an hour. After that, a good pattern is to ice for 10 minutes 3 times a day: in the morning, in the late afternoon after work or school, and about half an hour before bedtime. Also ice after any prolonged activity or vigorous exercise.

Always keep a damp cloth between your skin and the cold pack, and press firmly against all the curves of the affected area. Do not apply ice for longer than 10 minutes at a time, and do not fall asleep with the ice on your skin.

Heel Pain and Plantar Fasciitis

Plantar fasciitis is a condition that occurs when the thick, fibrous tissue that covers the bottom of your foot (plantar fascia) becomes inflamed and painful. Athletes, middle-aged people, and those who are overweight tend to develop plantar fasciitis. Prolonged standing and repetitive movements such as running and jumping can lead to heel pain and plantar fasciitis.

An excessive inward rolling of the foot (called pronation) during walking or running can also cause heel pain and plantar fasciitis. Pronation can be caused by wearing shoes that are worn out or have poor arch support, having tight calf muscles, or running downhill or on uneven surfaces.

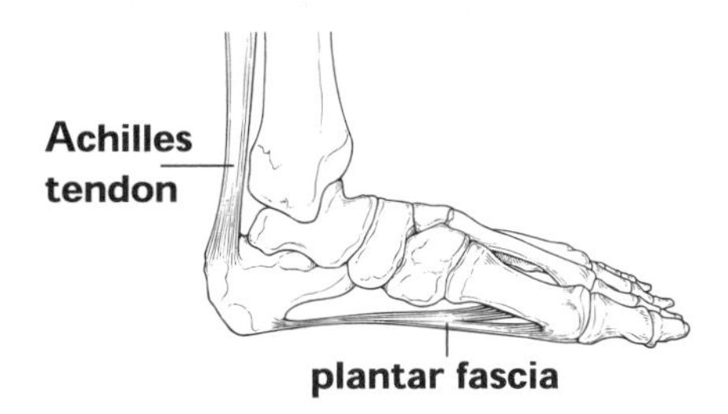

Foot or heel pain is often caused by inflammation of the plantar fascia or by Achilles tendinosis.

Achilles tendinosis can cause pain in the back of the heel. See Strains, Sprains, Fractures, and Dislocations on page 104 for information on torn or ruptured tendons.

A **heel spur** is a calcium buildup that most often develops where the plantar fascia attaches to the heel bone. Heel spurs usually do not cause pain and do not need to be treated. (Rarely, a painful heel spur may need to be surgically removed.) The pain many people attribute to heel spurs is in most cases caused by plantar fasciitis rather than by the heel spur itself.

Prevention

- Stretch your Achilles tendon and calf muscles several times a day (see page 348). Stretching is important for both athletes and non-athletes.
- Maintain a reasonable weight for your height.
- Always wear shoes with well-cushioned soles and good arch supports. Replace running shoes every 480 to 800 kilometres.
- Establish good exercise habits. If you are a runner, increase distance slowly, limit your training on hilly terrain, and run on softer surfaces (grass or dirt) rather than concrete. Cross-train by alternating running with different sports.

Home Treatment

Treat heel pain when it first appears to keep plantar fasciitis or other problems from becoming chronic.

- Reduce all weight-bearing activities to a pain-free level. Try low-impact activities such as cycling or swimming to speed healing. You may need to check with your doctor about when you can gradually resume high-impact activities.
- Apply ice to your heel. See Ice and Cold Packs on page 167.
- Try putting non-prescription arch supports in your shoes.
- Do not go barefoot until the pain is completely gone. Wear shoes or arch-supporting sandals during all weight-bearing activities, even going to the bathroom during the night.
- Take Aspirin, ibuprofen, or naproxen sodium to relieve pain. Do not give Aspirin to anyone younger than 20.
- Stretch your calf muscles. See page 348.
- For Achilles tendinosis or plantar fasciitis, try putting heel lifts or heel cups in both shoes. Use them only until the pain is gone (continue other home treatment).

When to Call a Health Professional

- If heel pain occurs with fever, redness, or heat in your heel, or if there is numbness or tingling in your heel or foot.
- If a heel injury results in pain when you put weight on your heel.
- If pain continues when you are not standing or bearing any weight on your heel.
- If heel pain persists for 1 to 2 weeks despite home treatment.

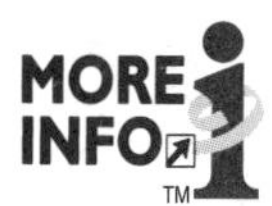

Your doctor may recommend other treatments for plantar fasciitis, such as taping, exercises, shoe inserts, or steroid injections. Surgery is usually done only as a last resort when other treatments fail to relieve pain.

Knee Problems

The knee is a vulnerable joint. It is basically just two long leg bones held together with ligaments and muscles. Problems develop when you put too much stress on the joint. The following are the three most common knee problems:

- Sprained knee ligaments (such as the medial collateral ligament) usually occur when the knee is twisted in a direction that it does not normally go. Sometimes knee ligaments (such as the anterior cruciate ligament) are torn. When this happens, knee cartilage (such as a meniscus) may also be damaged.
- Kneecap pain, also known as patellofemoral pain, occurs around or behind the kneecap (patella) when you run downhill, go up or down stairs, or after you sit for long periods of time.
- Patellar tendinosis, also known as jumper's knee, affects the tendon that attaches the kneecap to the shin bone (tibia). It is common among basketball and volleyball players.

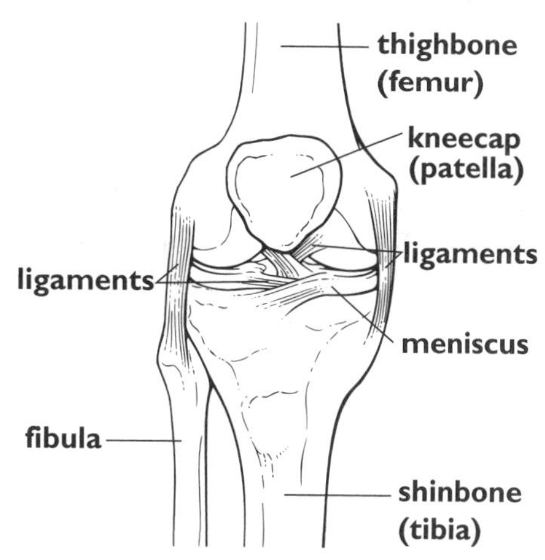

Knee problems can develop when the structures that support the joint are injured or become inflamed.

Prevention

- The best way to prevent knee problems is to strengthen and stretch the leg muscles evenly, especially those in the front and back of the thigh (quadriceps and hamstrings). See page 348.
- Avoid deep knee bends.
- Avoid running downhill unless you are fully conditioned.
- Avoid wearing shoes with cleats when playing contact sports.
- Wear shoes with good arch supports. Replace running shoes every 480 to 800 kilometres.
- Avoid wearing high-heeled shoes.

Home Treatment

- Apply ice to your knee. See Ice and Cold Packs on page 167.
- Rest your knee, and reduce by at least 50 percent the activities that cause pain.

- Ask your health professional about wearing a brace, an elastic or neoprene sleeve, or a band with a hole for the kneecap that holds the kneecap in place to help ease pain during activity. You can buy one at a pharmacy or sporting goods store.
- Stretch the front and back of your thigh muscles (quadriceps and hamstrings) after exercise, when they are warm. See pages 150 and 348.
- Also see Strains, Sprains, Fractures, and Dislocations on page 104 and Bursitis and Tendinosis on page 161.
- If knee pain is not related to exercise or a recent or past injury, see Arthritis on page 157.

When to Call a Health Professional

- If your knee gives out or won't bear weight.
- If you felt or heard a "pop" in your knee at the time of an injury.
- If your knee begins to swell within 30 minutes of an injury.
- If you have signs of damage to the nerves or blood vessels, such as numbness, tingling, a pins-and-needles sensation, or pale or bluish skin below the injury.
- If your knee looks deformed.
- If you are unable to straighten or bend the knee, or if the joint locks.
- If the knee is red, hot, swollen, or painful to touch.
- If pain is severe enough that you are limping, or if it does not improve within 2 days.

Fibromyalgia

Fibromyalgia is a condition that causes chronic muscle and soft tissue pain and tenderness on both sides of the body, above and below the waist. Fibromyalgia does not damage the body, destroy the joints, or cause any internal organ problems, but the pain may be severe enough to interfere with work and other activities.

The cause of fibromyalgia is not known. People who have fibromyalgia have many tender spots in specific areas of their bodies (tender points). They often have trouble sleeping. There may also be stiffness, weakness, and fatigue. Fibromyalgia is more common in women than in men.

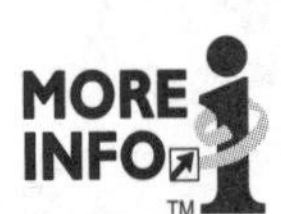

Regular exercise, such as walking, biking, or swimming, is the cornerstone of treatment for fibromyalgia. Doctors sometimes prescribe medications to help treat the symptoms. If stress makes your symptoms worse, see page 384.

Muscle Cramps and Leg Pain

Leg pain and muscle cramps ("charley horse" or "stitch") are common. They often occur during exercise, especially during hot weather, or at night. Dehydration, low levels of potassium in the body, or using a muscle that is not stretched well may cause cramps.

Shin splints cause pain in the front of the lower leg. Their cause is unclear, but they tend to develop when the legs are overused in high-impact activities.

Arthritis can also cause leg pain (see page 157). Leg pain that extends from the buttocks down the back of the leg and into the foot may be caused by sciatica. See page 145.

Phlebitis, an inflammation of a vein, also causes leg pain, usually in the calf of one leg. This condition can be serious if blood clots form in a deep vein, break loose, and lodge in the lungs. Phlebitis is most common after surgery or prolonged bed rest.

Decreased blood flow to the leg muscles caused by hardening of the arteries (atherosclerosis) is another possible cause of leg cramps. This is called **intermittent claudication**. Symptoms may include cramping pain in the calf that comes on with activity or exertion and is relieved by rest. Symptoms often occur after you walk a certain distance.

Growing Pains

Children age 6 to 12 often develop harmless "growing pains" in their legs at night. Other than growth itself, the cause is unknown. A heating pad, acetaminophen, or gentle massage of the legs may help.

Prevention

- Warm up well and stretch before any activity. Also stretch after exercise to keep hot muscles from shortening and cramping.
- Drink extra fluids before and during exercise, especially during hot or humid weather.
- Include plenty of potassium in your diet. Bananas, orange juice, and potatoes are good sources.
- To avoid stomach muscle cramps ("stitches") during exercise, do side stretches before exercising and learn to breathe with your lower lungs. See Roll Breathing on page 386.
- If leg cramps wake you at night, take a warm bath and do some stretching exercises before going to bed. Keep your legs warm while sleeping.

Home Treatment

- If there is pain, swelling, or heaviness in the calf of only one of your legs, or if you have other symptoms that cause you to suspect phlebitis (see When to Call a Health Professional), call your doctor before you try home treatment.

- Gently stretch and massage the cramping muscle.
- Drink more fluids. Cramps are often related to dehydration.
- For shin splints, apply ice and use pain relievers (ibuprofen or acetaminophen) while you take 1 to 2 weeks of rest from high-impact activity. Return to exercise gradually.

When to Call a Health Professional

- If you have any of the following symptoms of phlebitis:
  - Continuous leg or calf pain
  - Swelling of one leg
  - Any redness in the leg or calf that is tender to the touch
  - Fever
- If you have signs of impaired blood flow such as:
  - Pain that comes on after you walk a certain distance and that goes away with rest.
  - Sudden onset of moderate to severe pain with coldness or pale skin in the lower part of the leg.
  - Pale or blue-black colour to the skin of one or both legs or feet or the toes.
- If muscle cramps are not relieved by home treatment.

Osteoporosis

Osteoporosis is a disease that causes a person's bones to become so weak that they can break during normal daily activities. Osteoporosis affects millions of older adults. Women are four times more likely to develop osteoporosis than men are.

Osteoporosis is more common after menopause, when estrogen levels decline. Risk factors for osteoporosis include family history of osteoporosis, lack of weight-bearing exercise, slender body frame, and Asian or European heritage. Women who smoke or drink are also at greater risk. Elevated thyroid hormone (hyperthyroidism) may also cause osteoporosis.

Osteoporosis usually develops over many years without symptoms. The first signs of osteoporosis include loss of height, developing a curved upper back (dowager's hump), back pain, or broken bones.

Prevention

Weakening bones are a natural part of growing older. But if you start healthy habits early in life, you may be able to delay the development of osteoporosis.

- Get regular weight-bearing exercise, such as walking, jogging, climbing stairs, dancing, or weight lifting. Weight-bearing exercise helps keep bones strong.

- Eat a healthy diet that includes plenty of calcium and vitamin D. Both are needed for building healthy, strong bones. See page 359 for tips on getting more calcium in your diet. You can get a boost of vitamin D by drinking fortified milk or by spending 10 to 15 minutes in the sun each day. (If you have dark skin, you will need more time in the sun.) Take supplements of calcium and vitamin D if you think you are not getting enough in your diet.
- Don't smoke.
- Limit your alcohol intake to 1 drink per day or less.
- Cut down on caffeine. Caffeine increases calcium loss from your body and puts you at risk for osteoporosis.
- There are medications, including estrogen, that can help prevent osteoporosis. Talk with your doctor about whether these are appropriate for you. Also see Hormone Therapy on page 312.

If you already have osteoporosis, these healthy habits can help slow the disease process and possibly reduce your risk of broken bones.

When to Call a Health Professional

- If you think you have a broken bone; if you notice swelling; or if you cannot move a part of your body normally.
- If you have sudden, severe pain or problems bearing weight on the injured part of your body.
- If you notice that one of your arms or legs is misshapen. This may mean you have a broken bone.
- If you want to discuss your risk for developing osteoporosis.

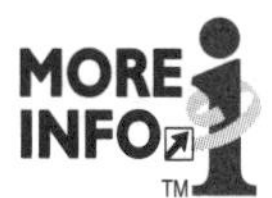

Special X-rays that measure bone density can tell you how much bone loss has occurred as a result of osteoporosis. If you are at high risk for osteoporosis, or if you are a woman over 65, a bone density measurement may provide you with important information to help you and your doctor decide whether you need treatment for osteoporosis.

Sports Injuries

Injuries are common among physically active people. Muscle aches and pains are likely to develop when you start a new activity (or resume an activity after taking a break from it), because the muscles used for the activity need time to build strength and endurance. Most sports injuries are caused by either accidents or overuse. Overuse injuries can be avoided if you train properly for activities and use appropriate equipment.

Prevention

- Warm up before exercising. Cold, stiff muscles and ligaments are more prone to injury. Cool down and stretch after activities. See page 348.
- Increase the intensity and duration of activities gradually. As your fitness level improves, you will be able to do increasingly strenuous exercise without injury.
- Use proper sports techniques and equipment. For example, wear supportive, well-cushioned shoes for running, aerobics, and walking; use a two-handed tennis backhand stroke; wear protective pads for in-line skating. Make sure that your bicycle is adjusted properly for your body. Wear a sport-specific helmet for your activity.
- Alternate hard workouts with easier ones to let your body rest. For example, if you run, alternate long or hard runs with shorter or easier ones. If you lift weights, don't work the same muscles 2 days in a row.
- Cross-train (do several activities regularly) to rest different muscle groups. Alternate days of walking or running with biking or swimming.
- Don't ignore aches and pains. When you feel the first twinge of pain, rest or reduce your activity for a few days. Apply ice and other home treatment, and you may avoid more serious problems.

Home Treatment

The biggest home treatment challenge for most people with sports injuries is to get enough rest to allow healing without losing overall conditioning.

- Maintain your fitness level by cross-training with activities that don't stress the injured area: swimming for sore ankles or feet; walking or biking for sore shoulders or elbows. Don't return to the activity that caused the injury too quickly.
- Resume your regular activity gradually. Start with a slow, easy pace, less weight (if you're lifting weights), fewer repetitions, or a shorter duration of activity, and increase only if you have no pain.
- Break your sport down into components. If you can throw a ball a short distance without pain, try increasing the distance. If you can walk comfortably, try jogging. If you can jog without pain, try running.

When to Call a Health Professional

Information on specific injuries can be found on the following pages:

- Bursitis and tendinosis, page 161.
- Tennis elbow and golfer's elbow, page 162.
- Patellar tendinosis, page 169.

- Achilles tendinosis and plantar fasciitis, page 167.
- Strains, sprains, fractures, and dislocations, page 104.

Temporomandibular (TM) Disorder

The temporomandibular joint (TMJ) is the joint in front of the ear that connects the lower jawbone (mandible) to the skull. Pain and discomfort in the jaw muscles and temporomandibular joint is called temporomandibular disorder (TM disorder).

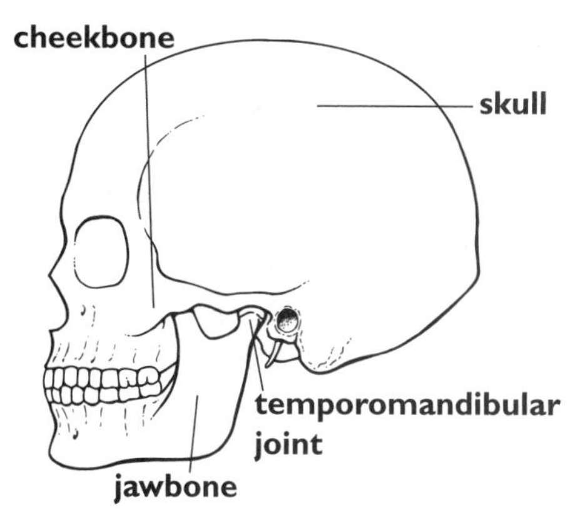

Pain and discomfort in the jaw muscles and jaw joint is called temporomandibular disorder.

The symptoms of TM disorder can include:

- Pain in one or both jaws when chewing or yawning.
- Painful clicking, popping, or grating in the jaw joint.
- Locking of the jaw in an open or closed position, or inability to "open wide."
- Headache, neck pain, facial pain, or shoulder pain.

The most common cause of TM disorder is tension in the jaw, neck, and shoulder muscles. This can be brought on by stress or by habits such as clenching or grinding your teeth. TM disorder can also occur when there is a problem, such as arthritis, in the joint itself.

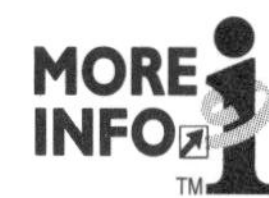

Home treatment and non-surgical treatments will successfully relieve most symptoms of TM disorder.

Your doctor may recommend use of a plastic mouth plate (splint), physical therapy, or prescription pain relievers. Surgery is rarely needed and may cause further problems.

Prevention

The key to preventing TM disorder is reducing muscle tension in your jaw.

- Relax. If you have a lot of stress and anxiety in your life, try relaxation techniques (see page 386).
- Do not bite your nails or cradle the telephone receiver between your shoulder and jaw.
- Stop chewing gum or tough foods at the first sign of pain or discomfort in your jaw muscles.
- Change your diet. Eat softer foods, and use both sides of your mouth to chew your food.

- Maintain good posture. Poor posture may disturb the natural alignment between your facial bones and muscles and cause pain.
- Get regular dental checkups.

Home Treatment

- Continue the prevention tips.
- Avoid opening your mouth too wide.
- Rest your jaw, keeping your teeth apart and your lips closed. (Keep your tongue on the roof of your mouth, not between your teeth.)
- Put an ice pack on the joint for 10 minutes, 3 times a day. Gently open and close your mouth while the ice pack is on. If the jaw muscle is swollen, apply ice 6 times a day.
- Take ibuprofen or acetaminophen to reduce swelling and pain.
- If there is no swelling, apply moist heat to your jaw for 10 to 15 minutes, 3 times a day. Gently open and close your mouth while the heat is on. Alternate heat with the cold pack treatments.
- Seek help if you are under severe stress or suffer from anxiety or depression. See Mental Health, Addictions, and Mind-Body Wellness starting on page 365.

When to Call a Health Professional

- If the pain is severe.
- If TM symptoms occur after an injury to the jaw.
- If your jaw locks in certain positions.
- If any jaw problem or pain lasts longer than 2 weeks without improvement.
- If you have noticed a change in the way your teeth fit together when you close your mouth.

Weakness and Fatigue

Weakness is a lack of physical or muscle strength and a feeling that extra effort is required to move your arms, legs, or other muscles.

Fatigue is a feeling of tiredness, exhaustion, or lack of energy.

Unexplained muscle weakness is usually more serious than fatigue. It may be caused by diabetes (see page 285), thyroid problems, stroke, or other problems related to the brain and spinal cord. Call your doctor immediately if you have sudden, unexplained muscle weakness.

Fatigue, on the other hand, can usually be treated with self-care. Most fatigue is caused by lack of exercise, stress or overwork, lack of sleep, depression, worry, or boredom. Colds and flu may cause fatigue and weakness, but the symptoms disappear as the illness runs its course.

Chronic Fatigue Syndrome

Chronic fatigue syndrome (CFS) is a flu-like illness that causes severe fatigue lasting longer than 6 months. The fatigue does not improve with rest. Other symptoms may include memory problems, headaches, sore throat, painful lymph glands, muscle and joint pain, and sleep problems.

CFS is difficult to diagnose. There are no definitive lab tests. Many other illnesses, such as depression, thyroid disorders, or mononucleosis, cause similar symptoms. A CFS diagnosis is made only after fatigue and other symptoms continue for at least 6 months and other possible causes have been ruled out.

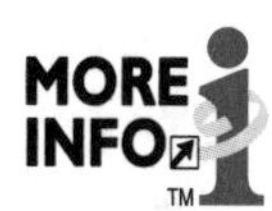

Treatment is focused on adequate rest, balanced diet, and gentle exercise. No medications are known to cure chronic fatigue syndrome, but many people may improve on their own over time. Treatment of the individual symptoms can be effective. For treatment of depression, which is common in people with CFS, see page 372.

Call your doctor if unexplained fatigue is severe and persistent and interferes with your activities for more than 2 weeks despite home treatment and rest.

Prevention

- Regular exercise is your best defence against fatigue. If you feel too tired to exercise vigorously, try a short walk.
- Eat a well-balanced diet.
- Make sure you are getting enough sleep. See page 376.
- Deal with emotional problems instead of ignoring or denying them. See page 365.
- Take steps to control your stress and workload. See page 384.

Home Treatment

- Follow the prevention guidelines and be patient. It may take a while before you feel energetic again.
- Listen to your body. Alternate rest with exercise.
- Limit medications that might contribute to fatigue. Tranquilizers and cold and allergy medications are particularly suspect.
- Reduce your use of caffeine, nicotine, and alcohol.
- Cut back on watching television and working or playing on the computer. Spend that time with friends, try new activities, or travel to break the fatigue cycle.

When to Call a Health Professional

- If you have unexplained muscle weakness in one area of your body.

- If severe or persistent fatigue causes you to limit your usual activities for longer than 2 weeks despite home treatment.
- If you experience sudden, unexplained weight loss or gain.
- If you do not feel more energetic after 4 weeks of home treatment.
- If fatigue gets worse despite home treatment.

Life is made up of sobs, sniffles, and smiles,
with sniffles predominating.
O. Henry

9

Chest and Respiratory Problems

Chest and respiratory problems can be as simple as a minor cold or as life-threatening as a heart attack. For most respiratory problems, including allergies, colds, sore throats, sinusitis, and tonsillitis, this chapter will help you decide what to do at home and when to call your doctor.

Look at the chart on the next page. If you don't find what you're looking for, please check the index.

Allergies

Allergies come in many forms. The most common causes of allergies are particles in the air. Hay fever (allergic rhinitis) is the most common allergic disease. Allergy symptoms include itchy, watery eyes; sneezing; runny, stuffy, or itchy nose; and fatigue. The symptoms are a lot like cold symptoms, but they usually last longer. Dark circles under the eyes (allergic shiners) or post-nasal drip may also accompany hay fever.

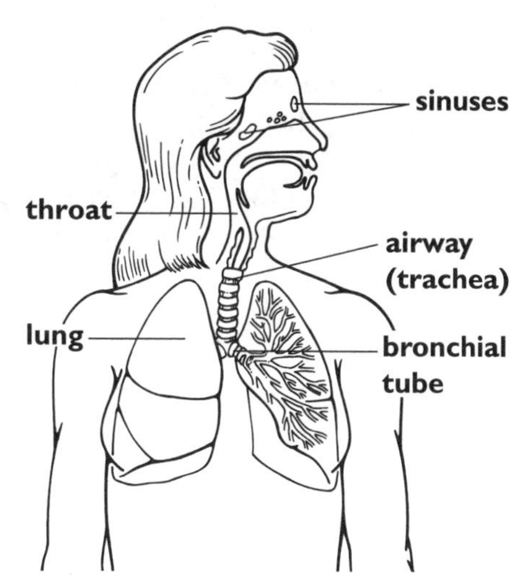

Respiratory problems can occur in the upper respiratory tract (nose, sinuses, throat, or trachea) or in the lower respiratory tract (bronchial tubes or lungs).

Chest, Respiratory, Nose, and Throat Problems

Symptoms	Possible Causes
Chest and Respiratory	
Wheezing or difficult (rapid, shallow, laboured) breathing	Allergies, p. 179; Asthma, p. 184; Bronchitis, p. 188.
Cough, fever, yellow-green or rust-coloured sputum, and difficulty breathing	Bronchitis, p. 188; Pneumonia, p. 188.
Chest pain or discomfort with sweating or rapid pulse	Possible heart attack. Call for help. See p. 86. Chest Pain, p. 190.
Burning, pain, or discomfort behind or below the breastbone	Heartburn, p. 121; Chest Pain, p. 190.
Coughing	Coughs, p. 195.
Pounding or racing heartbeat; heart skipping or missing a beat	Heart Palpitations, p. 198.
Nose and Throat	
Stuffy or runny nose with watery eyes, sneezing	Allergies, p. 179; Colds, p. 194.
Cold symptoms with fever, headache, severe body aches, fatigue	Influenza, p. 199.
Thick green, yellow, or grey nasal discharge with fever and facial pain	Sinusitis, p. 202.
Foul odour from nose; swollen, inflamed nasal tissue	Objects in the Nose, p. 96; Sinusitis, p. 202.
Sore throat	Sore Throat, p. 204; Tonsillitis, p. 204.
Sore throat with white spots on tonsils, swollen lymph nodes, fever of 38.3°C or higher	Strep Throat, p. 204.
Swollen tonsils, sore throat, fever	Tonsillitis, p. 204.
Swollen lymph nodes in the neck	Swollen Lymph Nodes, p. 208; Tonsillitis, p. 204.
Hoarseness, loss of voice	Laryngitis, p. 201.

You can often discover the cause of an allergy by noting when symptoms occur. Symptoms that occur at the same time each year (especially during spring, early summer, or early fall) are often caused by tree, grass, or weed pollen. Allergies that persist all year long may be due to dust, microscopic mites in household dust, cockroaches, mould spores, or animal dander. An animal allergy is often easy to detect: symptoms clear up when you stay away from the animal or its bedding.

Allergies seem to run in families. Parents with hay fever often have children with allergies. Hay fever may develop in children but is more common in teens and adults.

Life-Threatening Allergic Reactions

A few people have severe allergies to insect stings, nuts or other foods, or drugs, especially antibiotics such as penicillin. For these people, the allergic reaction is sudden and severe and may cause breathing difficulty and a drop in blood pressure. This type of reaction is called anaphylactic shock, or anaphylaxis.

An anaphylactic reaction is a medical emergency, and prompt care is needed. If you have ever had a severe allergic reaction, your doctor may suggest that you carry an epinephrine syringe (such as EpiPen or Ana-Kit) designed for giving yourself a shot that will decrease the severity of the reaction. If you have had an allergic reaction to a drug, wear a medical identification bracelet that will tell health professionals about your allergy in case you cannot.

Food Allergies

About 2 percent of adults have true food allergies. Most adverse reactions to foods are due to food intolerances, reactions to food additives, or food poisoning. Most true food allergies are to nuts, fish, shellfish, eggs, soy, wheat, and milk. An allergic reaction to a food can result in anaphylactic shock. See When to Call a Health Professional on page 183.

From 2 percent to 8 percent of infants have food allergies. By gradually introducing simple solid foods into your child's diet, you will be able to identify possible food allergies. Children often outgrow allergies to wheat, milk, eggs, and soy between the ages of 3 and 5. Allergies to nuts, fish, and shellfish usually persist into adulthood. If your child was allergic to a food when younger, you may be able to reintroduce it as he or she gets older. Talk to a health professional before trying to reintroduce the food. A child with a severe food allergy may have a life-threatening reaction to even a tiny amount of that food.

Prevention

- If practical, avoid the substance that causes allergy attacks. See page 181 for more information about food allergies.
- Allergy shots (immunotherapy) may help control symptoms of allergies and asthma or may reduce the risk of having an anaphylactic reaction. (See Life-Threatening Allergic Reactions on page 181.)

Home Treatment

If you can discover the source of your allergies, avoiding that substance may be the best treatment. Keep a record of your symptoms and the plants, animals, foods, medications, or chemicals that seem to trigger them.

Here are some general tips for avoiding irritants:

- Avoid yard work (raking, mowing), which stirs up both pollen and mould. If you must do yard work, wear a mask and take an antihistamine beforehand.
- Don't smoke, and avoid inhaling other people's smoke.
- Don't use aerosol sprays, perfumes, room deodorizers, cleaning products, or other substances that may trigger allergy symptoms.

If your symptoms are seasonal and seem to be related to pollen:

- Keep your house and car windows closed. Keep bedroom windows closed at night.
- Limit the time you spend outside when pollen counts are high. Dogs and other pets may bring large amounts of pollen into your house, so either leave them outside or wash them frequently.

If your symptoms are year-round and seem to be related to dust:

- Keep your bedroom and other places where you spend a lot of time as dust-free as possible.
- Avoid carpeting, upholstered furniture, and heavy draperies that collect dust. Vacuuming doesn't pick up house dust mites.
- Cover your mattress and box spring with dustproof cases and wipe them clean weekly. Avoid wool or down blankets and feather pillows. Wash all bedding in hot water once a week.
- Consider using an air conditioner or air purifier with a special HEPA filter. Rent one before buying to see if it helps.

If your symptoms are year-round and are worse during damp weather, they may be related to mould or mildew:

- Keep your home well ventilated and dry. Keep the humidity below 50 percent. Use a dehumidifier during humid weather.
- Use an air conditioner, which removes mould spores from the air. Change or clean heating and cooling system filters regularly.
- Clean bathroom and kitchen surfaces often with bleach to reduce mould growth.

What About Allergy Shots?

Allergy shots (immunotherapy) are a series of shots given to desensitize your body to substances that trigger allergic reactions (allergens). You may need to receive shots for 3 to 5 years before you stop having allergic reactions.

Immunotherapy is effective only if skin sensitivity testing has identified the specific allergy trigger. It is very effective against allergies to bee stings and other insect venom. For most people, immunotherapy is effective against grass, tree, and weed pollens, as well as house dust and house dust mites.

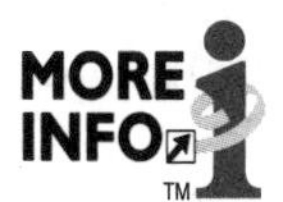

Because of the time and expense involved, you need a realistic idea of the benefits before you agree to immunotherapy. Discuss these with your doctor. Allergy shots may be worthwhile for you if:

- You cannot avoid allergy triggers, or avoiding them has not helped.
- Your symptoms have bothered you a lot for at least 2 years.
- Home treatment has not been successful.
- Neither prescription nor non-prescription medications bring you relief.
- Immunotherapy has been shown to be effective for the allergens identified by your skin tests.

If you are allergic to a pet:

- Keep the animal outside, or at least out of your bedroom.
- If your symptoms are severe and your efforts to reduce dander exposure do not help, the best solution may be to find a new home for the pet.

Decongestants and antihistamines may relieve some allergy symptoms. Use caution when taking these drugs. See pages 406 and 407.

For more information about allergies, including immunotherapy, contact your doctor, your public health unit, the BC Lung Association, or the Allergy/Asthma Information Association (AAIA).

When to Call a Health Professional

Call 911 or other emergency services immediately if you develop signs of a severe allergic reaction (anaphylaxis). The following severe symptoms may occur soon after you take a drug, eat a certain food, or are stung by an insect:

- Light-headedness (feeling like you might pass out) or confusion
- Swelling around the lips, tongue, or face that is interfering with breathing or getting worse
- Wheezing or difficulty breathing

Call a health professional:

- If your face, tongue, or lips are swollen, even if you are not having difficulty breathing and the swelling is not getting worse.

- If there is significant swelling around the site of an insect sting (for instance, the entire arm or leg is swollen).
- If you develop a skin rash, itching, a feeling of warmth, or hives.

Call your doctor if allergy symptoms worsen over time and home treatment doesn't help. Your doctor may recommend stronger medication or allergy shots (immunotherapy). See page 183.

Asthma

Asthma is a condition that causes long-term inflammation of the airways. The inflammation makes the airways overreact to certain particles in the air. During an asthma episode, the muscles in the tubes that carry air into the lungs (bronchial tubes) go into spasm; the mucous lining of the lungs swells; and secretions build up in the lungs, suddenly making breathing difficult.

A person who is having an asthma episode (attack) may make a wheezing or whistling sound while breathing. The person usually coughs a great deal and may spit up mucus. Sometimes a chronic, dry cough, especially at night or early in the morning, is the only symptom of mild asthma.

Many things can trigger asthma, including allergens such as dust mites, dust, pollen, cockroaches, and animal dander. Viral respiratory infections, such as colds, are common triggers of asthma. Other triggers include exercise, cold air, cigarette or wood smoke, chemical vapours, pain relievers (especially Aspirin), food preservatives and dyes, and emotional stress.

Asthma usually develops during childhood but may also begin later in life. The first episode often follows a cold or the flu. Asthma is more common in children who are exposed to cigarette smoke in the home. Some children outgrow asthma symptoms as they get older, but the symptoms may return later in life.

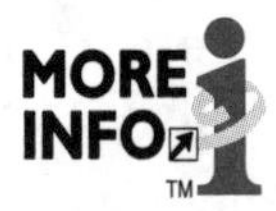

Most children and adults can control their asthma by avoiding triggers that cause attacks and using medications to manage symptoms. Severe attacks can usually be treated with inhaled or injected medications. Asthma attacks are rarely fatal if they are treated promptly and appropriately.

Prevention

There is no way to prevent asthma. However, you may be able to limit the length and severity of asthma episodes if you can avoid or control your exposure to things that trigger asthma symptoms.

- Review home treatment for allergies on page 182.
- Control cockroaches. Do not leave food or garbage in open containers. Use poison bait and traps to kill cockroaches. Avoid chemical sprays, which can trigger an asthma attack.
- Avoid smoke of all kinds. If you smoke cigarettes, stop. See pages 25 to 28 for tips on quitting. Avoid places where other people may be smoking, and make sure your home is a smoke-free environment. Don't use wood-burning stoves.
- Avoid irritants in the air. Stay indoors when the air pollution or pollen count is high. Try to avoid strong odours, fumes, and perfume.
- Avoid breathing cold air. In cold weather, breathe through your nose, and cover your nose and mouth with a scarf or a cold-weather mask.
- Aspirin, ibuprofen, and similar pain medications can cause severe asthma attacks in some people. Discuss the use of these medications with your doctor, and use them with caution. If these medications bother you, don't use them. Try acetaminophen instead.
- Do not use non-prescription cold and cough medications unless your doctor tells you to do so.
- Stress may be a factor in triggering asthma attacks. Practise the relaxation exercises on page 386.
- Reduce your risk of colds and flu by washing your hands often and getting a flu shot each year.
- If you use a humidifier, clean it thoroughly once a week.
- Build up the strength of your lungs and airways. Get regular exercise. Swimming or water aerobics may be good choices because you are less likely to have an asthma attack when you breathe moist air. If vigorous exercise triggers your asthma attacks, talk with your doctor. Adjusting your medication and your exercise routine may help.
- Work with your doctor to develop an asthma action plan so you can manage your symptoms at home. Make sure family members and friends know about your plan so they can help you during an asthma episode. See Asthma Action Plan on page 186.
- When you aren't having symptoms, follow your plan to treat ongoing airway inflammation. Get regular checkups to make sure your asthma action plan is working well for you.
- Learn to use a peak flow meter to monitor your ability to exhale. Used regularly, this device will give you an idea of how your lungs normally function. It also helps you tell when an asthma attack may be coming so you can take steps to prevent or treat it.

Since triggers for asthma attacks are often not known, you need to monitor your symptoms so you can prevent or treat asthma attacks before they become severe. Using an asthma action plan developed by a doctor to guide your home treatment, you may be able to prevent emergency room visits or admissions to the hospital for asthma symptoms.

Home Treatment

Once an asthma attack begins, prompt home treatment can provide relief.

- Learn to use a metered-dose inhaler. Inhalers help get the right amount of medication to your airways. A device called a spacer is now recommended for use with an inhaler. Ask your doctor or pharmacist to watch you use your inhaler and spacer to make sure you are doing it right. With practice, most people can use an inhaler and spacer correctly.
- Drink plenty of fluids, especially water, to thin the mucus in the bronchial tubes.
- Be confident that your home treatment will control the severity of the attack.
- Keep a diary outlining your asthma attacks. After you've had an attack, write down what triggered it, what helped end it, and any concerns you have about your asthma action plan. Take your diary when you see your doctor for your regular checkups. Ask questions you may have about your plan or medication.

Asthma Action Plan

An asthma action plan is a written plan that tells you how to manage your asthma symptoms at home. It helps take the guesswork out of treating your asthma. The plan will outline the medication you will take for your asthma symptoms and when to take it, depending on the zone you are in (green, yellow, or red). In order to determine what zone you are in, you need to know how to use a peak flow meter to measure your ability to exhale. The plan may also tell you when to talk to your health professional about your asthma symptoms.

The asthma action plan zones include:

- Green zone plan: Routine care to keep asthma symptoms from starting.
- Yellow zone plan: How to stop asthma symptoms and keep an asthma episode (attack) from getting worse. This may involve taking other medications in addition to the ones you usually take to control your asthma.
- Red zone plan: What to do for a severe asthma episode. This is a medical emergency.

Tuberculosis (TB)

Tuberculosis is a contagious disease caused by bacteria that usually infect the lungs (pulmonary TB). When a person who has pulmonary TB coughs, sneezes, or laughs, TB-causing bacteria are released into the air where other people can inhale them. This is how TB is spread. Children and people with weak immune systems are particularly prone to TB.

Most people who are exposed to TB never develop symptoms, because their immune systems are able to stop the disease. People who develop symptoms of TB, such as persistent cough, weight loss, fatigue, night sweats, and fever, need drug treatment to stop the disease from progressing and to reduce the risk of spreading TB to others. Treatment, which consists of several medications, may last from 6 months to 2 years.

People who have weak immune systems because of AIDS or other diseases, who are affected by problematic substance use, or who have a chronic lung disease called silicosis are at high risk for developing progressive TB, which can damage the lungs or spread to other parts of the body.

To prevent TB infection, avoid close contact with people who have TB if possible. If you live with someone who has TB, ask your doctor what you can do to protect yourself from TB infection and whether you need to be tested for TB.

When to Call a Health Professional

Always follow your asthma action plan if you have one. **Call 911 or other emergency services** if you are having severe asthma symptoms and:

- You are having severe difficulty breathing.
- Your medications have not helped after 20 minutes.

Call a health professional:

- If you have symptoms that may indicate heart problems, such as chest pain or shortness of breath. See page 190.
- If you are having a severe asthma attack (peak flow is less than 50 percent of your best), even if your medications have relieved some symptoms.
- If your asthma symptoms don't get better after you follow your asthma action plan.
- If you are coughing up yellow, dark brown, or bloody mucus.
- If acute asthma symptoms (wheezing, coughing, difficulty breathing) have happened for the first time.
- To discuss exactly what to do when an attack begins. Once you understand and have confidence in your asthma medication, you can often handle mild attacks without professional help.
- If you begin to use your asthma medication more often than usual. This may be a sign that your asthma is getting worse.

- If you or the people who live with you have not been educated about immediate treatment for asthma attacks.
- If the medication required to treat an asthma attack is not available.
- To talk about adjusting your medication. Your doctor needs your feedback to figure out the best medicine and the right dosage for you.
- To assess allergies, which may worsen asthma attacks.
- To get a referral to an asthma educator and perhaps a support group. You can get good information by talking with others who have asthma. This may boost your confidence in dealing with the problem.

Bronchitis and Pneumonia

Bronchitis is an inflammation and irritation of the airways that lead to the lungs. Viruses are the usual cause of bronchitis, but it can also be caused by bacteria or by exposure to cigarette smoke or air pollution. The inflammation caused by acute bronchitis is not permanent. It goes away when the infection or irritation goes away.

Symptoms of bronchitis usually begin 3 to 4 days after an upper respiratory infection, such as a cold. Symptoms often include a dry cough that may become productive (producing sputum), mild fever, fatigue, discomfort or tightness in the chest, and wheezing.

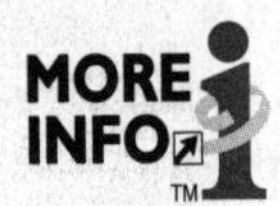

Frequent lung infections, especially in a person who smokes, may lead to the development of chronic bronchitis. Tobacco smokers are also at high risk for developing emphysema. Chronic bronchitis, emphysema, and other lung conditions are known as chronic obstructive pulmonary disease (COPD).

Pneumonia is an infection or inflammation that affects the bronchial tubes and lungs. Pneumonia is usually caused by bacteria, but viruses and other organisms can cause it as well. It may also develop as a complication of another viral illness, such as measles or chicken pox.

Pneumonia sometimes follows a viral respiratory infection, such as a cold or bronchitis. Having bronchitis and another lung disease, such as asthma, may increase your risk for pneumonia.

A person who has bacterial pneumonia is usually very sick. Symptoms may include:

- Productive cough with yellow, green, rust-coloured, or bloody sputum (mucus coughed up from the lungs).
- Fever and shaking chills.
- Rapid, shallow breathing.
- Chest-wall pain that is often made worse by coughing or taking a deep breath.

MORE INFO For more information, see the back cover.

- Rapid heartbeat.
- Fatigue that is worse than you would expect from a cold.

Prevention

- Get a pneumococcal vaccination if you are over 65. If you are younger than 65 and have a chronic disease or have had your spleen removed, you may need to be vaccinated. Talk to your doctor. See page 19.
- Get a yearly flu shot. See page 200.
- Give proper home care to minor respiratory problems such as colds and flu. See pages 194 and 199.
- Stop smoking. People who smoke or are around smokers have more frequent bouts of bronchitis.
- Avoid polluted air.
- Keep up your resistance to infection by eating a healthy diet, getting plenty of rest, and exercising regularly.

Home Treatment

Here is what you can do at home to prevent complications from bronchitis or pneumonia and feel better.

- Take the entire course of all prescribed medications. Although most cases of bronchitis can be managed with home treatment, severe or persistent symptoms may require prescription medication. Treatment for pneumonia almost always involves antibiotics.
- Drink plenty of fluids, especially water. Extra fluids help thin the mucus in the lungs so it can be coughed out.
- Get some extra rest. Let your energy go to healing.
- Take Aspirin, ibuprofen, or acetaminophen to reduce fever and relieve body aches. Do not give Aspirin to anyone younger than 20.
- Use a non-prescription cough suppressant that contains dextromethorphan to help quiet a dry, hacking cough so you can sleep. Avoid cough preparations that contain more than one active ingredient. See Cough Preparations on page 407.
- Breathe moist air from a humidifier, a hot shower, or a sink filled with hot water. The heat and moisture will thin mucus so it can be coughed out.
- If you have classic flu symptoms, call your doctor to talk about antiviral medications for the flu. See Influenza (Flu) on page 199.

When to Call a Health Professional

Any of the following symptoms may mean that your lung infection is getting worse or that you are developing a bacterial lung infection. Call if you develop:

- A cough that:
  - Occurs with wheezing or difficulty breathing that is new or different.
  - Brings up bloody sputum.

- Frequently produces yellow, green, or rust-coloured sputum from the lungs (not post-nasal drainage) and occurs along with a fever of 38.3°C or higher.
- Lingers more than 7 to 10 days after other symptoms have cleared, especially if it is productive (bringing up sputum). A dry, hacking cough may last several weeks after a viral illness such as a cold.

- A fever of 40.5°C or higher that does not go down after 30 to 60 minutes of home treatment.
- A fever of 40°C or higher that does not go down after 2 hours of home treatment.
- A fever higher than 38.3°C with shaking chills and a productive cough.
- A fever that persists despite home treatment. Many viral illnesses cause fevers of 38.8°C or higher for short periods of time (up to 12 to 24 hours). Call a doctor if the fever stays high:
  - 38.8°C or higher for 2 full days
  - 38.3°C or higher for 3 full days
  - 38°C or higher for 4 full days
- Laboured, shallow, or rapid breathing with shortness of breath.
- Significant chest-wall pain (pain in the muscles of the chest) when you cough or breathe.
- Fatigue that is worse than what you would expect from a cold.

Also call if:

- You are unable to drink enough fluids to avoid becoming dehydrated or you are unable to eat.
- The sick person is an infant, an older adult, or someone who is chronically ill, especially with lung problems.
- Any cough lasts longer than 2 weeks.

Chest Pain

Call 911 or other emergency services immediately if you think you may be having a heart attack. See Am I Having a Heart Attack? on page 191.

Call your doctor if you have continuous chest discomfort or pain and there is no obvious cause.

If the person who is having heart attack symptoms loses consciousness, follow the Rescue Breathing and CPR guidelines on page 68.

Angina is pain, pressure, heaviness, or numbness behind the breastbone or across the chest. It occurs when there is not enough oxygen reaching the heart muscle. It is a symptom of coronary artery disease. The pain caused by angina may radiate to the upper back, neck, jaws, shoulders, or arms. Angina may be brought on by stress or exertion and is relieved by rest and the use of prescribed medication.

A **heart attack** (myocardial infarction) is caused by blocked blood flow to the heart muscle. The pain of a heart attack is usually more severe than angina, lasts longer, and does not go away with rest or by taking medication that was previously effective for angina. Other symptoms that may be present include sweating, nausea, shortness of breath, weakness, or indigestion.

The following factors may increase your risk of a heart attack:

- Smoking
- Family history of heart disease
- Diabetes
- High blood pressure
- High cholesterol
- Inactive lifestyle
- High stress levels

Chest pain is a key warning sign of a heart attack, but it may also be caused by other problems.

If chest pain increases when you press your finger on the painful site, or if you can pinpoint the spot that hurts, it is probably chest-wall pain, which may be caused by strained muscles or ligaments or by a broken rib. An inflammation of the cartilage in the chest wall (called costochondritis) can also cause chest-wall pain. Chest-wall pain usually lasts only a few days. Aspirin or ibuprofen may help. Do not give Aspirin to anyone younger than 20.

A shooting pain that lasts a few seconds, or a quick pain at the end of a deep breath, is usually not a cause for concern. Hyperventilation (see page 89) can also cause chest pain.

Am I Having a Heart Attack?

You may be having a heart attack if you have chest discomfort or pain that:

❑ Lasts longer than 20 minutes and is not relieved by rest or nitroglycerine.

❑ Feels like pressure, tightness, squeezing, crushing, intense burning, or aching in your chest.

In addition to chest pain, you may also have:

❑ Pain spreading to your back, shoulder, neck, jaw or teeth, arm, or wrist.

❑ Sweating.

❑ Shortness of breath.

❑ Dizziness.

❑ Fainting.

❑ Nausea or vomiting.

❑ Unusual weakness.

❑ Fast or irregular heartbeat.

❑ Sense of doom.

The more boxes you check, the more likely it is that you are having a heart attack. There may be other explanations for chest pain, but you need to **call 911 or other emergency services immediately** if you think you could be having a heart attack.

Chest pain caused by pleurisy (inflammation of the membrane that surrounds the lungs) or pneumonia (see page 188) will get worse when you take a deep breath or cough. An ulcer (see page 134) can cause chest pain, usually below the breastbone, that is worse when your stomach is empty. Gallstones (see page 126) may cause pain in the right side of the chest or around the shoulder blade. The pain may worsen after a meal or in the middle of the night. Heartburn (see page 121) can also cause chest pain. Shingles (page 253) may cause a sharp, burning, or tingling pain that feels like a tight band around one side of the chest.

Home Treatment

For chest-wall pain caused by strained muscles or ligaments or a broken rib:

- Use pain relievers such as Aspirin, ibuprofen, or acetaminophen. Do not give Aspirin to anyone younger than 20.
- Use an ice pack to help relieve pain the first few days after an injury.
- After applying ice during the first 72 hours (or until the swelling has gone down), apply heat (a hot water bottle, warm towel, or heating pad) to help relieve pain. Use heat that is no warmer than bath water or the low setting on a heating pad. To prevent burns, do not go to sleep with a heating pad turned on.
- Use products such as Ben-Gay or Icy-Hot to help soothe sore muscles.
- Avoid any activity that strains the chest area. As your pain gets better, slowly return to your normal activities.

When to Call a Health Professional

Call 911 or other emergency services immediately if symptoms of a heart attack are present (see page 191).

If a doctor has diagnosed the cause of your chest pain and prescribed a home treatment plan, follow it. **Call 911 or other emergency services** if the pain worsens and may be caused by a heart problem, or if you develop any of the heart attack symptoms listed on page 191.

Call a health professional:

- If you suspect that you have angina and your symptoms have not been diagnosed.
- If symptoms of angina do not respond to your prescribed treatment, or if the pattern of your angina changes.
- If minor chest pain occurs without the symptoms of a heart attack and you have any of the following:
    - A history of heart disease or blood clots in the lungs.
    - Chest pain that is constant, nagging, and not relieved by rest.

- Chest pain that occurs with symptoms of pneumonia. See page 188.
- Mild chest pain that lasts longer than 2 days without improvement.

Viral or Bacterial?

Viral infections:

- Usually produce symptoms in several parts of the body at once: sore throat, runny nose, headache, muscle aches. In the digestive system, viruses cause nausea, vomiting, or diarrhea.
- Typically include colds, flu, bronchitis, and stomach flu.
- Cannot be cured by antibiotics.

Bacterial infections:

- Sometimes follow viral infections.
- Usually affect one area of the body: sinuses, lungs, an ear.
- May be cured by antibiotics.

Call a health professional if you develop any of the following symptoms of a bacterial infection:

- Fever of 40°C or higher that does not go down after 2 hours of home treatment.
- Fever higher than 38.3°C with shaking chills and productive cough (cough that brings up sputum).
- Fever that persists despite home treatment. Many viral illnesses cause fevers of 38.8°C or higher for short periods of time (up to 12 to 24 hours). Call a doctor if the fever stays high:
  - 38.8°C or higher for 2 full days
  - 38.3°C or higher for 3 full days
  - 38°C or higher for 4 full days
- Laboured, shallow, rapid breathing with shortness of breath.
- Yellow, green, rust-coloured, or bloody sputum and fever, cough, or fatigue that is worsening. Sputum that is coughed up from the lungs is more significant than mucus that has drained down the back of the throat (post-nasal drip).
- Nasal discharge that changes from clear to coloured (yellow or green) after 5 to 7 days of a cold, with other worsening symptoms such as sinus pain or fever. If nasal discharge is coloured from the start of a cold, call if it lasts longer than 7 to 10 days.
- Cough that lingers more than 7 to 10 days after other symptoms have cleared, especially if it is productive (bringing up sputum). A dry, hacking cough may last several weeks after a viral illness such as a cold.

Colds

The common cold is brought to you by any one of 200 viruses. The symptoms of a cold include runny nose, red eyes, sneezing, sore throat, dry cough, headache, and general body aches. There is a gradual 1- or 2-day onset. As a cold progresses, the nasal mucus may thicken. This is the stage just before a cold completes its course. A cold usually lasts a week or two.

Colds occur throughout the year but are most common in late winter and early spring. The average child has six colds a year; adults have fewer.

Using a mouthwash will not prevent a cold, and antibiotics will not cure a cold. There is no cure for the common cold. If you catch a cold, treat the symptoms.

Sometimes a cold will lead to a bacterial infection (see page 193) such as bronchitis or pneumonia. Good home treatment of colds can help prevent complications.

If a person seems to have a cold all the time, or if cold symptoms last 2 weeks or longer, suspect allergies (see page 179) or sinusitis (see page 202).

Prevention

- Eat well and get plenty of sleep and exercise to keep up your resistance.
- Try to avoid people who have colds.
- Keep your hands away from your nose, eyes, and mouth, but cover your mouth when you cough or sneeze.
- Wash your hands often, particularly when you are around people who have colds.
- Don't smoke.

Home Treatment

Home treatment for a cold will help relieve symptoms and prevent complications.

- Get extra rest. Slow down just a little from your usual routine. It isn't necessary to stay home in bed, but take care not to expose others to your cold.
- Drink plenty of liquids. Hot water, herbal tea, or chicken soup will help relieve congestion.
- Take Aspirin, ibuprofen, or acetaminophen to relieve aches. Do not give Aspirin to anyone younger than 20, because of the risk of Reye's syndrome (see page 268).
- Humidify your bedroom and take hot showers to relieve nasal stuffiness.
- Check the back of your throat for post-nasal drip. If you see streaks of mucus, gargle with warm water to prevent a sore throat.

- Use disposable tissues, not handkerchiefs, to reduce the chance of spreading the cold virus to others.
- If your nose is red and raw from rubbing it with tissues, put a dab of petroleum jelly on the sore area.
- Avoid cold remedies that contain a combination of drugs to treat many different symptoms. Treat each symptom separately. Take a decongestant for stuffiness, a cough medicine for a cough. See Home Treatment for coughs on page 196.
- Do not use nasal decongestant sprays for more than 3 days in a row. Continued use may lead to a "rebound" effect, causing the mucous membranes to become more swollen than they were before you used the spray. See page 406 to learn how to make nose drops at home.
- Avoid antihistamines. They are not an effective treatment for colds.
- If you have classic flu symptoms, call your doctor to talk about antiviral medications for the flu. See Influenza (Flu) on page 199.

When to Call a Health Professional

- If you develop signs of a bacterial infection (see Viral or Bacterial? on page 193).
- If you develop facial pain, fever, and other signs of sinusitis (see page 202).

Coughs

Coughing is the body's way of removing foreign material or mucus from the lungs. Coughs have distinctive traits that you can learn to recognize.

Productive coughs produce phlegm or mucus (sputum) that comes up from the lungs. This kind of cough generally should not be suppressed. It is needed to clear mucus from the lungs.

Non-productive coughs are dry coughs that do not produce sputum. A dry, hacking cough may develop toward the end of a cold or after exposure to an irritant, such as dust or smoke. Dry coughs that follow viral illnesses may last up to several weeks and often get worse at night.

A chronic, dry cough, especially at night or early in the morning, may be the only sign of mild asthma. See page 184.

Chronic coughs are often caused by the backflow (reflux) of stomach acid into the lungs and throat. If you suspect that problems with stomach acid reflux may be causing your cough, see Heartburn on page 121.

Prevention

- Don't smoke. See page 25 for tips on quitting. Avoid other people's smoke. A dry, hacking "smoker's cough" means your lungs are constantly irritated.

- Drink plenty of fluids every day. You are drinking enough if you are urinating more often than usual.

Home Treatment

- Drink lots of water. Water helps loosen phlegm and soothe an irritated throat. Also try drinking hot tea or hot water with honey or lemon juice in it. Do not give honey to children younger than 1 year of age.
- Cough drops can soothe an irritated throat. Expensive, medicine-flavoured cough drops are not any better than inexpensive, candy-flavoured ones or hard candy.
- Elevate your head with extra pillows at night to ease a dry cough.
- Avoid cold remedies that combine drugs to treat many symptoms. It is generally better to treat each symptom separately. See Cough Preparations on page 407.
- Use cough suppressants wisely. Coughing is useful because it brings up mucus from the lungs and helps prevent bacterial infections. People with asthma and other lung diseases need to cough. If you have a dry, hacking cough that does not bring anything up, ask your health professional about an effective cough suppressant medication.
- Do not take anyone else's prescription cough medication.
- Avoid exposure to dust, smoke, and other irritants, or wear an appropriate mask to protect yourself from the irritant.

Description and Treatment of Coughs	
Type of Cough	**Possible Causes**
Loud cough like a seal's bark	Croup, p. 273.
Dry cough in the morning that gets better as the day goes on	Dry air; cigarette smoking. Increase fluids. Humidify the bedroom. Stop smoking. Also see Coughs, p. 195.
Hacking, dry, non-productive cough; may be worse at night	Common for several weeks following a viral illness. May be due to post-nasal drip, smoking, or mild asthma. Increase fluids. Try a decongestant. Stop smoking. Also see Coughs, p. 195; Asthma, p. 184.
Productive cough following a cold or flu	Bronchitis, p. 188; Pneumonia, p. 188; Sinusitis, p. 202.
Dry, sudden-onset cough after a choking episode, most often in an infant or toddler	Foreign object in the throat. See Preventing Choking, p. 67.

When to Call a Health Professional

- If you develop signs of a bacterial infection (see Viral or Bacterial? on page 193).
- If a cough lingers more than 7 to 10 days after other symptoms have cleared, especially if the cough is productive (bringing up sputum). A dry, hacking cough may last several weeks after a viral illness such as a cold.
- If any cough lasts longer than 2 weeks.

Fever

A fever is a high body temperature. It is a symptom, not a disease. A fever is one way your body fights illness. A temperature of up to 39°C can be helpful, because it helps the body respond to infection. Most healthy adults can tolerate a fever as high as 39.4° to 40°C for short periods of time without problems.

For specific fever guidelines for children younger than 4 years of age, see page 278.

Home Treatment

- Drink plenty of fluids, especially water. You are drinking enough if you are urinating more often than usual.
- Take acetaminophen, Aspirin, or ibuprofen to lower fever. Do not give Aspirin to anyone younger than 20, because of the risk of Reye's syndrome (see page 268).
- Take and record your temperature whenever symptoms change.
- Take a sponge bath with lukewarm water if a fever causes discomfort.
- Watch for signs of dehydration. See page 118.
- Dress lightly.
- Eat light, easily digested foods, such as soup.
- If you have classic flu symptoms, call your doctor to talk about antiviral medications for the flu. See Influenza (Flu) on page 199.

When to Call a Health Professional

- If you have a fever of 40°C or higher.
- If you have a fever of 39.4° to 40°C that does not come down after 12 hours of home treatment.
- If you have a persistent fever. Many viral illnesses cause fevers of 38.8°C or higher for short periods of time (up to 12 to 24 hours). Call a doctor if the fever stays high:
  - 38.8° to 39.4°C for 1 full day
  - 38.3° to 38.8°C for 3 full days
  - 38° to 38.3°C for 4 full days
- If body temperature rises to 39°C or higher, all sweating stops, and the skin becomes hot, dry, and flushed (possible heatstroke, see page 87).
- If a fever occurs with other signs of a bacterial infection (see page 193).

- If a fever occurs with any of the following symptoms:
  - Very stiff neck and headache (see Encephalitis and Meningitis on page 201).
  - Shortness of breath and cough (see Bronchitis and Pneumonia on page 188).
  - Pain above the eyes or the cheekbones (see Sinusitis on page 202).
  - Pain or burning when urinating (see Urinary Tract Infections on page 138).
  - Abdominal pain, nausea, and vomiting (see Stomach Flu and Food Poisoning on page 133, or Appendicitis on page 115).
- If a fever is accompanied by disturbing symptoms, such as confusion, decreased alertness, or unusual behaviour.
- If you develop a fever after you start taking a new medication.

Heart Palpitations

Heart palpitations are an uncomfortable sensation that your heart is beating rapidly or irregularly. Heart palpitations can feel like:

- Your heart is pounding, or there is a fluttering in your chest.
- Your heart is doing a "flip-flop," or like it is skipping or missing a beat.
- Your heart is racing, or like there is an extra heartbeat.
- Your heart is beating in your neck.

Although palpitations may be caused by a heart problem, they often occur because of stress, fatigue, or overuse of alcohol or stimulants (caffeine, nicotine). People who experience severe anxiety may have heart palpitations. See Anxiety on page 370. Many medications, including diet pills, antihistamines, decongestants, and some herbal products, can cause heart palpitations.

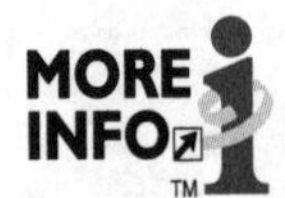

Nearly everyone has heart palpitations from time to time. There is usually no cause for concern. However, if you have heartbeat changes that are new and different or that occur with chest pain, shortness of breath, or light-headedness, or if you have risk factors for heart disease (smoking, high blood pressure, high cholesterol, inactive lifestyle, or high stress levels), see your doctor to have your condition evaluated.

Prevention

- Stop smoking.
- Avoid caffeine and alcohol or limit your intake.
- If you take prescription or non-prescription medications regularly, ask your pharmacist if the drugs you take can cause heart palpitations.

- If anxiety or stress may be causing heart palpitations, see Anxiety on page 370 and try the relaxation exercises on page 386.
- Make physical activity a daily habit. (If you frequently have heart palpitations, talk to your doctor before starting an exercise program.)
- See your doctor for regular check-ups if you have risk factors for heart attack (see page 191). Early detection and management of heart problems is the best way to prevent serious illness.

Home Treatment

- Take deep breaths and try to relax. This may slow a racing heart.
- If you start to feel light-headed (like you might pass out), lie down to avoid injuries that might result if you pass out and fall down.
- Keep a record of the date and time; your pulse; your activities when the irregular heartbeats happened; how long the irregular beats lasted; how many "skipped" beats there were; and any other symptoms.
- Follow the prevention guidelines.

When to Call a Health Professional

Call 911 or other emergency services immediately if symptoms of a heart attack are present (see page 191).

Call a health professional:

- If heart palpitations occur with any of the following symptoms:
  - Weakness or fatigue
  - Light-headedness (feeling like you might pass out)
  - Confusion
  - Feeling as if something bad is going to happen
  - Feeling like your heart beats irregularly all the time
- If heart palpitations are new or different than before and are not relieved by home treatment.

Influenza (Flu)

Influenza, or flu, is a viral illness that commonly occurs in the winter and affects many people at once. British Columbia is preparing for an outbreak of pandemic influenza, in which whole communities could get sick within days or weeks. A prepared community is a resilient community, better able to handle the outbreak. You can do your part by being prepared for a health emergency (see Disasters and Public Health Threats starting on page 51). Learn how to stay healthy, practise self-care, and care for others if they get sick.

Flu is not the same as the common cold— the symptoms of flu are usually more severe and come on quite suddenly. Symptoms include fever, shaking chills, body aches, muscle pain, headache, pain when you move your eyes, fatigue, weakness, and runny nose. Symptoms may last up to 10 days. Most other viral illnesses have milder symptoms that don't last as long.

Although a person with the flu feels very sick, the illness seldom leads to more serious complications. However, flu can be dangerous for babies, older adults, and people with certain chronic conditions.

Antiviral medications are recommended for people at high risk for complications from the flu. These drugs can reduce the severity and duration of some types of influenza if they are taken before or soon after symptoms develop. People at low risk for complications may choose to take medication for the flu so that they feel better faster. These medications work best if taken within 48 hours after symptoms first appear.

Prevention

- You can get a free flu shot each autumn if you are 65 or over; if you have a chronic illness, such as asthma, heart disease, or diabetes; if you live in a nursing home; if you live with or care for anyone at high risk; if you are a health care worker or an emergency responder; or if you are in your third trimester of pregnancy and are expected to deliver during flu season. Flu shots are also recommended for all children ages 6 to 23 months and for anyone who cares for a child age 0 to 23 months.
- Consider buying an annual flu shot if you or your family members are likely to be exposed to the disease at work, school, or daycare, or if you just want to reduce the chance that you and your family will catch the disease. The vaccine can be given to anyone over 6 months of age as long as he or she is not allergic to the vaccine or its components. Call your public health unit for more information.
- Keep up your resistance to infection by eating a healthy diet, getting plenty of rest, and exercising regularly.
- Avoid exposure to the flu virus. Wash your hands often and keep your hands away from your nose, eyes, and mouth.
- Stop smoking to lower your risk of complications from the flu.

Home Treatment

- Get plenty of rest.
- Drink extra fluids to replace those lost from fever, to ease a scratchy throat, and to keep nasal mucus thin. Hot tea with lemon, plain water, fruit juice, and soup are all good choices.
- Take acetaminophen, Aspirin, or ibuprofen to relieve fever, headache, and muscle aches. Do not give Aspirin to anyone younger than 20, because of the risk of Reye's syndrome (see page 268).

When to Call a Health Professional

It is common for adults with influenza to have high fevers (up to 40°C) for 3 to 4 days. When trying to decide if you need to see a health professional, consider the likelihood that you have the flu versus a possible bacterial infection. If it is the flu season and many people in your community have similar symptoms, it is likely that you have the flu. Call a health professional:

- If you want to take antiviral medication to reduce the severity of the flu. Medication is recommended for babies, older adults, and people with chronic health problems.
- If you develop signs of a bacterial infection (see page 193).
- If you seem to get better, then get worse again.

Laryngitis

Laryngitis is an infection or irritation of the voice box (larynx). The most common cause is a viral infection such as a cold. Other causes include allergies; excessive talking, singing, or yelling; cigarette smoke; and the backflow (reflux) of stomach acid into the throat. Heavy drinking or smoking can lead to chronic laryngitis.

Symptoms include hoarseness or loss of voice, the urge to clear your throat, fever, tiredness, throat pain, and cough.

Prevention

To prevent hoarseness, lower your voice as soon as you feel minor pain. Give your vocal cords a rest.

Encephalitis and Meningitis

Encephalitis is an inflammation of the brain that may occur during or after a viral infection, such as chicken pox, flu, West Nile fever, measles, mumps, mononucleosis, cold sores, or genital herpes. Mosquitoes and ticks spread encephalitis in some parts of the world, including North America.

Meningitis is a viral or bacterial illness that causes inflammation in the tissues that surround the brain and spinal cord. It may follow an infection, such as an ear or sinus infection, or a viral or bacterial illness.

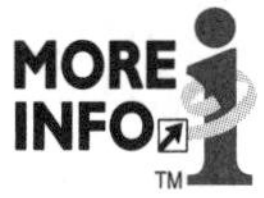

Encephalitis and meningitis are serious illnesses that have similar symptoms. Call a health professional immediately if any of the following symptoms develop, especially after a viral illness or after you are bitten by mosquitoes:

- Severe headache with stiff neck, fever, nausea, and vomiting
- Drowsiness, lack of energy, confusion, memory problems, or unusual behaviour

Home Treatment

- Your voice box will usually heal in 5 to 10 days. Medication does little to speed recovery.
- If hoarseness is caused by a cold, treat the cold (see page 194). Hoarseness may last up to 1 week after a cold goes away.
- Rest your voice. Talk as little as possible. Don't shout, and avoid clearing your throat.
- Stop smoking and avoid other people's smoke. See page 25 for tips on quitting.
- Humidify your bedroom or your whole house if possible. Try standing in the steam from a hot shower.
- Drink plenty of fluids, especially water. You are drinking enough if you are urinating more often than usual.
- To soothe the throat, gargle with warm salt water (5 g of salt in 240 ml of water), or drink weak tea or hot water with honey or lemon juice in it. Do not give honey to children younger than 1 year of age.
- If you suspect that problems with stomach acid reflux may be contributing to your laryngitis, see Heartburn on page 121.

When to Call a Health Professional

- If you develop signs of a bacterial infection (see page 193).
- If hoarseness persists for 3 to 4 weeks.

Sinusitis

Sinusitis is an inflammation or infection of the mucous membranes lining the sinuses and nasal passages. The sinuses are hollow spaces in the head. Sinusitis causes the sinuses to become blocked, leading to pain and pressure in the face.

Sinusitis most often follows a cold and may also be associated with allergies, an infected tooth (dental abscess), air pollution, and other factors. Sinusitis can occur in infants and children as well as adults.

The key symptom of sinusitis is pain over the cheekbones and upper teeth, in the forehead over the eyebrows, or around and behind the eyes. There may also be headache, swelling around the eyes, fever, stuffy nose, coughing, or mucus draining down the back of the throat (post-nasal drip). In children, coughing and nasal discharge that last more than 7 to 10 days along with complaints of headache and facial pain are signs that the problem may be sinusitis, not just a cold.

If your symptoms are severe or continue for more than 10 to 14 days, you may need to take antibiotics. A sinus infection can lead to chronic sinusitis if it does not respond to home treatment or antibiotics, or if it is not treated at all.

Prevention

- Treat nasal congestion caused by colds promptly. See page 194.
- Avoid cigarette, cigar, and pipe smoke in your home and workplace. Smoke irritates inflamed membranes in your nose and sinuses.
- If you have allergies, avoid the things that trigger your allergy attacks.

Home Treatment

Home treatment can often relieve early symptoms of sinusitis, such as facial pressure and stuffiness, and get your sinuses draining normally again so that you may not need antibiotic treatment.

- Drink extra fluids to keep mucus thin. Drink at least 8 to 10 glasses of water or juice per day.
- Apply moist heat (a warm towel or gel pack) to your face several times a day for 5 to 10 minutes at a time.
- Breathe warm, moist air from a steamy shower, a hot bath, or a sink filled with hot water.
- Increase the humidity in your home, especially in the bedrooms. Avoid cold, dry air.
- Take an oral decongestant, try a decongestant nasal spray, or use a mucus-thinning agent (see page 406). Do not use a nasal decongestant spray for more than 3 days in a row. Avoid products that contain antihistamines unless your symptoms may also be related to allergies.
- Take Aspirin, acetaminophen, or ibuprofen to relieve facial pain and headache. Do not give Aspirin to anyone younger than 20, because of the risk of Reye's syndrome (see page 268).
- Check the back of your throat for post-nasal drip. If you see streaks of mucus, gargle with warm water to prevent a sore throat.
- Blow your nose gently. Do not close one nostril when blowing your nose.
- Salt water (saline) irrigation helps wash mucus and bacteria out of the nasal passages. Use non-prescription saline nose drops or a homemade solution (see page 406):
    - Use a bulb syringe to gently squirt the solution into your nose, or snuff the solution from the palm of your hand, one nostril at a time.
    - The salt water should go in through your nose and come out your mouth.
    - Blow your nose gently afterward. Repeat the salt water wash 2 to 4 times a day.

When to Call a Health Professional

- If cold symptoms last longer than 10 to 14 days or worsen after the first 7 days.

- If you have a severe headache that is different from a "normal" headache and is not relieved by acetaminophen, Aspirin, or ibuprofen.
- If you have facial swelling, or if your vision changes or gets blurry.
- If nasal discharge changes from clear to coloured (yellow or green) after 5 to 7 days of a cold and other symptoms (sinus pain, fever) worsen. If nasal discharge is coloured from the start of a cold, call if it lasts longer than 7 to 10 days.
- If facial pain (especially in one sinus area or along the ridge between the nose and lower eyelid) persists after 2 days of home treatment.
- If sinusitis symptoms persist after you have taken a full course of antibiotics.

Sore Throat, Strep Throat, and Tonsillitis

Most sore throats are caused by viruses and may occur with a cold or after a cold. A mild sore throat may be caused by dry air, smoking, air pollution, or yelling. People who have allergies or stuffy noses may breathe through their mouths while sleeping, which can cause a mild sore throat.

Sore throats can also be caused by inflammation of the tonsils (tonsillitis) or adenoids (adenoiditis). This is common in children. Tonsillitis and adenoiditis are usually caused by a virus. In addition to sore throat, symptoms of tonsillitis or adenoiditis include fever, swollen lymph nodes, and tiredness along with cold symptoms such as runny nose and a cough. It may be painful to swallow, and the tonsils are often bright red, spotted with pus, and swollen. Adenoiditis can also cause headache and vomiting. Chronically inflamed adenoids may block the passageway between the ears and the throat (eustachian tubes), contributing to ear infections. See page 225.

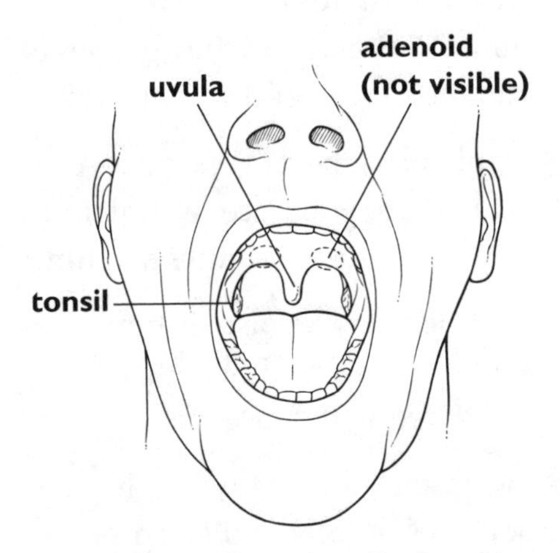

Location of tonsils and adenoids

Strep throat is a sore throat caused by streptococcal bacteria. It is most common in children from 3 to 15 years of age. You can get strep throat even if your tonsils have been removed.

Tonsillectomy and Adenoidectomy

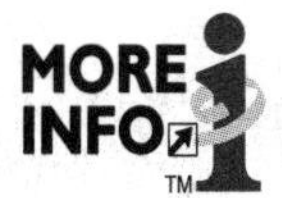

It was once common to remove children's tonsils and adenoids. Because of the risks, costs, and limited benefits, tonsillectomy and adenoidectomy are now done less often, and only when the benefits greatly outweigh the risk, inconvenience, and pain.

Tonsillectomy may be recommended if at least one of the following criteria is met:

- There have been at least 4 to 6 severe tonsillitis infections caused by strep bacteria in the past year despite treatment with at least 2 different antibiotics.
- The enlarged tonsils cause severe breathing difficulty or sleep disturbance.
- There are deep pockets of infection in the tonsils that haven't responded to drug treatment.

Adenoidectomy may be recommended if at least one of the following criteria is met:

- The enlarged adenoids are blocking the airway, causing breathing difficulty and sleep disturbance.
- The adenoids are believed to cause persistent ear infections, despite antibiotic treatment.

If your doctor recommends surgery but your case does not meet the above criteria, consider getting a second opinion. See page 13.

In general, the more cold-like your symptoms are, the less likely it is that you have strep throat or another bacterial infection. Strep throat causes some or all of these symptoms:

- Severe and sudden sore throat
- Fever of 38.3°C or higher
- Swollen lymph nodes in the neck
- White or yellow coating on the tonsils

Strep throat is treated with antibiotics to prevent rheumatic fever. Antibiotics are effective in preventing rheumatic fever if started within 9 days of the onset of the sore throat.

Another cause of persistent sore throat is mononucleosis (mono, or "the kissing disease"), which is caused by the Epstein-Barr virus. Mono is most common in older teens and young adults. In addition to a severe sore throat, fever, and fatigue, mono symptoms often include weakness, body aches, and swollen lymph nodes in the neck. A less common symptom is pain in the upper left part of the abdomen, caused by enlargement of the spleen. Mono is diagnosed with a blood test called the monospot test.

Most people recover from mono after several weeks. However, for some people it may take several months to get their normal energy level back, and it is normal for the lymph nodes to remain enlarged for up to 1 month (see Swollen Lymph Nodes on page 208). There is no specific treatment for mono except rest, plenty of fluids, salt water gargles for throat pain, and Aspirin or acetaminophen for body aches. Do not give Aspirin to anyone younger than 20, because of the risk of Reye's syndrome (see page 268).

A less common cause of sore throat is the backflow (reflux) of stomach acid into the throat. Although reflux is often associated with heartburn or an "acid" taste in the mouth, sometimes a sore throat is the only symptom. If you think stomach acid reflux may be causing your throat pain, see Heartburn on page 121.

Snoring

Up to 50 percent of all adults snore occasionally, and about 25 percent of all adults are habitual snorers. Snoring is caused by blockage of the airways in the back of the mouth and nose. These airways can be blocked for many reasons, such as excess neck tissue caused by being overweight or a stuffy nose caused by allergies or a cold. Some people who snore have sleep apnea. Sleep apnea is present when a person repeatedly stops breathing for 10 to 15 seconds or longer during sleep.

Snoring can disrupt a person's sleep patterns, so he or she may be sleepy and less alert during the day. A person's snoring can also disrupt the sleep of family members or roommates. Here are some tips for people who snore:

- Exercise daily to maintain a healthy body weight and improve muscle tone. Avoid exercise within 2 hours of bedtime, because exercise may make it harder to fall asleep.
- Avoid heavy meals, alcohol, sleeping pills, and antihistamines before bedtime.
- Sleep on your side rather than your back. (Sew a pocket onto the back of your pyjama top, and put a tennis ball inside the pocket. This will keep you from sleeping on your back.)
- Establish regular sleeping patterns. Go to bed at the same time every night, even on weekends.
- Let the person who doesn't snore fall asleep first.

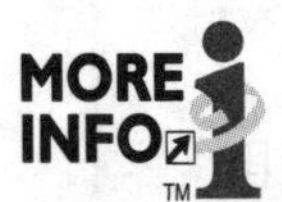

If snoring becomes a problem for you or affects your household, see a health professional. An examination of the nose, mouth, and neck may be needed. Your doctor may also want to do a sleep study to see if sleep apnea is one of the reasons why you snore. Treatment will depend on what is causing you to snore.

Prevention

- Identify and avoid irritants that cause sore throat (such as smoke, fumes, or yelling). For tips on quitting smoking, see page 25.
- Avoid contact with people who have strep throat. People who have strep throat should stay home from work, school, or daycare until 24 hours after starting antibiotic treatment.
- If you have mono, try to keep from spreading the virus: don't share eating or drinking utensils; avoid kissing; and do not donate blood until your symptoms are gone and you are feeling better.

Home Treatment

Home care is usually all that is needed for viral sore throats and tonsillitis. If you are taking antibiotics for strep throat, these tips will also help you feel better.

- Gargle with warm salt water (5 g of salt in 240 ml of water). The salt reduces swelling and discomfort.
- If you have post-nasal drip, gargle often to prevent more throat irritation.
- Drink more fluids to soothe your sore throat. Honey and lemon in hot water or in weak tea may help. Do not give honey to children younger than 1 year of age.
- Stop smoking, and avoid other people's smoke.
- Acetaminophen, Aspirin, or ibuprofen will relieve pain and reduce fever. Do not give Aspirin to anyone younger than 20, because of the risk of Reye's syndrome (see page 268).
- Some non-prescription throat lozenges (such as Sucrets Extra Strength or Chloraseptic) are safe and effective and have a local anaesthetic to soothe pain. Regular cough drops or hard candy may also help.

When to Call a Health Professional

- If any one of the following symptoms develops:
  - Difficulty swallowing.
  - Excessive drooling caused by inability to swallow.
  - Laboured or difficult breathing.
- If you develop a severe sore throat after being exposed to strep throat.
- If a sore throat occurs with 2 of these 3 symptoms of strep throat:
  - Fever of 38.3°C or higher.
  - White or yellow coating on the tonsils.
  - Swollen lymph nodes in the neck.
- If a rash occurs with sore throat. **Scarlet fever** is a rash that may occur when there is a strep throat infection. Like strep throat, scarlet fever is treated with antibiotics.

- If you cannot trace the cause of a sore throat to a cold, allergy, smoking, overuse of your voice, or other irritation.
- If a mild sore throat lasts longer than 2 weeks.
- If a child has at least 4 to 6 episodes of tonsillitis in 1 year despite antibiotic treatment.
- If a child persistently breathes through his or her mouth, snores, or has a very nasal- or muffled-sounding voice. These are signs of chronic adenoid inflammation.

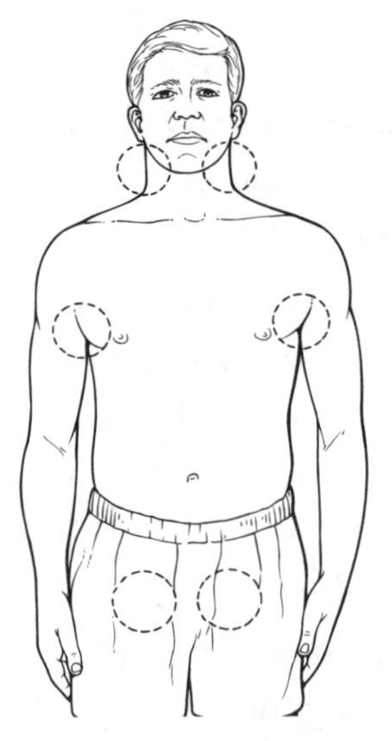

Swollen lymph nodes may be felt in the areas shown.

Swollen Lymph Nodes

The lymph nodes are small glands located throughout the body. The most noticeable lymph nodes are those in the neck. The lymph nodes swell as the body fights minor infections from colds, insect bites, or small cuts. More serious infections can cause the lymph nodes to greatly enlarge and become very firm and tender.

Swelling in the lymph nodes on either side of the neck is common with a cold or sore throat. The lymph nodes in the groin may swell if there is a vaginal or other pelvic infection, or if there is a cut or sore on the leg or foot.

Lymph nodes may remain hard long after the initial infection goes away. This is especially true in children, whose lymph nodes may get smaller but remain hard and visible for several weeks.

Home Treatment

- There is no specific home treatment for swollen lymph nodes. Continue treating the cold or other infection that is causing the lymph nodes to swell.
- Your child may develop hard, swollen lymph nodes following a cold or minor infection. If the lymph nodes near the site of the infection are not tender and are not getting larger, you can monitor them at home and report them at the child's next regular visit to the doctor.

When to Call a Health Professional

- If the lymph nodes are large, very firm, red, and very tender.
- If swollen lymph nodes are associated with other signs of infection in a nearby cut or sore. See page 100.
- If you develop swollen lymph nodes after travelling in wilderness areas or abroad.
- If swollen lymph nodes continue to get bigger, or appear without apparent cause and persist for 2 weeks or longer.
- If swollen lymph nodes appear in areas other than the ones shown on page 208.

West Nile Virus

West Nile virus is an infection spread to humans by mosquitoes. Mosquitoes get infected when they bite infected birds, and then they transmit the virus to humans and other animals by biting them.

Most people who get the West Nile virus have no symptoms. When symptoms do occur, they appear 3 to 14 days after the bite and include fever, headache, body aches, and sometimes a skin rash. This is called **West Nile fever**. It is usually mild and lasts several days.

Rarely, West Nile infection may affect the brain, causing encephalitis, meningitis, or sudden paralysis. This is called **West Nile neurologic syndrome**. It can be life-threatening. People who get this serious illness usually need care in hospital until they recover. The illness can also cause long-lasting problems such as seizures, memory loss, personality changes, walking or balance problems, tremors, and brain damage.

Anyone at any age who is exposed to infected mosquitoes can get West Nile virus. Older adults who get it are more likely to develop severe illness. British Columbia monitors mosquitoes and crows to identify the presence of West Nile virus so that health authorities can inform the public of any risk.

Prevention

You can avoid West Nile virus by avoiding mosquito bites.

- Stay indoors at dusk and dawn and in the early evening. Mosquitoes that carry the virus are most active at these times.
- Wear long sleeves and pants when you are in an area with mosquitoes.
- Do not keep open containers of water near your home. Standing water is a breeding site for mosquitoes.
- Spray clothing with DEET after you are sure the fabric will not be damaged. (DEET can damage some synthetic fabrics as well as plastic watch crystals and eyeglasses frames.) Mosquitoes can bite through thin clothing.

- Use only registered insect repellents. DEET is a very effective product. Health Canada says DEET should be used in concentrations according to age and length of time outdoors. For example, if you are 23 and going outside for 5 hours, use 15%. If a child is 10 years old and going outside for 5 hours, use 10% and apply it again after 3 hours. Follow these safety tips when using DEET:
  - For children under 2 years, do not use DEET at all.
  - For children age 2 to 11 years, use a repellent with 10% DEET or less.
  - People 12 years and older may use up to 30% DEET.
  - Within the limits above, do not use a higher concentration of DEET than you need to. Higher concentrations of DEET give you longer, not better, protection.

When to Call a Health Professional

Call your doctor right away if you have been exposed to mosquitoes in the past 2 weeks and have any of these symptoms:

- Fever, headache, stiff neck, and confusion
- Muscle weakness or inability to move parts of your body
- Mild fever, rash, body aches, or swollen lymph glands that last more than 2 or 3 days

Keep in mind that you might not know you were bitten.

How Can You Learn More?

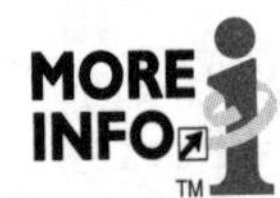

For the latest information on West Nile virus, contact your local health authority, public health unit, or the BC NurseLine (see the phone numbers on the back of this book). You can also find information at BC HealthGuide OnLine and in the BC HealthFiles at www.bchealthguide.org; the BC Centre for Disease Control at www.bccdc.org; or Health Canada's Pest Management Regulatory Agency's Web site at www.pmra-arla.gc.ca.

You can observe a lot just by watching.
Yogi Berra (naturally)

10

Eye and Ear Problems

From dry eyes to pink eye and earaches to earwax, your eyes and ears can cause you trouble. With home care and patience, most of these problems will clear up. This chapter explains what you can do at home and when to get professional help.

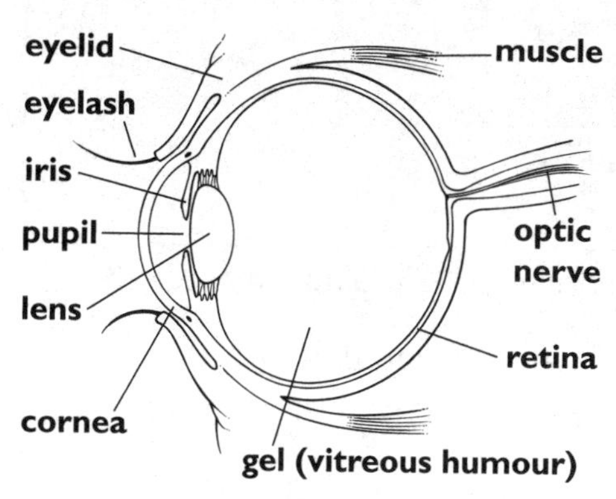

The structures at the front of the eye (lens, pupil, cornea, iris) let light into the eye. Light hits the back of the eye (retina) and is changed into nerve signals that are carried to the brain by the optic nerve. The brain reads the signals from the optic nerve as images that you "see."

Blood in the Eye

Sometimes blood vessels in the whites of the eyes break and cause a red spot or speck. This is called a subconjunctival hemorrhage. The blood may look alarming, especially if the spot is large, but it is usually not a cause for concern. The red spot will go away in 2 to 3 weeks. Older adults may want to check their blood pressure. (Call your doctor if it is over 140/90.)

Call a health professional immediately if your eye is bloody and painful; if there is blood in the coloured part of the eye; or if the bleeding followed a blow or injury to the eye. Also call if bleeding in the eye occurs often; occurs after you begin taking blood thinners (anticoagulants); or covers more than one-fourth of the white of the eye.

Eye Problems

Symptoms	Possible Causes
Red, itchy, watery eyes	Allergies, p. 179. Think about allergy to eye care products, makeup, or smoke. Possible contact lens problem, p. 215.
Excessive discharge from eye; red, swollen eyelids; sandy feeling	Eye Inflammations, p. 215. Possible contact lens problem, p. 215.
Pimple or swelling on eyelid	Styes, p. 222.
Pain in the eye	Chemical Burns, p. 75; Migraine Headaches, p. 238; Cluster Headaches, p. 241; Objects in the Eye, p. 95; Possible contact lens problem, p. 215; Eye Inflammations, p. 215.
Severe eye pain, blurred vision, reddened eyeball	**See a doctor now!**
Sudden onset of vision changes such as flashes of light, partial blindness, or shadow across part of visual field	Call a health professional immediately! Possible retinal detachment, p. 219.
Gradual onset of cloudy, filmy, or fuzzy vision; difficulty seeing close objects	Presbyopia, p. 219; Cataracts, p. 213.
Tunnel vision (gradual loss of side or peripheral vision)	Glaucoma, p. 218.
Halos around lights	Cataracts, p. 213; Glaucoma, p. 218.
Distorted vision, dark spot in centre of vision; straight lines appear wavy	Macular Degeneration, p. 220.
Red spot on white of eye	Blood in the Eye, p. 211.
Black eye	Bruises, p. 72.
Dry, scratchy eyes	Dry Eyes, p. 214.
Drooping eyelids; excess tearing	Eyelid Problems, p. 217.

Cataracts

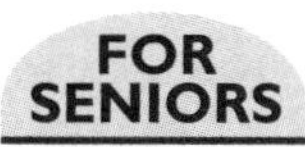

A cataract is a painless, cloudy area in the lens of the eye. A cataract blocks the passage of light through the lens to the nerve layer (retina) at the back of the eye, and it may cause vision problems.

Cataracts are very common in older adults and can result from normal age-related changes in the lens. They can also occur after an eye injury, as a result of eye disease, as a side effect of certain medications, or as a result of medical conditions such as diabetes.

Symptoms of cataracts include cloudy, fuzzy, or filmy vision; decreased night vision; problems with glare; and double vision. You may see spots or halos around lights. Your eyeglasses prescription may change frequently.

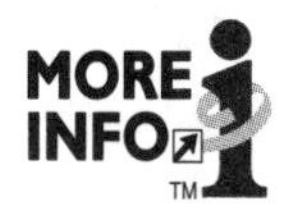

Without treatment, some cataracts can become larger or denser over time, making your vision problems worse. However, cataracts do not always need to be removed. The vision loss that results from cataracts often develops slowly and may never become severe. Many people with cataracts get along very well with the help of eyeglasses, contact lenses, and other vision aids and are able to avoid or delay surgery. The decision whether to have cataract surgery often depends on how much cataracts are interfering with a person's ability to do daily activities.

Prevention

There is no proven way to prevent cataracts. However, certain health habits may help slow cataract development. These include:

- Not smoking.
- Wearing a hat or sunglasses when you are in the sun and avoiding sunlamps and tanning booths.
- Eating a diet rich in vitamins C and E.
- Limiting your alcohol intake.
- Avoiding the use of steroid medications when possible.
- Keeping high blood pressure and diabetes under control.

Home Treatment

Home treatment will not cure cataracts, but it may help you avoid or delay surgery. There are many things you can do to make the gradual changes in your vision easier to live with.

- Reposition room lights and use window shades to prevent glare on TV and computer screens.
- Use table or floor lamps for close reading and other fine work.
- Put more lights or use higher-watt bulbs over steps and in hallways.

- Use contrasts in colour and brightness to make things easier to find at home. For example, if you have light-coloured walls, use dark switch plates to mark the location of switches. Use coloured, high-contrast labels to "colour code" medications, spices, stove dials, and other items.
- Keep your eyeglasses prescription current. Update your prescription before considering surgery.
- Try reading large-print books and newspapers. Also, bank cheques, medication labels, and other items are often available in large print. Magnifying glasses may help you read some things, but only if the type is very clear. Magnified blurry print will be larger but will still be blurry.

When to Call a Health Professional

- If you have severe eye pain.
- If you have a change in your vision, such as vision loss, double vision, or blurred vision.
- If your eyeglasses prescription changes frequently.
- If daytime glare is a problem.
- If you have difficulty driving at night because of glare from oncoming headlights.
- If vision problems are affecting your ability to do daily activities.

Dry Eyes

Eyes that don't have enough moisture in them may feel dry, hot, sandy, or gritty. Low humidity, smoke, the natural aging process, certain diseases, and certain medications (such as antihistamines, decongestants, some antidepressants, or birth control pills) can cause dry eyes.

Home Treatment

- Give your eyes a rest. While reading, watching television, or using a computer, take frequent breaks and close your eyes. If you can, blink your eyes more often.
- If possible, avoid smoke and other eye irritants.
- Try a non-prescription artificial tear solution, such as Tears Naturale or HypoTears. Do not use eyedrops for reducing redness (such as Visine) to treat dry eyes, because your eyes may become even redder and your symptoms worse when you stop using the drops.

When to Call a Health Professional

Call a health professional if your eyes are persistently dry and artificial tears do not help.

Contact Lenses

If you wear contact lenses, these tips will help you avoid problems.

Follow the cleaning instructions for your lenses. Keep your lenses and anything that touches them (hands, storage containers, solution bottles, makeup) very clean. Wash your hands before handling your contacts.

Use a commercial contact lens solution. (Generic brands are just as good as name brands.) Homemade solution is easily contaminated with bacteria. Never wet your lenses with saliva, which contains bacteria that may cause an eye infection.

Insert your contacts before applying eye makeup. Do not apply makeup to the inner rim of the eyelid. Replace eye makeup every 3 to 6 months to reduce the risk of contamination.

When worn for long periods of time, extended-wear lenses are more likely to cause severe eye infections. If you choose to wear them, follow the wearing and cleaning schedule your eye care professional recommends.

Symptoms of a possible problem with your contacts include unusual redness, pain, or burning in the eye; discharge; blurred vision; or extreme sensitivity to light. Remove your lenses, disinfect them, and do not reinsert them until your symptoms are gone. If symptoms last longer than 2 to 3 hours after you remove your contacts, call your eye care professional.

Visit your eye care professional as directed or at least once a year to check the condition of your lenses and the health of your eyes.

Eye Inflammations

Conjunctivitis, or pink eye, is an inflammation of the membrane (conjunctiva) that lines the eyelid and covers the surface of the eye. Bacteria and viruses (which can be very contagious), allergies, dry air, and irritants in the air such as smoke, fumes, or chemicals can cause pink eye. When bacteria or a virus is involved, the condition is more commonly called an infection.

The symptoms of pink eye may include redness in the whites of the eyes, red and swollen eyelids, lots of tears, itching or burning, a sandy feeling in the eyes, and sensitivity to light. There may be a discharge that causes the eyelids to stick together during sleep. Antibiotic ointment or drops may be needed if the discharge is yellow (you may have an infection).

Prevention

- Do not share towels, handkerchiefs, pillows, eye makeup, or contact lens equipment or solutions.

- Wash your hands before and after treating pink eye in your own eyes or someone else's.
- Wear safety glasses when working with chemicals. If a chemical gets into your eye, immediately flush the eye with water. See page 75.

Home Treatment

Although most cases of pink eye will clear up on their own in 7 to 10 days, viral pink eye can last many weeks. Pink eye caused by allergies or pollution will last as long as you are exposed to the irritating substance. Good home care will speed healing and ease discomfort.

- Apply cold or warm compresses several times a day to relieve discomfort.
- Gently wipe the edge of the eyelid with moist cotton or a clean, wet face cloth to remove encrusted matter. Wipe from the inside corner (next to the nose) to the outside. Use a clean surface for each wipe.
- Don't wear contact lenses or eye makeup until the inflammation is gone. Discard eye makeup after an eye infection, and clean your contacts and storage case. Replace disposable contacts with a new pair.
- If eyedrops are prescribed, insert them as follows:
  - For older children and adults: Pull the lower lid down with two fingers to create a little pouch. Put the drops there. Close the eye for 30 to 60 seconds to let the drops move around.
  - For younger children: Ask the child to lie down with eyes closed. Put a drop in the inner corner of the eye. When the child opens the eye, the drop will run in.
  - Be sure the bottle tip is clean and does not touch the eye, eyelid, or eyelashes. If the tip does touch any of these surfaces, throw the bottle away and replace it.

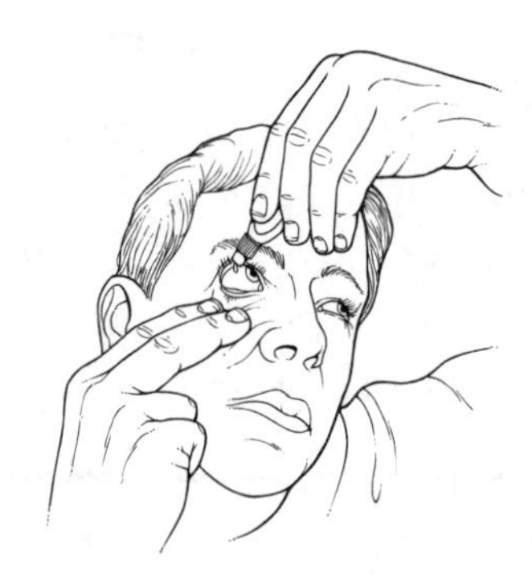

Inserting eyedrops

- Putting antibiotic ointment in the eye can be tricky, especially with children. If you can get it on the eyelashes, it will melt and get into the eye.
- Make sure any non-prescription medicine you use is ophthalmic (for eyes), not otic (for ears).
- Wash your hands thoroughly before and after treating pink eye.

When to Call a Health Professional

- If there is pain in the eye (rather than irritation), blurring, or loss of vision that is not cleared even momentarily by blinking.
- If the eye is painfully sensitive to light.
- If the skin around the eye or the eyelid is red.
- If it feels like there is a foreign object in the eye.
- If the eye is red and there is a yellow or bloody discharge that does not begin to go away in 24 hours.
- If there is a new difference between the sizes of the pupils.
- If symptoms of an eye infection last longer than 7 days.
- If your eye symptoms have not improved within 48 hours after you start using antibiotics.
- If you wear contact lenses and you have had pink eye more than once.

Eyelid Problems

FOR SENIORS

One of the most common eye problems in older adults is a skin condition called **blepharitis**. Symptoms include redness, irritation, and scaly skin at the edges of the eyelids. The scales may be dry or greasy. Eyelashes may fall out as well. The cause of blepharitis is not known, but it is more common in people who have dandruff, skin allergies, or eczema and in those who often have styes. The problem is often chronic.

Another common age-related eye change is drooping eyelids. Drooping is the result of reduced muscle tone in the muscles that control the eyelids. If your lower eyelids droop low enough (**ectropion**), they may no longer be able to protect your eyes, and your eyes may become dry and irritated. If your upper eyelids droop low enough (**ptosis**), they may interfere with your vision.

Drooping eyelids can prevent tears from draining normally, so tears may run down your cheeks. Excessive tearing can also be a sign of increased sensitivity to light or wind, an eye infection, or a blocked tear duct. If your eyes tear when they are exposed to bright light or wind, wear protective glasses.

Home Treatment

To treat blepharitis at home, wash your eyelids, eyebrows, and hair daily with baby shampoo. To wash your eyelids, put a few drops of shampoo in a cup of water, dip a cotton ball, cotton swab, or face cloth in the solution, and gently wipe your eyelids. Rinse well with clear water.

When to Call a Health Professional

- Blepharitis often requires antibiotic treatment. Call a health professional:
  - If your eye is painful.

- If your eyelids are bleeding.
- If the problem is not improving after 1 week of home treatment.

- If your eyelids suddenly start to droop.
- If drooping eyelids interfere with your vision.
- If your eyes are dry and irritated, or if your eyelids do not close completely when you sleep.
- If your eyelashes start to rub on your eyeball.

Glaucoma

Glaucoma causes damage to the optic nerve that results in the loss of eyesight. The optic nerve, which is located at the back of the eye, carries signals from the eye to the brain. The brain translates those signals into images that you see. In a person with glaucoma, increased pressure inside the eye may be part of the reason why the optic nerve becomes damaged. The pressure increase is caused by the buildup of fluid inside the eye.

There are two types of glaucoma that can occur in adults:

- **Open-angle glaucoma**, the most common form of glaucoma, is usually painless and can develop gradually over several years without being detected. Both eyes can be affected at the same time. However, one eye may be affected more than the other. Open-angle glaucoma often affects side (peripheral) vision first. By the time you notice a change in your vision, the damage is permanent.
- **Closed-angle glaucoma** comes on suddenly and can lead to permanent eye damage in a matter of hours. Symptoms of closed-angle glaucoma include severe eye pain, blurred vision, redness in the eye, and possibly nausea and vomiting. Call a health professional immediately if you develop these symptoms.

Untreated glaucoma is a leading cause of blindness in older adults. African Americans, people who have high pressure in their eyes (intraocular pressure), and those who have a family history of glaucoma are at increased risk for developing glaucoma.

Prevention

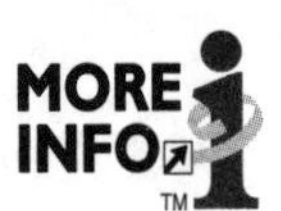

Regular eye examinations, including glaucoma tests, will help detect glaucoma before it affects your eyesight. Talk to your doctor about how often you should be tested for glaucoma. If there is a history of glaucoma in your family or you have other risk factors for glaucoma, talk with your health professional about having more frequent eye examinations. If you are at increased risk for glaucoma, you need to have regular eye examinations by an eye specialist (ophthalmologist).

Home Treatment

If you have been diagnosed with glaucoma, use your prescribed medications exactly as directed.

When to Call a Health Professional

Call 911 or other emergency services immediately:

- If your vision in one eye suddenly becomes severely blurred.
- If there is severe pain and redness in the affected eye.
- If you see coloured halos around lights.
- If you have nausea or vomiting in addition to the above symptoms.

Call a health professional:

- If you have noticed blind spots in your side (peripheral) vision in one or both eyes.
- If you have noticed that over time you are having more difficulty seeing.
- If you have a family history of open-angle glaucoma and you have not had an eye examination in more than a year.

Presbyopia

Presbyopia is a condition that affects almost everyone sometime after age 40. As the eyes age, the lenses become less flexible, which makes it harder for them to focus on close objects or small print. You may find that you have to hold objects at arm's length to see them clearly. (People with presbyopia sometimes say that they don't need glasses; they just need longer arms.)

Home Treatment

Glasses or contact lenses can usually give you clear vision again. If you already wear glasses, you may need bifocals, which will allow you to see objects that are close up and those that are far away. Non-prescription reading glasses may be appropriate for some people.

When to Call a Health Professional

Presbyopia usually develops gradually, over months to years. If your vision changes more quickly, over just a few weeks, call your doctor. This may be an early symptom of another condition, such as diabetes.

Retinal Disorders

The retina is a thin membrane made up of nerve cells that lines the back of the eyeball. The nerve cells in the retina detect light and send signals to the brain about what the eye sees. Problems with the retina can lead to impaired vision or blindness.

Torn or Detached Retina

Retinal detachment occurs when the retina becomes separated from the wall of the eye. Once the retina becomes detached, it stops working properly. This causes vision loss in the affected area of the retina. Although retinal detachment may occur at any age, older people, those who are nearsighted, and those with a family history of retinal detachments are at higher risk. Most retinal detachments are caused by age-related changes in the gel-like substance (vitreous) that fills the eye. A blow to the head or eye may also cause the retina to detach. Symptoms of a retinal tear or detachment may include seeing floaters or flashes of light or seeing a new shadow or "curtain" across part of your field of vision.

Many retinal tears do not require treatment. Tears that occur with symptoms, such as floaters or flashes of light, are more likely to require surgical treatment to prevent retinal detachment and vision loss.

Treatment for retinal detachment always involves surgery. In most cases, good vision can be restored if surgery is done soon after retinal detachment occurs.

Macular Degeneration

Macular degeneration is an eye disease that destroys central vision by damaging the macula. The macula is the part of the retina that provides clear, sharp central vision that you use to focus on what's in front of you. Macular degeneration may occur in one or both eyes. Signs of the disease may range from dim or fuzzy vision to a blank or dark spot in the centre of your visual field. Straight lines (such as in the Amsler grid on page 221) may appear wavy, and colours may appear faded or dim.

As the condition progresses, central vision is lost. Peripheral (side) vision is not affected, and many people function well despite the loss of central vision, although walking, reading, driving, and other activities that require central vision are much more difficult.

Floaters and Flashes

Floaters are spots, specks, and lines that float across your field of vision. They are caused by stray cells or strands of tissue that float in the vitreous humour, the gel-like substance that fills the eyeball. Floaters can be annoying but are not usually serious. However, if you see floaters or flashes of light for the first time, or if you have a sudden change in the size or amount of floaters or flashes, call a health professional immediately. These are signs of possible retinal detachment, which may require immediate treatment. If you have had floaters for some time, or if you have occasional flashes, mention it at your next routine eye examination.

Smoking increases your risk for macular degeneration. There is some evidence that eating plenty of dark, leafy green vegetables, such as spinach and collard greens, may reduce your risk for macular degeneration.

Laser surgery may prevent or delay further loss of vision in one type of macular degeneration if the condition is detected early.

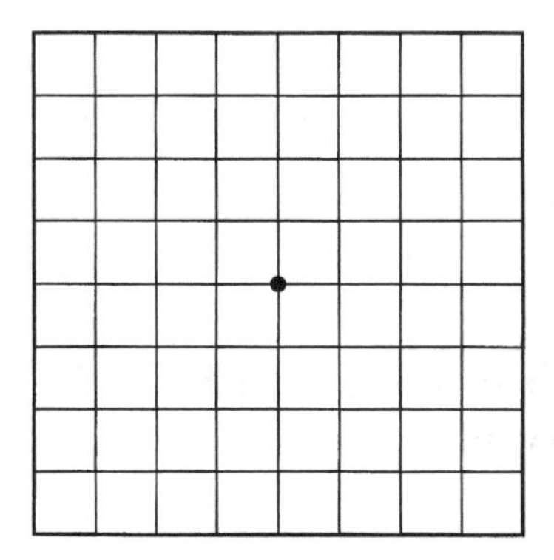

Amsler grid: Cover one eye and look at the grid above. Repeat with the other eye covered. If the lines around the centre dot look wavy or distorted, you may have a macular problem.

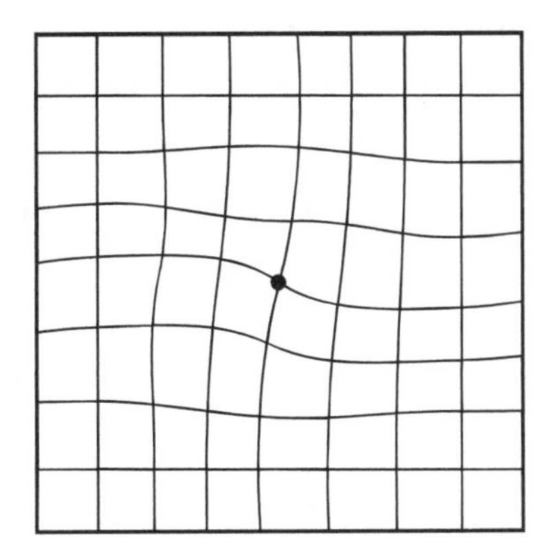

This is how the first grid might look to someone who has macular degeneration.

Diabetic Retinopathy

Diabetic retinopathy develops when the blood vessels that supply blood to the retina are damaged by diabetes. It often has no symptoms until it is quite advanced. If it is not treated, diabetic retinopathy can lead to blindness. Regular eye examinations can detect this problem early, when it can be more successfully treated. Keeping your blood sugar levels in a safe range is important to help reduce your risk for retinal changes. See Diabetes on page 285.

When to Call a Health Professional

Call a health professional immediately if you have a sudden onset of vision disturbances, such as floaters and flashes of light, partial blindness, or dark spots in your field of vision.

Call your doctor:

- If straight lines appear wavy or curved, or the size or shape of objects begins to look different or distorted.
- If you often see new floaters or flashes of light.

If you are at high risk for macular degeneration or diabetic retinopathy, have eye examinations according to the schedule recommended by your doctor and report any new changes in your vision as soon as possible.

PRK and LASIK

PRK and LASIK are two different surgical procedures that can correct vision problems such as nearsightedness, farsightedness, and astigmatism. For each procedure, a surgeon uses laser instruments to reshape the cornea (the clear tissue that covers the iris and pupil) in a way that allows improved vision. These procedures take 15 to 30 minutes to complete. If both eyes need correction, they can be treated at the same time, although some doctors prefer to treat one eye at a time.

Some people may still need to wear glasses or contact lenses after the surgery, especially when light is dim and at night (usually the prescription is not as strong). A person may see halos around lights for up to 6 months after having corrective eye surgery.

PRK and LASIK cannot prevent or restore vision loss caused by cataracts or macular degeneration. Nor can they prevent or correct the age-related vision changes that make reading glasses necessary (presbyopia).

Styes

A sty is a non-contagious infection of the eyelash follicle. It looks like a small, red bump, much like a pimple, either in the eyelid or on the edge of the lid. It comes to a head and breaks open after a few days.

Styes are very common and are not a serious problem, although they can be painful. Most will go away on their own with home treatment and don't require removal.

Home Treatment

- Do not rub your eye, and do not squeeze or open the sty.
- Apply warm, moist compresses for 10 minutes, 3 to 6 times a day, until the sty comes to a head and drains.
- Do not wear eye makeup or contact lenses until the sty heals.

When to Call a Health Professional

- If the sty is very painful, grows larger quickly, or continues to drain.
- If the sty interferes with your vision.
- If the sty gets worse despite home treatment or doesn't heal within 1 week.
- If the redness and swelling around the sty spread to involve the entire eyelid or the eyeball.

Dizziness and Vertigo

Dizziness is a word often used to describe two different sensations: light-headedness and vertigo. Knowing the difference can help you and your health professional narrow down the list of possible problems.

Light-headedness is a feeling that you are about to pass out (faint). Although you may feel unsteady, there is no sensation of movement. Light-headedness usually improves when you lie down. If light-headedness gets worse, it can lead to fainting and nausea or vomiting.

Light-headedness usually does not indicate a serious problem. It is common to feel light-headed occasionally. Light-headedness is often caused by a momentary drop in blood pressure and reduced blood flow to the brain when you get up too quickly from a seated or lying position. This is called **orthostatic hypotension**, which may be caused by dehydration or medications such as water pills (diuretics), high blood pressure medications, and certain heart medications.

Eye Twitches

Eye twitches or muscle spasms around the eye are most often associated with fatigue or stress. Twitches will usually stop on their own in a short time, and they will improve with rest or reduced stress.

Call a health professional if eye twitches occur with redness, swelling, discharge from the eye, or fever; if twitches last longer than 1 week; or if the twitching involves other facial muscles.

Light-headedness is common when you have the flu, a cold, or allergies. Vomiting, diarrhea, and fever can cause dehydration and light-headedness. Other common causes of light-headedness include hyperventilation, stress, anxiety, drinking alcohol, or using illegal drugs. A more serious cause of light-headedness is bleeding. If a person is bleeding internally, light-headedness and fatigue may be the first noticeable symptoms of blood loss.

An uncommon cause of light-headedness is an abnormality in your heart rhythm that reduces blood flow. This can cause recurrent episodes of light-headedness and can lead to fainting (cardiac syncope). Unexplained fainting needs to be evaluated by a health professional. See Unconsciousness on page 110.

Vertigo is a sensation that you or your surroundings are spinning or moving when there is no actual movement. Vertigo is often related to inner ear problems. It may occur with nausea and vomiting. Standing or walking may be impossible when you have severe vertigo.

The most common form of vertigo is triggered by changes in the position of your head, such as when you move your head from side to side, bend your head back to look up, or lie down. This is called **benign positional vertigo**.

Ear Problems	
Symptoms	**Possible Causes**
Earache and fever; pulling at ears by infants and small children, especially with inconsolable crying	Ear Infections, p. 225.
Pain while chewing; headache	TM Disorder, p. 175.
Pain when ear is wiggled or while chewing; itching or burning in ear	Swimmer's Ear, p. 230.
Discharge from ear	Swimmer's Ear, p. 230; eardrum rupture, p. 225.
Feeling of fullness in ear, with runny or stuffy nose, cough, fever	Colds, p. 194; Ear Infections, p. 225.
Feeling of something moving or "bumping around" in ear	Objects in the Ear, p. 94.
Hearing loss; inattentiveness	Hearing Loss, p. 229; Earwax, p. 227; fluid in the ear (effusion), p. 226.
Ringing or noise in the ears	Tinnitus, p. 232.

Vertigo may also be caused by labyrinthitis, an inflammation in the part of the inner ear that controls balance. Labyrinthitis is usually caused by a viral infection and sometimes follows a cold or the flu.

Other underlying problems that can cause vertigo are Ménière's disease (a balance problem believed to be caused by a buildup of fluid in the inner ear), migraine headaches, multiple sclerosis, stroke, and in rare cases a brain tumour.

Home Treatment

Light-headedness is usually not a cause for concern unless it is severe or persistent or occurs with other symptoms such as an irregular heartbeat or fainting. The greatest danger of light-headedness or vertigo is the injury that might result if you fall.

- When you feel light-headed, lie down for a minute or two. This lets more blood flow to your brain. Then sit up slowly and remain sitting for 1 to 2 minutes before slowly standing up.
- If you have a cold or the flu, rest and drink extra fluids.
- Do not drive, operate machinery, or put yourself in any other potentially dangerous situation while you are having vertigo or feeling light-headed.

- When you are having vertigo, avoid lying flat on your back. Propping yourself up slightly may help relieve the spinning sensation. Keep your eyes open.

When to Call a Health Professional

Call 911 or other emergency services immediately:

- If vertigo is accompanied by severe headache, confusion, loss of speech or sight, weakness in the arms or legs, or numbness in any part of the body.
- If light-headedness occurs with chest pain that is squeezing or crushing, or occurs with any other symptoms of a heart attack (see page 191).
- If someone who is feeling dizzy loses consciousness and you are unable to wake the person.
- If vertigo or loss of balance occurs with other signs of serious illness, such as headache with severe stiff neck, fever, irritability, confusion, or a seizure.
- If severe, persistent light-headedness occurs with a sudden change in heart rate.

Call a health professional:

- If light-headedness or vertigo develops after an injury.
- If you have vertigo that is severe (may cause vomiting) or that occurs with hearing loss.
- If you suspect your dizziness may be a side effect of a medication.
- If you experience vertigo that:
  - Occurs frequently and has not been diagnosed.
  - Lasts longer than 5 days.
  - Differs significantly from other episodes.
- If you have repeated spells of light-headedness over a few days.
- If you feel light-headed and your pulse is less than 50 or more than 150 beats per minute. See page 103 to learn how to take your pulse.

Ear Infections

Ear infections most often occur in the middle ear or the ear canal. For information about infections in the ear canal, see Swimmer's Ear on page 230.

A middle ear infection (otitis media) often develops during a cold. Colds can cause the eustachian tube, which connects the middle ear to the throat, to swell and close. When the eustachian tube is closed, fluid builds up in the middle ear. Bacteria or viruses then grow in the fluid, causing a middle ear infection.

The infected fluid that is trapped in the middle ear puts pressure on the eardrum. In some cases, the pressure may continue to build until the eardrum ruptures. A single **eardrum rupture** usually is not serious and rarely causes hearing loss. The eardrum usually heals on its own once the infection clears. However, repeated eardrum ruptures can lead to permanent hearing loss.

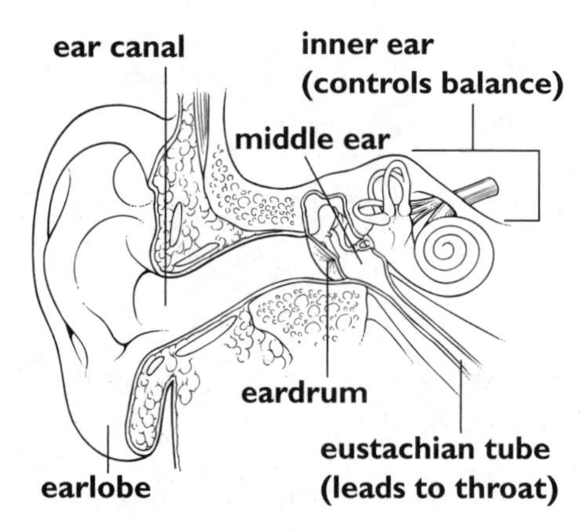

Ear infections can occur in the ear canal, middle ear, or inner ear. Dizziness can be caused by an inflammation of the middle or inner ear.

Symptoms of a middle ear infection include ear pain, dizziness, ringing or a feeling of fullness in the ear, hearing loss, fever, headache, and runny nose. Children who can't yet talk may tug on their painful ears. Drainage from the ear that is bloody or looks like pus may indicate a ruptured eardrum. Ear pain caused by a middle ear infection usually improves once an eardrum ruptures.

Fluid buildup in the middle ear is called **effusion**. There may be no symptoms, or there may be a muffling of sound, minor hearing loss, and mild discomfort. Effusion that persists after a middle ear infection is not a cause for concern and probably will not require treatment unless it lasts longer than 3 months and causes significant hearing loss. See Recurrent Ear Infections and Persistent Effusion on page 228.

Prevention

- Breast-feed your baby. Breast-fed babies have fewer ear infections. If you bottle-feed your baby, hold the baby in an upright position to prevent milk from getting into the eustachian tubes. Do not allow your baby to fall asleep with a bottle (however, it is all right to let a nursing baby fall asleep at the breast).
- Avoid exposing children to cigarette smoke, which is associated with more frequent ear infections.
- Limit your child's contact with children who have colds.
- Wean your child from his or her soother at about 6 months of age. Babies who continue to use their soothers after 12 months of age are more likely to develop ear infections.
- Wash your hands often, especially if you have a cold or other upper respiratory infection.
- Make sure your child is up to date with his or her immunizations.

Home Treatment

- Apply heat to the ear to ease the pain. Use a warm face cloth or a heating pad set on low. Don't use a heating pad on a baby or a child. Don't use a heating pad in bed; you may fall asleep and burn yourself.

- Acetaminophen, Aspirin, or ibuprofen will help relieve earache. Do not give Aspirin to anyone younger than 20, because of the risk of Reye's syndrome (see page 268).
- Drink more clear liquids.
- If dizziness occurs, see page 222.
- If an ear infection has caused the eardrum to rupture, avoid getting water in the ear until the eardrum heals (about 3 to 4 weeks).

When to Call a Health Professional

- If ear pain is severe or increases despite home treatment.
- If ear pain occurs with other signs of serious illness, such as headache with severe stiff neck, fever, irritability, or confusion. (See Encephalitis and Meningitis on page 201.)
- If your baby pulls or rubs his or her ear and appears to be in pain (crying, screaming).
- If your child has a fever over 38°C (taken in the armpit) with other signs of an ear infection.
- If an infant younger than 3 months has a fever of 37.4°C (taken in the armpit) or higher.
- If you suspect that the eardrum has ruptured or if there is bloody or pus-like drainage from the ear.
- If symptoms have not improved after 48 hours of treatment with an antibiotic.
- If your child has ear tubes and develops an earache or has drainage from the ear.
- If mild ear pain continues for longer than 3 to 4 days.
- If there is redness or swelling around or behind the ear.
- If you cannot move your facial muscles normally.

Earwax

Earwax is a protective secretion that filters dust, repels water, and keeps the ears clean. Normally, earwax is semi-solid, drains freely from the ears, and does not cause problems.

Occasionally, earwax will build up, harden, and cause some hearing loss or discomfort. Poking at the wax with cotton swabs, fingers, or other objects will only push the wax deeper into the ear canal and pack it against the eardrum. When wax is tightly packed, professional help is needed to remove it.

In general, it is best to leave earwax alone. You can handle most earwax problems that do occur by avoiding cotton swabs and following the home treatment tips.

Home Treatment

Do not use home treatment if you suspect that the eardrum is ruptured, if there is drainage from the ear that looks like pus or contains blood, or if the person has ear tubes.

To remove earwax safely:

- Soften and loosen the earwax with warm (body temperature) mineral oil. Place 2 drops of mineral oil in the ear twice a day for 1 or 2 days. Once the wax is loose and soft, use the spray from a warm, gentle shower or a bulb syringe to remove it. Direct the water into the ear, and then tip the head to let the wax drain out.
- Or, each night for the next 1 to 2 weeks, use a non-prescription wax softener, followed by gentle flushing with warm water from a bulb syringe. Putting cool or hot fluids in the ear may cause dizziness, so make sure the water is warm (body temperature).

Recurrent Ear Infections and Persistent Effusion

If your child has at least 3 ear infections in a 6-month period, or 4 infections in a 1-year period, talk to your family doctor or pediatrician about preventive antibiotic treatment. This is a low dose of antibiotics given daily throughout the season when your child is prone to ear infections.

However, there is growing debate among health professionals about the effectiveness of antibiotics in preventing ear infections. In addition, there is increasing concern that routine use of antibiotics may cause bacteria to change so that common antibiotics cannot kill them. As a result, ear tubes (tympanostomy tubes) may be recommended instead of antibiotics for recurrent infections.

In some children, fluid (effusion) remains in the middle ear more than 3 months after an ear infection clears up. If this occurs in your child, he or she should be given a hearing test, because long-lasting effusion can cause hearing loss or speech delays. If there is no hearing loss, you may choose to use home treatment for another 3 months. If the fluid has not gone away after those 3 months, your doctor may recommend ear tubes. If hearing tests show that your child has experienced a hearing loss, your doctor may recommend ear tubes or antibiotics.

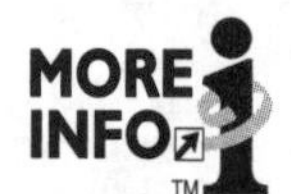

The decision about how to treat recurrent ear infections is made on a case-by-case basis. Ask your doctor about the long-term risks and benefits of all the available treatment options.

When to Call a Health Professional

- If the wax buildup remains hard, dry, and compacted after 1 week of home treatment.
- If earwax is causing ringing in your ears, a full feeling in your ears, or hearing loss.
- If earwax buildup occurs with other problems such as nausea or difficulty with balance.
- If an earwax problem develops in a person who has a ruptured eardrum or ear tubes or who has had previous ear surgery.

Hearing Loss

Millions of people cope with some degree of hearing loss. Most hearing loss is caused by problems in the inner ear or in the acoustic nerve, which sends sound signals to the brain. This is called **sensorineural hearing loss**. Damage to the inner ear can be the result of exposure to loud noise, certain medications (including high doses of Aspirin), or changes that come with age. In some cases, children are born with this type of hearing loss. People with sensorineural hearing loss may have trouble understanding the speech of others yet be very sensitive to loud sounds. They may also hear ringing, hissing, or clicking noises.

Hearing loss that develops when something prevents sound from reaching the inner ear is called **conductive hearing loss**. The most common cause is packed earwax in the ear canal, which can be easily treated (see page 227). Infection, abnormal bone growth, and excess fluid in the ear are other causes of conductive hearing loss.

People who have conductive hearing loss often say that their own voice sounds loud while other voices sound muffled. There may be a low level of ringing in the ear (tinnitus).

Depending on the underlying problem, conductive hearing loss is usually treated by ear flushing, medication, or surgery.

A more unusual form of hearing loss is caused by damage to the hearing centres in the brain. This is called **central deafness**, and it can occur after a head injury or stroke. The person's ear works normally, but his or her brain has difficulty interpreting sounds.

Some hearing loss may be the result of decreased blood flow to the inner ear or parts of the brain that help process information from the ear. If you have circulatory problems caused by heart disease, high blood pressure, or diabetes, be sure to follow your care plan for keeping those conditions under control.

Prevention

- Avoid loud noise whenever possible. If you know you are going to be exposed to it at work, at home, at the shooting range, or in other settings, wear earplugs or protective earmuffs. The noise generated by snowmobiles, motorcycles, lawn mowers, power tools and appliances, high-volume music, and other sources can permanently damage your hearing.

- Never use cotton swabs, hairpins, or other objects to remove earwax or to scratch your ears. They can damage the ear canal or eardrum. See page 227 for tips on removing earwax.
- Ask your pharmacist if any medications you are taking can affect your hearing. For example, the use of certain antibiotics, blood pressure medications, ibuprofen, and large doses of Aspirin (8 to 12 tablets per day) is linked to hearing loss.
- During air travel, swallow and yawn frequently when the plane is descending. If you have a cold, the flu, or a sinus infection, take a decongestant a few hours before the plane is scheduled to land.

When to Call a Health Professional

- If hearing loss develops suddenly (within a matter of days or weeks).
- If you have hearing loss in one ear only.
- If you develop a hearing problem while taking medication, including Aspirin or ibuprofen.
- If hearing loss occurs with vertigo or loss of movement in your face.
- If you are thinking about wearing hearing aids. Make an appointment with an ear specialist (otolaryngologist) if:
  - You often ask people to repeat themselves or have difficulty understanding words.
  - You have difficulty hearing when someone speaks in a whisper.
  - You cannot hear soft sounds, such as a dripping faucet, or high-pitched sounds.
  - You continuously hear a ringing or hissing background noise.
  - A hearing problem is interfering with your life.

Swimmer's Ear

Swimmer's ear (otitis externa) is inflammation or infection of the ear canal, the passage leading from the external ear to the eardrum. It often develops after water has gotten into the ear. Sand or other debris that gets into the ear canal may also cause swimmer's ear.

Other causes of inflammation in the ear canal include a cut inside the ear or an injury from a cotton swab or other object; prolonged use of earplugs; soap or shampoo buildup; and chronic skin conditions such as eczema and psoriasis.

Symptoms include pain, itching, and a feeling of fullness in the ear. The ear canal may be swollen. A more severe infection can cause increased pain, discharge from the ear, and possibly some hearing loss. Unlike a middle ear infection, the pain of an ear canal infection is worse when you chew, press on the "tag" in front of the ear, or wiggle your earlobe.

Prevention

- Try to keep water out of your ears. After swimming or showering, shake your head to remove water from the ear canals. Gently dry your ears with the corner of a tissue or towel, or use a blow-dryer on its lowest setting, held several inches from your ear.
- Put a few drops of rubbing alcohol, or alcohol mixed with an equal amount of white vinegar, in the ear after swimming or showering. Pull your ear up and back to let the liquid go deep into the ear canal; then tilt your head and let it drain out. You can also use non-prescription drops (such as Star-Otic) to prevent swimmer's ear.
- Never use cotton swabs, hairpins, or other objects to clean wax out of your ears. This can damage the ear canal or eardrum. See page 227 for tips on removing earwax.
- Avoid prolonged use of earplugs.
- Avoid getting soap and shampoo in the ear canal. To remove dirt or sand that gets into the ear while swimming, direct a gentle stream of warm water from the shower or a bulb syringe into your ear; then tip your head to let the water drain out.

Home Treatment

- Make sure there isn't an object or insect in the ear. See Objects in the Ear on page 94.
- If the eardrum may be ruptured or there is drainage from the ear that looks like pus or contains blood, do not insert eardrops or anything else into the ear unless a health professional has told you to do so.
- Gently rinse the ear using a bulb syringe and a solution of equal parts white vinegar and rubbing alcohol. Make sure the solution is at body temperature. Putting cool or hot fluids in the ear may cause dizziness.
- Avoid getting water in the ear until the irritation clears up. Cotton lightly coated with petroleum jelly can be used as an earplug. Do not use plastic earplugs.
- If your ear is itchy, try non-prescription swimmer's eardrops before and after getting your ears wet.
- To insert eardrops, have the person lie down, ear facing up. Warm the drops first by rolling the container between your hands. Place drops on the wall of the ear canal in small quantities so air can escape and drops can get into the ear. Wiggling the outer ear or pulling the ear up and back will help. See the illustration on page 232.

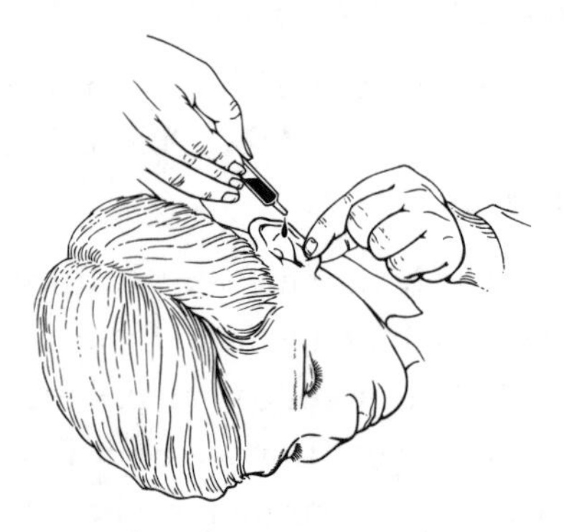

Never stick a dropper into the ear canal. Put drops on the outer ear near the opening of the ear canal, and gently wiggle the ear until the drops flow into the canal.

- To ease ear pain, apply a warm face cloth or a heating pad set on low. (Don't use a heating pad on an infant or a child. Never use a heating pad in bed; you may fall asleep and burn yourself.) There may be some drainage when the heat melts earwax. As long as the drainage does not contain pus or blood, it is not of concern.
- Acetaminophen or Aspirin may help relieve pain. Do not give Aspirin to anyone younger than 20, because of the risk of Reye's syndrome (see page 268).

When to Call a Health Professional

- If symptoms persist or worsen after 3 days of home treatment.
- If the ear canal is swollen, red, and very painful.
- If redness extends to the outer ear.
- If there is redness or swelling around or behind the ear.
- If there is bloody or pus-like discharge from the ear.
- If ear pain follows a cold.
- If dizziness or unsteadiness develops.

Tinnitus

Most people experience occasional ringing (or roaring, hissing, buzzing, or tinkling) in their ears. The sound usually lasts only a few minutes. If it becomes persistent, you may have tinnitus.

Tinnitus is often the result of damage to the nerves in the inner ear, usually caused by prolonged exposure to loud noise. Other causes include excess earwax, ear infection, dental problems, head or ear injuries, and medications, especially antibiotics and large amounts of Aspirin. Excessive alcohol or caffeine intake can also cause tinnitus or make existing tinnitus worse. In rare cases, tinnitus can be caused by a brain tumour.

Tinnitus that comes and goes usually does not require medical treatment. However, if tinnitus is accompanied by other symptoms, becomes persistent, or starts to localize to one ear, a visit to a health professional usually is needed. Often there is no cure for tinnitus, but your health professional can help you learn how to live with the problem.

Prevention

Follow the prevention tips for hearing loss on page 229.

Home Treatment

- Cut back on or eliminate alcohol and beverages containing caffeine.
- Limit your use of products containing Aspirin, ibuprofen, and other non-steroidal anti-inflammatory drugs (NSAIDs).
- If you think earwax may be causing your tinnitus, see Earwax on page 227.

When to Call a Health Professional

- If tinnitus develops suddenly and affects only one ear.
- If you have new tinnitus with other symptoms such as significant hearing loss, vertigo (see page 222), loss of balance, nausea, or vomiting.
- If tinnitus develops after an injury to the head or ear.
- If tinnitus lasts longer than 2 weeks despite home treatment.

I'm very brave generally, only today
I happen to have a headache.
Tweedledum in Alice in Wonderland

11

Headaches

Headaches are one of the most common health complaints. Some possible causes include tension, infection, allergy, injury, hunger, changes in the flow of blood in the vessels of the head, or exposure to chemicals.

Most headaches that occur without other symptoms will respond well to self-care. The majority of headaches are caused by tension and respond well to prevention measures and home treatment. See page 240.

An unusual headache that is very different from any you have had before, or a change in the usual pattern of your headaches, is a cause for concern. See Headache Emergencies on page 238. However, if you have had similar headaches before and your doctor has recommended a treatment plan for them, emergency care may not be needed.

Headaches that routinely occur during or after physical exertion, sexual activity, coughing, or sneezing may be a sign of a more serious disease and should be discussed with a health professional.

Headaches in Children

Migraine headaches (see page 238) often begin during childhood or adolescence and are the most common form of headache in children.

Children's headaches can also be related to stress about school, sports, relationships, or peer pressure. Even fun activities can be overdone and cause fatigue and headaches. Many times, just talking about a problem with your child may help. Encourage your children to talk openly about problems and stress.

Possible Headache Causes	
If headache occurs:	**Possible causes include:**
On awakening	Tension Headaches, p. 240; Allergies, p. 179; Sinusitis, p. 202; Neck Pain, p. 153; TM Disorder, p. 175.
In jaw muscles or in both temples	TM Disorder, p. 175; Tension Headaches, p. 240.
Each afternoon or evening; after hours of desk work; with sore neck and shoulders	Tension Headaches, p. 240; Neck Pain, p. 153.
On one side of the head, with visual disturbances or runny nose	Migraine Headaches, p. 238; Cluster Headaches, p. 241.
After a blow to the head	Head Injuries, p. 85.
After exposure to chemicals (paint, varnish, insect spray, cigarette smoke)	Chemical headache. Get into fresh air. Drink water to flush poisons.
With fever, runny nose, or sore throat	Flu, p. 199; Sore Throat, p. 204; Colds, p. 194; Sinusitis, p. 202.
With fever, stiff neck, nausea, and vomiting	Encephalitis and Meningitis, p. 201.
With runny nose, watery eyes, and sneezing	Allergies, p. 179.
With fever and pain in the cheek-bones or over the eyes	Sinusitis, p. 202.
On mornings when you drink less caffeine than usual	Caffeine-withdrawal headache. Cut back slowly, p. 240.
Following a stressful event	Tension Headaches, p. 240.
At the same time during the menstrual cycle	Premenstrual Syndrome, p. 315.
With new medication	Drug allergy. Contact your doctor.
With severe eye pain	Possible acute glaucoma, p. 218. **See a doctor now!**

Hunger can also cause headaches in children. A daily breakfast and a nutritious after-school snack may prevent headaches. Needing corrective lenses and not getting enough sleep are other possible headache causes. Children will often have headaches along with sore throats, colds, sinus problems, or other infections.

Treatment for headaches in children and teens is based on the same factors as adult headache treatment: how often the headaches occur; how severe the pain is and how long it lasts; and how much the headaches disrupt normal activities. However, in children there is an increased emphasis on non-drug treatments.

Although migraines in children can be managed in much the same way as migraines in adults, less is known about the long-term effects of migraine medications in children. Some medications are not recommended for young children.

Home Treatment

- If your child's doctor has prescribed a specific treatment for the child's headaches, begin treatment as soon as your child reports the headache.
- For headaches that are mild and occur only occasionally, let your child rest quietly in a darkened room with a cool compress on his or her forehead. If rest does not relieve your child's headache, try a non-prescription medication such as acetaminophen or ibuprofen. Follow the dosage directions on the package for your child's age group. Do not give Aspirin to anyone younger than 20, because of the risk of Reye's syndrome (see page 268).
- If your child tends to have mild headaches that occur frequently, encourage him or her to go on with normal activities. Do not allow your child to avoid chores or other activities unless his or her headache pain is moderate or severe. It is useful to "practise what you preach" in this area. When you have a headache, deal with it in a matter-of-fact way. Try to maintain your own usual activities when you have a headache, and adopt a calm approach to managing the pain. If your children see you successfully managing your headaches, they will be likely to do the same for themselves.
- Talk to your child. Let him or her know you care. Extra attention and quiet time may be enough to relieve the headache.

When to Call a Health Professional

- If a severe headache occurs with signs of encephalitis or meningitis (see page 201), especially if your child recently had a viral illness.
- If a headache is severe and is not relieved by relaxing or taking a non-prescription pain reliever.

- If a headache occurs with other symptoms, such as abdominal pain, nausea, or vomiting, and is not relieved by home treatment and a non-prescription pain reliever.
- If a child's headaches occur twice a week or more, or if you are using pain relievers to control a child's headaches more than once a week.
- If you cannot discover a reasonable cause for your child's headaches.
- If headaches awaken your child at night or are worse early in the morning.
- Also see Headache Emergencies on page 238.

Headache Emergencies

Call your doctor now if you have:

- A very sudden "thunderclap" headache.
- A sudden, severe headache unlike any you have had before.
- Headache with stiff neck, fever, nausea, vomiting, drowsiness, or confusion.
- Headache with weakness, paralysis, numbness, visual disturbances, slurred speech, confusion, behaviour changes, or seizures.
- Headaches following a recent fall or blow to the head. See page 85 for information on head injuries.
- Headache with severe eye pain.

Migraine Headaches

Migraine headaches are severe headaches that often occur with nausea, vomiting, and extreme sensitivity to light or sound. People often describe migraine headaches as throbbing or piercing. The pain may range from mild to terribly severe.

Migraine headaches are usually one-sided, but sometimes pain occurs on both sides of the head. In some people, the pain may switch sides each time they have a migraine.

Migraine headaches sometimes occur with an aura, a collection of symptoms that usually develop within an hour before a migraine headache begins. Visual disturbances, such as flashing lights, distortion in the size or shape of objects, or blind or dark spots in the field of vision, are the most common symptoms of an aura. An aura may also include symptoms that affect the nervous system, such as numbness or tingling in the face or arm, strange smells or sounds, or weakness on one side of the body. Some people have more vague symptoms, such as hunger, excessive thirst, or changes in mood or energy level, that appear 1 to 2 days before the headache develops.

Migraines are more common in females than in males. The headaches may begin during childhood, but most begin during the teens and early 20s. In women, they are often associated with menstrual periods.

Prevention

- Keep a diary of your headache symptoms. See Tracking Your Headaches on page 239. Once you know what events, foods, medications, or activities bring on your headaches, you may be able to prevent or limit their recurrence.
- Do what you can to manage stress. See Stress and Distress on page 384 for tips.

Tracking Your Headaches

If you have recurring headaches, keep a record of your symptoms. This record will help your doctor if medical evaluation is needed. Write down:

1. The date and time each headache started and stopped.

2. Any factors that seemed to trigger the headache: food, smoke, bright light, stress, activity.

3. The location and nature of the pain: throbbing, aching, stabbing, dull.

4. The severity of the pain.

5. Other physical symptoms: nausea, vomiting, visual disturbances, sensitivity to light or noise.

6. If you are a woman, note any association between your headaches and your menstrual cycle or your use of birth control pills or hormone replacement therapy.

Home Treatment

- At the first sign of a headache, try to go to a quiet, dark place and relax. Sleeping can relieve migraines.
- Some people find that taking a pain reliever such as acetaminophen or ibuprofen at the first sign of a headache brings relief. However, frequent use of pain relievers can cause rebound headaches (headaches that return as the effects of the pain relievers wear off).
- Apply a cold pack to the painful area or put a cool cloth on your forehead. Do not apply heat, because it may make a migraine worse.
- Have someone gently massage your neck and shoulder muscles, or give yourself a massage.
- Practise a relaxation exercise such as progressive muscle relaxation or roll breathing. See pages 386 and 387.
- If a doctor has prescribed medication for your migraines, take the recommended dose at the first sign that a migraine is starting.

When to Call a Health Professional

- If you suspect that your headaches are migraines.
- If headaches are becoming more frequent or more severe.

Also see Headache Emergencies on page 238.

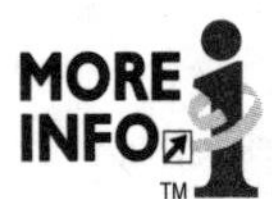

Professional diagnosis and treatment, combined with your self-care, can help decrease the impact of migraines on your life. Discuss relaxation and biofeedback techniques with your doctor. They help many people prevent migraines. If non-drug treatments are not effective, there are many new prescription drugs available that can make migraines less severe or prevent them.

Tension Headaches

Most headaches are tension headaches, which become more frequent and severe during times of emotional or physical stress. Tightness or pain in the muscles of the neck, back, and shoulders may accompany a tension headache. A previous neck injury or arthritis in the neck can also cause tension headaches.

A tension headache may cause pain all over your head, a pressure sensation, or a feeling like having a tight band around your head. Your head may feel like it is in a vise. Some people feel a dull, pressing, burning sensation above the eyes.

The pain may also affect the jaw, face, neck, shoulders, and upper back. You can rarely pinpoint the centre or source of pain.

Prevention

- Reduce emotional stress. Take time to relax before and after you do something that has caused a headache in the past. Try the progressive muscle relaxation or roll breathing exercises on pages 386 and 387.
- Reduce physical stress. When sitting at a desk, change positions often, and stretch for 30 seconds each hour. Make a conscious effort to relax your jaw, neck, shoulder, and upper back muscles.
- Evaluate your neck and shoulder posture at work and make adjustments if needed. See page 155.
- Exercise daily. It can help relieve muscle tension and reduce stress.
- Treat yourself to a massage. Some people find regular massages very helpful in relieving tension. See page 395.
- Limit caffeinated drinks to 1 or 2 per day. People who drink a lot of caffeine often develop a headache several hours after they have their last caffeinated drink; or they may wake with a headache that is relieved by drinking caffeine. Cut down slowly to avoid caffeine-withdrawal headaches.

Home Treatment

- Stop whatever you are doing and sit quietly for a moment. Close your eyes and inhale and exhale slowly. Try to relax your head and neck muscles.

- Take a stretch break or try a relaxation exercise. See page 386.
- Gently and firmly massage your neck muscles. See page 154 for neck exercises.
- Apply heat to the painful area with a heating pad, a hot water bottle, or a warm shower.
- Lie down in a dark room with a cool cloth on your forehead.
- Taking acetaminophen or ibuprofen often helps relieve a tension headache. However, using nonprescription or prescription headache medications too often may make headaches more frequent or severe when the medication wears off.

When to Call a Health Professional

- If a headache is severe and cannot be relieved with home treatment.
- If unexplained headaches continue to occur more than 3 times a week.
- If headaches become more frequent and severe.
- If headaches occur during or after physical exertion, sexual activity, coughing, or sneezing.
- If headaches awaken you from a sound sleep or are worse first thing in the morning.
- If you need help discovering or eliminating the source of your tension headaches.

Also see Headache Emergencies on page 238.

Cluster Headaches

Cluster headaches are sudden, very severe, sharp, stabbing headaches that occur on one side of the head, usually in the temple or behind the eye. They are much more common in men than in women.

During a cluster headache, the eye and nostril on the affected side may be runny, and the eye may also be red. The pain often begins at night and may last from a few minutes to a few hours.

Cluster headaches occur in periods of time called cluster periods, which may last days or months and then disappear for months or even years. During a cluster period, a person may have headaches several times a day. To prevent headaches during a cluster period, avoid alcohol and tobacco products, maintain a regular sleep schedule, and try to reduce your overall stress level.

See your doctor if you think you have cluster headaches or if you have persistent, severe headaches with no apparent cause. Also see Headache Emergencies on page 238.

I have a simple philosophy . . .
scratch where it itches.
Alice Roosevelt Longworth

12

Skin, Hair, and Nail Problems

Skin problems can be a nuisance, but they are rarely life-threatening. Diagnosing skin problems may require a doctor's help, especially the first time you have a particular ailment. Use the chart on the next page and the index to find the skin problem you're interested in. Also see Childhood Rashes on page 264.

Acne

Acne is the term for blemishes (pimples or blackheads) that commonly form on the face, chest, upper back, or shoulders. A pimple forms when an oil duct in the skin is blocked, and secretions and bacteria build up under the skin. Acne usually starts during the teen years and often persists into adulthood.

Many women get a few pimples just before their menstrual periods. Stress and some birth control pills may make acne worse. Fatty foods, such as chocolate and nuts, are not considered to be a cause of acne.

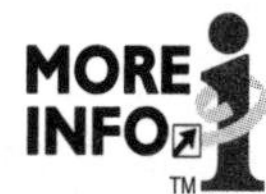

Many cases of acne will respond to home treatment, especially if they are mild. For severe or persistent cases, your doctor can prescribe stronger topical medication, antibiotics, or other drugs.

Prevention

- Gently wash your face with a mild soap, such as Dove, or one that contains benzoyl peroxide. Wash as often as necessary to keep your face clean (at least once a day), but do not scrub or overdry.
- While foods are no longer considered a significant cause of acne, eat a healthy diet and avoid any food that seems to cause pimples.

Skin Problems

Symptoms	Possible Causes
Raised, red, itchy welts or fluid-filled bumps after an insect bite or taking a drug	Allergies, p. 179; Hives, p. 255; Insect and Spider Bites and Stings, p. 91.
Red, painful, swollen bump under the skin	Boils, p. 248.
Red, flaky, itchy skin	Dry Skin, p. 252; Atopic Dermatitis, p. 246; Fungal Infections, p. 253; Rashes, p. 257.
Crusty, honey-coloured rash, most often between the nose and upper lip	Impetigo, p. 281.
Rash that develops after wearing new jewellery or clothing, being exposed to poisonous plants, eating a new food, or taking a new drug	Rashes, p. 257; Allergies, p. 179.
Red, itchy, blistered rash	Possible poison ivy, oak, sumac. See Rashes, p. 257; Chicken Pox, p. 269.
Painful blisters in a band around one side of the body	Shingles, p. 253.
Change in the shape, size, or colour of a mole, or a persistently irritated mole; a sore that does not heal	Skin Cancer, p. 258.
Cracked, blistered, itchy, peeling skin between the toes	Fungal Infections (athlete's foot), p. 253.
Red, itchy, weeping rash on the groin or thighs	Fungal Infections (jock itch), p. 253; Impetigo, p. 281.
Scaly, itchy, bald spots or sores on the scalp	Fungal Infections (ringworm), p. 253.
Flaky, silvery patches of skin, especially on the knees, elbows, or scalp	Psoriasis, p. 251.
Sandpapery skin rash with sore throat and a strawberry-textured tongue	Scarlet fever. See p. 207.
Sores on the lip or in the mouth	Canker Sores, p. 249; Cold Sores (fever blisters), p. 250.

Home Treatment

- Cleanliness is essential. Wash your face, shoulders, chest, and back with lukewarm (not hot) water and a very gentle soap, such as Aveeno, Cetaphil, or Neutrogena. Avoid drying soaps, such as deodorant soaps. Always rinse well.
- Keep long hair off your face and shoulders, and wash it daily.
- Avoid touching your face or other areas that have acne.
- Don't squeeze pimples. This can cause infection and scarring.
- Non-prescription benzoyl peroxide gel or cream is one of the best treatments for acne. Start with the lowest strength, and increase the strength if your skin is able to tolerate it. Apply a very thin layer of the medication once a day, half an hour after washing. It may take up to 2 months to work and may cause mild redness and dryness. Never use more than 5% benzoyl peroxide unless a doctor recommends that you do so.
- Use only water-based lotions and cosmetics that do not clog skin pores (non-comedogenic), and only if they don't aggravate acne.
- Controlling stress may help reduce acne flare-ups. See page 384.

Rosacea

Rosacea is a chronic skin disease that causes red patches, red lines (tiny blood vessels), and small pimples on the face, as well as burning and irritation in the eyes. It is often mistaken for acne. If treated early, rosacea may remain minor and be controlled fairly well. Left untreated, it can progress and eventually cause larger bumps on the nose and face (rhinophyma) and serious eye problems.

Rosacea most often affects adults. Fair-skinned people who blush easily or whose facial flushing produces a redness that lasts longer than is typical are most likely to develop rosacea. The condition tends to run in families.

Symptoms of rosacea may get worse in response to spicy foods; alcohol; exposure to sun, heat, or very cold temperatures; strenuous exercise; or certain skin care products, perfumes, or sunscreens.

If you have rosacea, try to identify and avoid things that trigger your symptoms and cause you to flush. Antibiotic creams and other medications can help control pimples and redness. Laser treatment can be used to treat the blood vessels on the surface of the skin and reduce redness in advanced cases.

When to Call a Health Professional

- If acne gets worse despite 6 to 8 weeks of home treatment.
- If you have severe red or purple inflammation, cysts, or nodules under the skin.
- If scars develop as acne heals.
- If you develop acne after starting a new medication.

Atopic Dermatitis

Atopic dermatitis (AD) is a chronic skin disorder that often develops in people who have asthma, hay fever, and other allergies. It causes an itchy, red, raised rash that may weep or ooze clear fluid. The rash may develop tiny blisters, which break and crust over. The blisters are prone to infection, especially if scratching is not controlled.

In children, AD appears most often on the face, scalp, arms, thighs, and torso. AD is often worse during infancy. It improves in many children by age 5 or 6. Most children have outgrown it entirely by their early teens.

In adults, it usually appears on the neck and in the bend of the elbows and knees. Adults whose hands or feet are often exposed to irritating substances, such as chemicals, develop AD on those areas.

Home Treatment

Helping the skin retain moisture is essential to the successful treatment of AD.

- Take brief, daily baths or showers with lukewarm (not hot) water. Use a gentle soap (such as Dove, Olay, or Neutrogena) or non-soap cleanser (such as Cetaphil or Aveeno). If possible, bathe without soap, or use soap in the armpits and groin area only.
- After bathing, pat skin dry and immediately apply a moisturizer (Lubriderm, Moisturel). The moisturizer may help keep your skin from drying out. Reapply it often.
- Use a humidifier in the bedroom or on your furnace.
- Taking an oral antihistamine (such as Benadryl) may help relieve itching and relax you enough to allow sleep. Avoid antiseptic and antihistamine creams and sprays, because they irritate the skin.
- Avoid contact with any irritants or allergens that cause problems. Wear gloves when working with irritating substances.
- Wash clothes and bedding in mild detergent and rinse at least twice. Do not use fabric softener if it irritates your skin. Avoid wools and scratchy fabrics.
- For more tips on relieving itching, see page 252.

When to Call a Health Professional

- If there are crusting or oozing sores, serious scratch marks, or skin discolouration. Also see Signs of Infection on page 100.
- If itching interferes with sleep, and home treatment is not working.
- If you cannot control atopic dermatitis with home treatment.

Calluses and Corns

Calluses and corns are hard, thickened skin that is exposed to friction and pressure. Calluses are common on the soles of the feet, the heels, and the hands. Corns usually form on the toes.

If a callus or corn becomes painful, soak your feet in warm water, and rub the callus or corn with a towel or pumice stone. You may need to do this for several days until the thickened skin is gone. Non-prescription products for removing calluses and corns are also available. If a callus or corn breaks open or becomes sore, see your doctor.

Do not try to cut or burn off corns or calluses. If you have diabetes or peripheral vascular disease, talk with your doctor before attempting to remove troublesome corns or calluses.

Blisters

Blisters are usually the result of persistent or repeated rubbing against the skin. Some illnesses, such as shingles, cause blister-like rashes (see Shingles on page 253). Burns can also blister the skin. See page 73.

Prevention

- Avoid shoes that are too tight or that rub your feet.
- Wear gloves to protect your hands when doing heavy chores.

Home Treatment

- If a blister is small and closed, leave it alone. Protect it from further rubbing by applying a loose bandage. Avoid the activity or shoes that caused the blister to form.
- If a small blister is in a weight-bearing area, protect it with a doughnut-shaped moleskin pad. Leave the area over the blister open.
- If a blister is larger than 2.5 cm across, it is usually best to drain it. The following is a safe method:
  - Wipe a needle with rubbing alcohol.
  - Gently puncture the edge of the blister.
  - Press the fluid in the blister toward the hole you have made so it can drain.

- Once you have opened a blister, or if it has torn open:
  - Wash the area with soap and water.
  - Do not remove the flap of skin covering a blister unless it is very dirty or torn, or if pus is forming under the skin flap. Gently smooth the skin flap flat over the tender skin underneath.
  - Apply an antibiotic ointment and a sterile bandage. Do not use alcohol or iodine on an open wound. They will delay healing.
  - Change the bandage once a day or anytime it gets wet or dirty to reduce the chance of infection.
  - Remove the bandage at night to let the area dry.

When to Call a Health Professional

- If blisters form often and you do not know the cause.
- If signs of infection develop. See page 100.
- If you have diabetes or peripheral vascular disease and blisters are forming on your hands, feet, or legs.

Boils

A boil is a red, swollen, painful bump under the skin, similar to an overgrown pimple. Boils are often caused by infected hair follicles. Bacteria from the infection form an abscess or pocket of pus. The abscess can become large and cause severe pain.

Boils occur most often in areas where there is hair and chafing. The face, neck, armpits, breasts, groin, and buttocks are common sites.

Prevention

- Wash boil-prone areas with soapy water. An antibacterial soap may help. Dry thoroughly.
- Avoid clothing that is too tight.

Home Treatment

- Do not squeeze, scratch, drain, or open the boil. Squeezing can push the infection deeper into the skin. Scratching can spread the bacteria to other parts of the body.
- Wash yourself well with an anti-bacterial soap to keep the infection from spreading.
- Apply hot, wet face cloths to the boil for 20 to 30 minutes, 3 to 4 times a day. Do this as soon as you notice a boil. The heat and moisture can help bring the boil to a head, but it may take 5 to 7 days. Applying a hot water bottle or a waterproof heating pad over a damp towel may also help.
- Continue using warm compresses for 3 days after the boil opens. Apply a bandage to keep draining material from spreading, and change the bandage daily.

When to Call a Health Professional

If needed, your doctor can drain the boil and treat the infection. Call the doctor:

- If the boil is on your face, near your spine, or in the anal area.
- If signs of worsening infection develop. See page 100.
- If any other lumps, particularly painful ones, develop near the infected area.
- If the pain limits your normal activities.
- If you have diabetes.
- If the boil is as large as a Ping-Pong ball.
- If the boil has not improved after 5 to 7 days of home treatment.
- If many boils develop over several months.

Canker Sores

Canker sores are painful, open sores that form on the inside of the mouth. Possible causes of canker sores include injury to the inside of the mouth, infection, certain foods, stress, genetic tendency to get canker sores, and female hormones. The sores usually heal in 7 to 10 days.

Prevention

- Avoid injuring the inside of your mouth:
  - Chew food slowly and carefully.
  - Use a soft-bristle toothbrush, and brush your teeth thoroughly but gently.
  - Don't chew on toothpicks, plastic straws, or other objects.
- Avoid foods that seem to cause sores.
- Don't smoke or chew tobacco products.

Home Treatment

- Avoid coffee, spicy and salty foods, nuts, chocolate, and citrus fruits when you have open sores in your mouth.
- Apply a non-prescription canker sore medication to protect the sore, ease pain, and speed healing.
- Rinse your mouth with an antacid (such as Maalox or Mylanta) or with a mixture of 15 ml of hydrogen peroxide in 240 ml of water.
- Applying a thin paste of baking soda and water to the sore may relieve pain.

When to Call a Health Professional

- If mouth sores develop after you start taking a medication.
- If a canker sore, or any sore, does not heal in 14 days, or if multiple sores appear.
- If a sore is very painful or recurs frequently.
- If white spots that are not canker sores appear in the mouth and are not improving after 1 to 2 weeks.

Birthmarks

Birthmarks are relatively common. Most are harmless. Over time they may fade, increase in size or thickness, or stay the same.

Macular stains (sometimes called salmon patches, angel kisses, or stork bites) are light pink birthmarks that appear on the upper lip, eyelids, forehead, and back of the neck. They usually fade within a few months.

Hemangiomas are soft, red, or blue lumps formed by clusters of blood vessels. They may be present at birth or appear during the first few months. They may grow for up to 6 months, stabilize for a short time, and then usually begin to recede and fade. Nearly all disappear by age 9.

Port-wine stains are pink or wine-coloured birthmarks that appear most often on the head and face. They are permanent, become darker as the child grows, and may need to be treated by a dermatologist or plastic surgeon to stop them from expanding.

Report any changes in birthmarks to your health professional. Birthmarks need to be removed if they interfere with breathing or vision or disfigure the face. If surgery is desired for cosmetic reasons, talk with your health professional about the best timing for surgery.

Cold Sores

Cold sores (fever blisters) are small, red blisters that usually appear on the lip and outer edge of the mouth. They often weep a clear fluid and scab over after a few days. They are sometimes confused with impetigo (see page 281), which usually develops between the nose and upper lip. The fluid that weeps from impetigo is cloudy and honey-coloured, not clear.

Cold sores are caused by a herpes virus. Herpes viruses (chicken pox is another kind) stay in the body after the first infection. Later, something triggers the virus to become active again. Cold sores may appear after colds, fevers, or exposure to the sun, after stressful times, or during menstruation. Sometimes they develop for no apparent reason.

Prevention

- Avoid kissing a person who has a cold sore. Also avoid direct skin contact with genital herpes sores (see page 333) or herpes sores elsewhere on the body.
- Use sunscreen on your lips and wear a hat if exposure to the sun seems to trigger cold sores.
- Reducing stress may help in some cases. Practise relaxation exercises often. See page 386.

Home Treatment

- Apply ice or a cool, wet towel to the area 3 times a day. This may help reduce redness and swelling.

- Apply petroleum jelly to ease cracking and dryness.
- Use a lip protector, such as Blistex, to ease the pain. Don't share the product with anyone else.
- Apply vitamin E gel or a product containing aloe vera, goldenseal, or bee propolis to the sore.
- Be patient. Cold sores usually go away in 7 to 10 days.

When to Call a Health Professional

Call if sores last longer than 2 weeks or if you have frequent outbreaks of cold sores. A prescription medication given within the first 48 hours of symptoms may reduce the severity of an outbreak.

Dandruff

Dandruff occurs when the skin cells of the scalp flake off. This flaking is natural and occurs all over your body. On the scalp, however, flakes can mix with oil and dust to form dandruff. Dandruff cannot be cured, but it can be controlled.

Home Treatment

- Try frequent and thorough shampooing with any shampoo. Wash hair daily if it controls dandruff.
- If dandruff is excessive and itchy, try a dandruff shampoo (such as Head & Shoulders, Sebulex, or Neutrogena T/Gel). Work the dandruff shampoo into your scalp and leave it on for several minutes before rinsing thoroughly.

When to Call a Health Professional

Call if frequent shampooing or shampooing with a dandruff shampoo doesn't control dandruff.

Psoriasis

Psoriasis is a chronic skin condition that causes raised red patches topped with silvery, scaling skin. These usually occur on the knees, elbows, scalp, and back. The fingernails, palms, and soles of the feet may also be affected. Psoriasis can also cause a form of arthritis.

The patches, called plaques, are made of dead skin cells that accumulate in thick layers. Normal skin cells are replaced about every 28 days. In people who have psoriasis, skin cells are replaced every 3 to 6 days.

Psoriasis is not contagious. It may come and go. Small patches of psoriasis can often be treated with regular use of hydrocortisone creams. Other products (lotions, gels, shampoos) may also be useful, although they may increase your skin's sensitivity to the sun. Limited exposure to the sun may also help, but be sure to protect unaffected skin with sunscreen.

Stress may contribute to psoriasis. Stress reduction may help in some cases. See page 384.

Call your doctor if psoriasis covers much of your body or is very red. Extensive or severe cases often need professional care.

Dry Skin

Dry, itchy, flaky skin is the most common skin problem, especially in the winter. It develops when the skin loses water to the air. Dry indoor air is a common cause, as is excessive bathing in hot water.

Prevention

- Avoid showers. They strip the natural oil that helps hold moisture in the skin. Baths are much kinder to the skin than showers are.
- Use bath oils in the bathwater. Be careful not to slip.
- Use mild soaps (such as Dove or Cetaphil). You may only need to use soap under your arms and in the groin area.
- Use a moisturizing lotion immediately after your bath.

Home Treatment

- Follow the prevention guidelines above.
- For very dry hands, try this for a night: Apply a thin layer of petroleum jelly and wear thin cotton gloves to bed. (Dry feet may benefit from similar treatment.)
- Avoid scratching, which damages the skin. If itching is a problem, see Relief From Itching on page 252.

When to Call a Health Professional

- If you itch all over your body but there is no obvious cause or rash.
- If itching is so bad that you cannot sleep, and home treatment is not helping.
- If you have open sores from scratching.

Relief From Itching

- Keep the itchy area well moisturized. Dry skin may make itching worse.
- Take an oatmeal bath to help relieve itching: Wrap 240 ml of oatmeal in a cotton cloth, and boil as you would to cook it. Use this as a sponge and bathe in tepid water without soap. Or try an Aveeno colloidal oatmeal bath.
- Apply calamine lotion to poison ivy or poison oak rashes.
- Try a non-prescription 1% hydrocortisone cream for small itchy areas. Use it very sparingly on the face or genitals. If itching is severe, your doctor may prescribe a stronger steroid cream or ointment.
- Try a non-prescription oral antihistamine such as Benadryl or Chlor-Tripolon.
- Cut nails short or wear gloves at night to prevent scratching.
- Wear cotton or silk clothing. Avoid wool and acrylic fabrics next to the skin.

Fungal Infections

Fungal infections of the skin most commonly affect the feet, groin, scalp, or nails. Fungi grow best in warm, moist areas of the skin, such as between the toes, in the groin, and in the area beneath the breasts.

Athlete's foot is the most common fungal skin infection. Symptoms include itching and cracked, blistered, and peeling areas between the toes and on the soles of the feet. Athlete's foot often recurs and must be treated each time.

Jock itch causes severe itching and moistness on the skin of the groin and upper thighs. There may be red, scaly, raised areas on the skin that weep or ooze pus or clear fluid.

Ringworm is a fungal infection that grows on the outer layer of skin, hair, or nails.

On the skin, ringworm appears as patches that are clear in the centre with edges that are red or peeling or have blister-like bumps. The skin is often very itchy, and the rash can spread quickly.

On the scalp and beard, ringworm appears as round or oval patches of baldness, which may be scaly, red, crusty, or swollen with little blister-like bumps. The hair on the scalp and beard may have flakes that look like dandruff.

Fungal infections of the **fingernails** and **toenails** cause discolouration, cracking, thickening, and often softening of the nails. They are difficult to treat.

Shingles

Shingles (herpes zoster) is caused by the reactivation of the chicken pox virus in the body years after the initial illness. The virus usually affects one or two of the large nerves that spread outward from the spine, causing pain and a rash in a band around one side of the chest, abdomen, or face. The rash will blister and scab, then clear up over the course of a few weeks.

No one knows what makes the virus active again. Shingles can affect anyone who has had chicken pox. However, older adults and people with weakened immune systems are more likely to get shingles. People with weakened immune systems include those who have had a bone marrow or organ transplant; those who have cancer, especially of the lymph system; or those infected with HIV.

Exposure to the shingles rash can cause chicken pox in a person who has not had chicken pox before.

If you suspect shingles, call your doctor or the BC NurseLine to discuss medication that can limit the pain and rash. If possible, call as soon as you notice the rash. Medication works best when it is started immediately.

Thrush is a yeast infection that occurs in the mouth, especially in babies. It causes a white coating inside the mouth, often on the inside of the cheeks, that may look like milk but is hard to remove. Thrush may develop after the use of antibiotics. (Yeast infections also develop in the vagina. See page 319.)

Prevention

- Keep your feet clean, cool, and dry. Dry well between the toes after swimming or bathing. Use antifungal powder to prevent infection or reinfection.
- Wear leather shoes or sandals that allow your feet to "breathe," and wear cotton socks to absorb sweat. Use powder on your feet and in your shoes. Give shoes 24 hours to dry between wearings.
- Wear thongs or shower sandals in public pools and showers.
- Keep your groin area clean and dry. Wash and dry well, especially after exercising. Wear cotton underclothes and avoid tight pants and panty hose.
- Teach children not to play with dogs or cats that have bald or mangy spots on their coats.
- Don't share hats, combs, brushes, or towels.

Home Treatment

- Follow the prevention guidelines.
- For athlete's foot and jock itch, use a non-prescription antifungal powder or lotion, such as Micatin. Always wash the affected area before applying the powder or lotion. Use the medication for 1 to 2 weeks after the symptoms clear up to prevent recurrence. Do not use hydrocortisone cream on a fungal infection.
- Ringworm on the body can be treated with an antifungal.

When to Call a Health Professional

- If signs of infection are present. See page 100.
- If you have diabetes and develop athlete's foot. People with diabetes are at increased risk for infection and may need professional care.
- If you experience a sudden loss of patches of hair, along with flaking, broken hairs, and inflammation of the scalp; or if several members of your household are experiencing hair loss.
- If ringworm is severe and spreading or is present on the scalp. Prescription medicine may be needed.

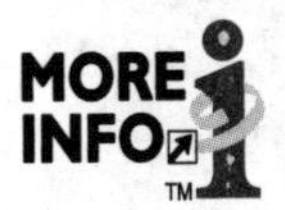

If a fungal infection does not improve after 2 weeks or clear up after 1 month despite home treatment, you may want to consider prescription medication. Discuss the options with your doctor.

Hives

Hives are raised, red, itchy, often fluid-filled patches of skin called wheals or welts that may appear and disappear at random. They range in size from less than 0.6 cm to 7.5 cm across or more, and they may last a few minutes or a few days.

A single hive commonly develops after an insect sting. Multiple hives often develop in response to a medication, food, or infection. Other possible causes of hives include plant allergies, inhaled allergens, stress, cosmetics, and exposure to heat, cold, sunlight, or natural rubber latex. Often a cause cannot be found.

Home Treatment

- Avoid the substance that causes hives.
- Apply cool-water compresses to help relieve itching. Also see Relief from Itching on page 252.
- Take an oral antihistamine (such as Benadryl or Chlor-Tripolon) to treat the hives and relieve itching. Once the hives have disappeared, decrease the dose of the medication slowly over 5 to 7 days.

When to Call a Health Professional

Call 911 or other emergency services if spreading hives occur with dizziness, wheezing, difficulty breathing, tightness in the chest, or swelling of the tongue, lips, or face.

Call a health professional:

- If hives develop soon after you start taking a new medication.
- If hives cover all or most of your body.
- If hives persist for 24 hours despite home treatment.

Ingrown Toenails

Ingrown toenails usually develop when an improperly trimmed toenail cuts into the skin at the edge of the nail or when you wear shoes that are too tight. Because the cut can easily become infected, prompt care is needed.

Prevention

- Cut toenails straight across and leave the nails a little longer at the corners so that the sharp ends don't cut into the skin.
- Wear roomy shoes, and keep your feet clean and dry.

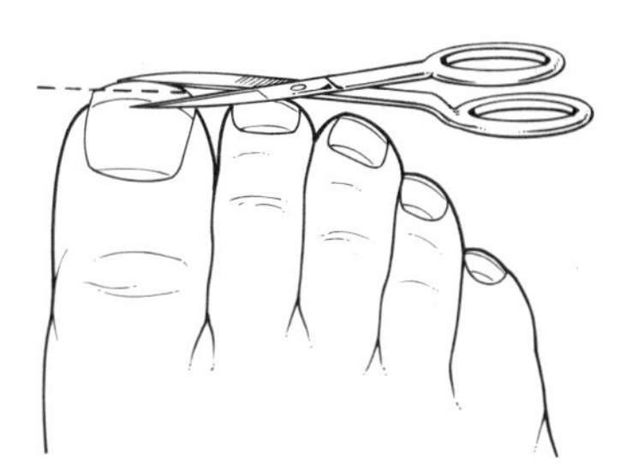

Cut toenails straight across.

Home Treatment

- Soak your foot in warm water for 15 minutes to soften the skin around the nail.

- To keep the nail from cutting the skin, wedge a small piece of wet cotton under the corner of the nail to cushion it and lift it slightly. Repeat daily until the nail has grown out and can be trimmed.
- Daily foot soaks in warm water will help relieve swelling or tenderness while toenails grow out.

When to Call a Health Professional

- If signs of infection develop. See page 100.
- If you have diabetes or circulatory problems and develop an ingrown toenail.

Lice and Scabies

Lice are tiny, white, wingless insects that may live on the skin, hair, or clothing. They feed by biting the skin and sucking blood. The bites itch and may cause an allergic rash. Head lice live in the hair on the head; body lice live on clothing; and pubic lice (also called crabs) live in the groin, underarms, and eyelashes.

Lice are spread by close physical contact or contact with the clothing, bedding, brushes, or combs of an infested person. Pubic lice can be spread through sexual contact.

Scabies are tiny mites that burrow under the skin and lay eggs. This burrowing causes an allergic rash that may itch intensely. Scabies are often found between folds of skin on the fingers and toes, wrists, underarms, and groin. The scabies mites are spread through close contact with an infested person or the person's bedding, clothing, or towels. Scabies are usually treated with a prescription medication that is applied over the entire body and left on overnight. Itching may last for several weeks after treatment.

Prevention

Be alert for signs of lice: itching and lice or tiny eggs (nits) attached to the hair shafts of the head. Prompt treatment can help prevent spreading lice to others.

People who have lice or scabies should avoid close contact with others to prevent spreading the insects or mites.

Home Treatment

- Nix, Kwellada-P, and R&C are non-prescription medications for lice. Follow the manufacturer's directions for use exactly. After treatment for head lice, comb the hair well with a fine-toothed nit comb to remove all nits. (Nit combs are available at most pharmacies and supermarkets.)
- On the day you start treatment, wash all dirty clothing, bedding, and towels in hot water to help get rid of lice, nits, and mites. Iron or dry-clean items that cannot be washed, or freeze them for 24 hours.
- Some schools have a "no nits" policy stating that children may not return to school until they are

free of lice nits. Children who have been treated for scabies can return to school after treatment is completed.

- Contact your pharmacist or public health nurse for more information about treatment and preventing reinfestation.

When to Call a Health Professional

Call if treatment with non-prescription medication is not successful. Stronger prescription drugs are available.

Rashes

A rash (dermatitis) is any irritation or inflammation of the skin. Rashes can be caused by illness, allergy, or heat, and sometimes by emotional stress. For rashes related to childhood illnesses, see page 264. If the rash developed after you were bitten by a tick, see page 109.

Poison ivy and other plant rashes are often red, blistered, and itchy and appear in lines where the leaves brushed against the skin.

When you first get a rash, ask yourself these questions to help determine the cause (also see pages 244 and 264):

- Did a rash that is contained to a specific area (localized) develop after you came in contact with anything new that could have irritated your skin: poison ivy, oak, or sumac; soaps, detergents, shampoos, perfumes, cosmetics, or lotions; jewellery or fabrics; new tools, appliances, latex gloves, or other objects? The location of the rash is often a clue to the cause.
- Have you eaten anything new that you may be allergic to?
- Are you taking any new medications, either prescription or non-prescription?
- Have you been unusually stressed or upset recently?
- Is there joint pain or fever with the rash?
- Is the rash spreading?
- Does the rash itch?

Prevention

- If you are exposed to poison ivy, oak, or sumac, wash your skin with rubbing alcohol or plenty of water within 10 to 15 minutes to get the allergy-causing oil off your skin. This may help prevent or reduce the rash. Use soap only after using plenty of water. Also wash your clothes, your dog, and anything else that may have come in contact with the plant.
- Avoid products that have caused a rash in the past, such as detergents, cosmetics, lotions, clothing, or jewellery.
- Use fragrance- and preservative-free or hypoallergenic detergents, lotions, and cosmetics if you have frequent rashes.

Home Treatment

- Wash affected areas with water. Soap can be irritating. Pat dry thoroughly.
- Apply cold, wet compresses to reduce itching. Repeat frequently. Also see page 252.
- Keep cool, and stay out of the sun.
- Leave the rash exposed to the air. Baby powder can help keep it dry. Avoid lotions and ointments until the rash heals. However, calamine lotion is helpful for plant rashes. Use it 3 to 4 times a day.
- Use hydrocortisone cream to provide temporary relief from itching. Use very sparingly on the face and the genital area.

When to Call a Health Professional

- If signs of infection develop. See page 100.
- If you suspect a medication reaction caused the rash.
- If a rash occurs with fever and joint pain.
- If a rash occurs with a sore throat. See information about scarlet fever on page 207.
- If a rash appears and you aren't sure what is causing it.
- If a rash does not clear up after 2 to 3 weeks of home treatment.

Skin Cancer

Skin cancer is the most common type of cancer. Most skin cancer is caused by sun damage and occurs on the face, neck, and arms, where sun exposure is greatest. Light-skinned, blue-eyed people are more likely to develop skin cancer. Dark-skinned people have less risk.

Most skin cancers are non-melanoma skin cancer, which includes basal cell and squamous cell carcinoma. Non-melanoma skin cancer is rarely life-threatening. Melanoma is a more serious type of skin cancer. It may affect only the skin, or it may spread (metastasize) to other organs and bones. Melanoma can be life-threatening.

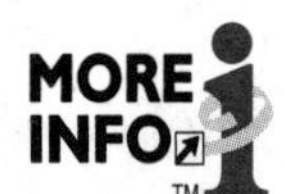

Most non-melanoma skin cancers are easy to treat if they are caught early. Early surgical removal of thin melanomas can cure the disease in most cases.

Skin cancers differ from non-cancerous growths in the following ways:

- They tend to bleed more than non-cancerous growths do and are often open sores that do not heal.
- They tend to be slow-growing. However, melanoma may appear suddenly and grow quickly.

Prevention

Most skin cancers can be prevented by avoiding excessive exposure to the sun (including sun lamps). Most damaging sun exposure has occurred by age 20, so keep your children protected (see page 259). Repeated sun exposure and severe sunburns are major factors in some types of skin cancer.

Home Treatment

Examine all areas of your skin with a mirror or with another person's help. Look for unusual moles, spots, bumps, or sores that won't heal. Pay special attention to areas that get a lot of sun exposure: hands, arms, back, chest, neck (especially the back of the neck), face, ears. Report any changes to your doctor.

When to Call a Health Professional

Call your doctor if you notice any unusual skin changes or growths, especially if they bleed and continue to change.

If your moles do not change over time, there is little cause for concern. If you have a family history of malignant melanoma, let your doctor know, because you may be at higher risk for malignant melanoma. Call your doctor if you notice any of the following "ABCD" changes in a mole or other skin growth:

- **A**symmetrical shape: One half does not match the other half.
- **B**order irregularity: The edges are ragged, notched, or blurred.
- **C**olour not uniform: Watch for shades of red and black, or a red, white, and blue mottled appearance.
- **D**iameter: A mole is larger than a pencil eraser. (Harmless moles are usually smaller than this.)

Asymmetrical shape

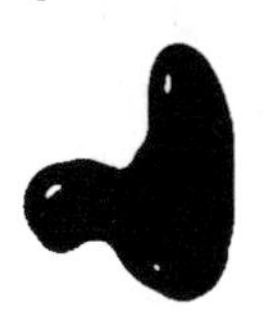

Border irregular

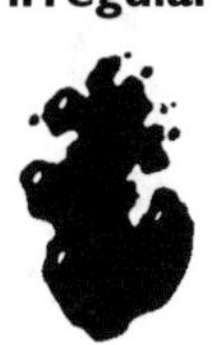

Colour varied

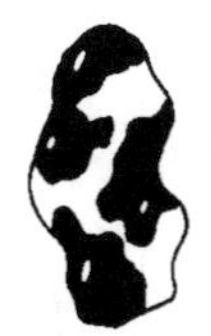

Diameter larger than a pencil eraser

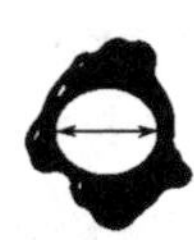

Watch for these "ABCD" mole changes.

Also call if you notice:

- Scaliness, oozing, bleeding, or spreading of pigment into surrounding skin.
- Appearance of a bump or nodule on the mole, or any change in the appearance of the mole.
- Itching, tenderness, or pain.

Sunburn

A sunburn is usually a first-degree burn that involves the outer surface of the skin. Sunburns are painful but can usually be treated at home unless they are extensive. Severe sunburns can be serious in infants, small children, and older adults.

Repeated sun exposure and sunburns increase your risk for skin cancer (see page 258).

Prevention

If you are going to be outdoors for more than 15 minutes, take the following precautions:

- Wear light-coloured, loose-fitting, long-sleeved clothes, and a broad-brimmed hat to shade your face. Wear sunglasses that provide ultraviolet (UV) protection.
- Use a sunscreen that has a sun protection factor (SPF) of 15 or higher. Sunscreens labelled "broad spectrum" can protect the skin from the two types of harmful sun rays (UVA and UVB).
- Apply the sunscreen at least 30 minutes before you will be exposed to the sun.
- Apply sunscreen to all the skin that will be exposed to the sun, including the nose, ears, neck, scalp, and lips. It needs to be applied evenly over the skin.
- Reapply sunscreen every 2 to 3 hours while in the sun and more often if you are swimming or sweating a lot.
- Older adults have sensitive skin and should always use a sunscreen with an SPF of 30 or higher.
- Drink lots of water. Sweating helps cool the skin.
- Avoid the sun between 10 a.m. and 4 p.m., when the burning rays are strongest. Seek shade whenever possible.
- Don't forget the kids. Sun exposure may be very hard on their tender skin. Teach your young children safe sun habits—hats and sunscreen—early. Use a sunscreen with an SPF of 30 or higher to protect babies' and children's very sensitive skin. Keep babies younger than 6 months out of the sun.

Home Treatment

- Drink plenty of water and watch for signs of dehydration (especially in infants or children). See page 118. Also watch for signs of heat exhaustion. See page 87.
- Cool baths or compresses can be very soothing. Take acetaminophen or ibuprofen for pain. Don't give Aspirin to anyone younger than 20, because of the risk of Reye's syndrome.
- A mild fever and headache can accompany a sunburn. Lie down in a cool, quiet room to relieve headache.
- There is nothing you can do to prevent peeling; it is part of the healing process. Lotion can help relieve itching.

When to Call a Health Professional

- If you develop signs of heatstroke (red, hot, dry skin; confusion). See page 87.
- If symptoms of heat exhaustion (dizziness, nausea, headache) persist after you have cooled off.

- If you develop signs of severe dehydration. See When to Call a Health Professional on pages 119 to 120.
- If you have severe blistering (over 50 percent of the affected body part) or severe pain with fever, or if you feel very ill.
- If you have a fever of 38.8°C or higher.

Warts

Warts are skin growths that are caused by a virus. They can appear anywhere on the body. Warts are not dangerous, but they can be bothersome.

Genital and anal warts are transmitted through sexual contact. Certain types increase a woman's risk for cervical cancer. See page 334.

Plantar warts appear on the soles of the feet. Most of the wart lies under the skin surface and may make you feel like you are walking on a pebble.

Warts appear and disappear spontaneously. They can last a week, a month, or even years. Warts seem to come and go for little reason; it's possible that they are reacting to slight changes in the immune system. Some people are more susceptible to warts than others.

When necessary, your doctor can remove warts. Unfortunately, they often come back.

Home Treatment

- Try the least expensive method of treating warts first. You may save a trip to your doctor. If you find a treatment that works for you, stick with it.
- If you have diabetes or peripheral vascular disease, talk to your health professional before trying home treatment to remove the wart.
- If the wart bleeds a little, cover it with a bandage and apply light pressure to stop the bleeding.
- If you are sure that your skin growth is a wart, you can treat it with a non-prescription product containing salicylic acid. Follow the instructions supplied with the medication. Salicylic acid may take weeks to months to cure a wart.
- You can also try covering the wart with up to 5 layers of waterproof tape.
    - Use enough tape to cover the whole wart, and make sure the covering is watertight.
    - Leave the tape on for 5 days; then take it off for 12 hours. Repeat the process until the wart is gone. If the wart is not gone in 2 months, consider trying a different treatment.
- If treatment with salicylic acid or tape causes the area to become tender or irritated, take a 2- to 3-day break from the treatment.

- Rub the wart with a pumice stone or file to remove dead tissue. Don't use these items for any other purpose or you may spread the wart-causing virus; both the debris from the wart and the area of the pumice stone or file that touched the wart can be infectious. Wash your hands with soap after you touch the debris from the wart or the pumice stone or file.
- For plantar warts, apply a doughnut-shaped pad to cushion the wart and relieve pain. Before you go to bed, apply salicylic acid to the wart, and cover the wart with a bandage (or wear a sock). Wash the medication off in the morning.
- Don't cut or burn off a wart.

When to Call a Health Professional

- If a wart looks infected after being irritated or knocked off.
- If a plantar wart is painful when you walk, and foam pads do not help.
- If you have warts in the anal or genital area. See page 334.
- If a wart develops on your face and is a cosmetic concern.

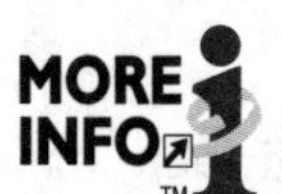

A wart that causes continual discomfort or warts that are numerous enough to be a problem may need to be surgically removed. Talk with your doctor about the risks and benefits of removing warts surgically.

Hair Loss

Many people lose hair as they grow older. Such hair loss is natural and is largely the result of heredity. Balding poses no health risks other than sunburn, which you can prevent by wearing a hat and using sunscreen when outdoors. While men tend to lose hair from the hairline and crown of the head, women's hair becomes thinner all over.

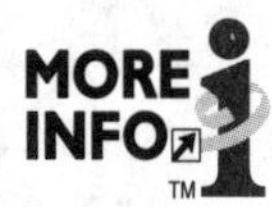

If you are thinking about medication (such as minoxidil) or surgical treatment for hair loss, make sure you understand the risks of treatment, how many treatments you will need, and how long the results will last.

Bald spots are not the same as baldness. Wearing tight braids or habitually tugging or twisting your hair may cause bald spots. Ringworm is a fungal infection that causes scaly bald spots. See page 253. A condition called alopecia areata causes patchy hair loss that may require treatment with prescription medications.

Thinning hair can signal problems such as thyroid disease or lupus. Emotional or physical stress can cause short-term hair loss, as can changes in hormone levels during pregnancy and menopause.

If hair loss is sudden, or if it develops after you start taking a new medication, call your doctor.

My mother had a great deal of trouble with me,
but I think she enjoyed it.
Mark Twain

13

Infant and Child Health

When your children get sick or hurt, you are usually the first person to provide care. Your calmness, confidence, and competence in caring for your children's health problems will help them enjoy good health and learn the importance of self-care for their own use as they mature.

Virtually every health problem in this book can affect children. However, a few are almost exclusively childhood concerns. For convenience, these problems are grouped here in a single chapter. If the problem you are looking for is not in this chapter, please look for it in the index. You can also get a free copy of BC's *Baby's Best Chance* at your public health unit.

Facts About Infants and Young Children

The following brief notes are of particular concern to parents. This information may help dispel some unnecessary fears and give you some guidance.

Umbilical Cords and Belly Buttons

Keep the cord dry and do not give your baby a tub or pan bath until the cord has fallen off and the navel is healed. Fold diapers below and shirts above the cord to promote drying.

The cord will drop off and the navel will heal within several weeks. After the cord comes off, there may be a moist or bloody oozing for a few days. This does not need special treatment.

Call your doctor if there is redness or swelling around the navel or a large amount of foul-smelling discharge from the navel.

The appearance of the belly button is not affected by the way the cord is tied off. A small lump of tissue sometimes remains after the cord falls off. If the lump is small, treatment is usually not needed. If it is larger and does not fall off after 2 weeks, call your doctor.

Childhood Rashes	
Rashes that come with childhood illnesses are hard to tell apart. Review all symptoms before deciding what to do.	
Description	**Possible Illness**
Red, pimple-like spots that turn to blisters; fever	Chicken Pox, p. 269.
Rash in diaper area only	Diaper Rash, p. 274.
Red rash on face that looks like slapped cheeks; pink rash that comes and goes on torso; possible fever	Fifth Disease, p. 284.
Red or pink dots on head, neck, shoulders; more common in infants	Prickly Heat, p. 283.
Sudden high fever for 2 to 3 days followed by rose-pink rash on torso, arms, and neck after fever goes down	Roseola, p. 284.
Fine pink rash that starts on face and covers whole body; swollen glands behind ears	Rubella (rare), p. 18.
Fever, runny nose, hacking cough; red eyes 2 to 3 days before spotty red rash covers whole body	Measles (rare), p. 18.
High fever, sore throat, sandpapery rash, and strawberry-textured tongue	Scarlet fever, p. 207.
Blisters on mouth and tongue appearing 1 to 2 days after onset of fever and sore mouth or throat; painless, blistering rash on fingers, hands, feet	Hand-Foot-and-Mouth Disease, p. 271.

Breast-Feeding

Breast milk is the ideal food for babies up to 6 months of age. The Canadian Paediatric Society Nutrition Committee, Dietitians of Canada, and Health Canada recommend breast-feeding for the first 6 months and for up to 2 years. However, the length of time that breast-feeding should continue differs for each mother and her child. Although breast-feeding is best, babies can also get good nutrition from formula.

Breast milk contains substances that help your baby resist infections and other diseases. Breast-fed babies have fewer colds and ear infections, less diarrhea, and less vomiting. Breast milk is easier to digest than formula.

Getting some instruction helps ensure that you can breast-feed successfully. If possible, take a breast-feeding class. Your local public health nurse, the La Leche League, and Health Canada are all good sources of breast-feeding information, advice, and support.

Circumcision

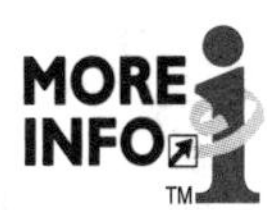

Circumcision is surgery to remove the foreskin of a newborn boy's penis. There are both benefits and risks associated with circumcision. Discuss them with your doctor. The decision is entirely up to you. Circumcision is not an insured service in British Columbia.

If you do choose to have your baby circumcised, one benefit is that circumcision makes it easier to keep the penis clean, which reduces your baby's risk for urinary tract infections. Later in life, a circumcised male has a slightly lower chance of getting a sexually transmitted disease than an uncircumcised male.

The risks of circumcision are slight. Complications of local infection or bleeding occur in about 2 of every 1,000 cases. Local anaesthetic reduces the pain of circumcision and is now recommended. Generally, circumcision is not recommended for sick infants.

If you have your son circumcised, after the procedure apply petroleum jelly liberally to the head of the penis at each diaper change to prevent the scab from sticking to the diaper. Wash the penis by dripping warm water over it (do not use alcohol or baby wipes). Pat dry with a soft towel. Some redness at the circumcision site is normal. Call your doctor if the redness extends down the shaft of the penis, or if there is more than a small amount of blood on the diaper.

If you choose not to have your son circumcised, wash his penis as you would any other body part. Do not try to pull back (retract) the foreskin before age 3, and never forcibly retract the foreskin. Most boys' foreskins are fully retractable by age 5, but some may not fully retract until puberty. Once the foreskin is fully retractable, teach your son to wash his penis well at every bath and to gently retract and wash beneath the foreskin. After puberty he should wash the area under the foreskin daily.

Toilet Training

Every child has a unique timetable for becoming toilet-trained. Most children are ready to begin toilet training between 24 and 30 months of age. Your child may be ready if he or she:

- Passes stools at about the same time each day.
- Is able to have a dry diaper for at least 2 hours at a time during the day.
- Makes certain facial expressions when urinating or passing stools.
- Lets you know when a diaper is dirty and asks to have it changed.
- Seems eager to please and can follow simple instructions.
- Tells you that he or she wants to use the toilet or wear adult underwear.

If you think your child is ready to begin toilet training, the following tips may make it go more smoothly:

- Get your child a potty chair. Let the child get used to using the chair by having him or her sit on it with a diaper on when he or she is passing stools or urinating.
- Let your child watch you or a sibling of the same sex use the toilet. Talk with your child about what you are doing.

Child Car Seats

Infant and child car seats save lives. Many provinces require them for all children under age 4 and those weighing less than 18 kg (40 lb). Children who are not in car seats can be seriously injured or killed during crashes or even by abrupt stops at low speeds. For maximum safety, follow the manufacturer's recommendations for car seat use.

All children under age 12 should be in the backseat, especially if the car has air bags.

Infants under 9 kg (20 lb), regardless of age: Use an infant car seat that reclines and faces the rear.

Infants younger than 1 year, regardless of weight: Use an infant car seat that reclines and faces the rear.

Children over 9 kg (20 lb) and older than 1 year: Use a toddler seat that faces the front of the car and has a shield or harness. Some infant seats can be converted to toddler seats.

Children over 18 kg (40 lb) and over age 4: Use a booster seat that raises the child so that the regular lap and shoulder belts fit properly. Adjust the shoulder belt to fit across the shoulder, not the neck. Use the booster seat until your child is big enough to use the seat belt properly.

Set a good example for your children by always wearing your own seat belt, and always insist that they buckle up.

- Select clothing for your child that is easy to take off. Clothes with elastic waistbands or easy-to-open fasteners, such as Velcro, work best. Pull-on diapers are also helpful.
- Reward every success with hugs and words of praise. Accidental wetting and soiling are common in the first few weeks, but don't scold or punish your child when they happen. Keep a casual attitude.

Bladder control may take longer than bowel control. If the child is aware of when his or her bladder is full, try putting the child on the potty chair every 30 to 60 minutes. Praise the child for success, and give gentle encouragement when the child wets his or her pants.

Sleep Habits

Babies have both deep and light sleep cycles. In each sleep cycle, there are 60 minutes of light sleep, 60 to 90 minutes of deep sleep, and another 30 minutes of light sleep. At the end of this cycle, the baby is semi-alert and can be wakened easily.

Parents can help their baby sleep through the night by helping the baby learn to soothe him- or herself back to sleep during the light sleep cycles.

For babies age 4 to 6 months:

- Put the baby in the crib when he or she is drowsy but awake.
- Make middle-of-the-night feedings short and boring.
- As the baby gets older, delay the middle-of-the-night feeding, and discontinue it sometime after age 6 months.

It is safer for a baby to sleep on his or her back to prevent sudden infant death syndrome (SIDS). Do not force a baby into a sleeping position. Babies are capable of moving themselves.

Bedwetting

Bedwetting (enuresis) in children who have never been dry is common, but most children will outgrow it by age 5 or 6. In almost all cases, bedwetting is really not a disease, but rather a normal variation in development.

In some cases, a child who has been dry for several months or longer may start to wet the bed again. This can happen without a clear cause, or it may be caused by a urinary tract infection or emotional problems.

Home Treatment

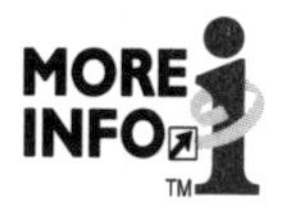

There are a number of ways to deal with bedwetting. Ask your doctor for advice in managing bedwetting until your child outgrows it.

- Do not punish, embarrass, or blame your child. Praise and reward your child for dry nights.

- Have your child empty his or her bladder before bed.
- Remind the child to get up during the night to urinate. Providing a bedside potty chair and night-light may help.
- Do not force your child to wear diapers at night. Try waterproof, extra-absorbent underwear instead. A thick pad or a vinyl mattress cover will protect the mattress.
- Encourage the child to take responsibility for changing his or her clothes after wetting, for putting a dry towel down on the bed, and for helping wash the bed linens.
- Add 120 ml vinegar to the wash water to eliminate odour in clothing and bedding.

When to Call a Health Professional

Your doctor can rule out or treat any physical causes of bedwetting and help you and your child manage the problem. Call your doctor:

- If bedwetting occurs with pain or burning during urination or other signs of a urinary tract infection. See page 138.
- If bedwetting occurs in a child older than 6 years, and home treatment is not successful after 4 to 5 weeks.
- If bedwetting becomes more frequent or severe despite home treatment.

Reye's Syndrome

Reye's syndrome is a rare, serious disease that can develop in anyone under age 20. It occurs most often in children 6 to 12 years old. The cause of Reye's syndrome is unknown. It usually occurs after Aspirin is given to a child who has a viral illness such as chicken pox or flu. Reye's syndrome is not contagious.

Reye's syndrome causes changes in the body that affect all the organs but are most harmful to the brain and liver.

Symptoms of Reye's syndrome include:

- Sudden onset of persistent vomiting that is not related to having flu.
- Drowsiness and lack of energy.
- Rapid, deep breathing (hyperventilation).
- Behaviour changes such as extreme irritability, aggressiveness, or confusion.

If Reye's syndrome is not treated immediately, it can lead to seizures, coma, and, in severe cases, death.

Early treatment of Reye's syndrome increases the chance for full recovery. Most people have no long-lasting complications and gradually get better after a few weeks. However, some people may have permanent brain damage.

To prevent Reye's syndrome, never give Aspirin to anyone younger than 20 unless your health professional directs you to do so.

- If bedwetting occurs in a child who had previously been dry for several months.
- If a child age 4 or older is wetting the bed and leaking stool.
- If a child over age 3 has daytime bladder control problems after having been toilet-trained.

Chicken Pox

Chicken pox (varicella) is a common, contagious viral infection. In otherwise healthy children, it is usually a relatively minor illness. For the first couple of days, your child will feel ill and have fever, loss of appetite, headache, and fatigue. Then a rash of red, pimple-like spots will appear. A child may have as few as 30 spots, but usually there are hundreds. The rash may cover the child's entire body, including the throat, mouth, ears, groin, and scalp.

The spots turn into clear blisters that become cloudy, break open, and crust over. The rash itches a lot. Spots continue to appear for 1 to 5 days and subside over 1 to 2 weeks.

Chicken pox is very contagious. After exposure to the chicken pox virus, symptoms usually appear in 14 to 16 days. The contagious period starts up to 5 days before the rash appears and lasts until 5 days after the rash appears or all the spots have crusted over. Children can usually return to school or daycare after the sixth day of the rash as long as any blisters that have not crusted over are covered with clothing.

Serious complications from chicken pox are rare and may include pneumonia, encephalitis (see page 201), and bacterial skin infection. Certain groups are at increased risk for complications. If they are exposed to chicken pox and are not immune (because of vaccination or having already had chicken pox), there are two options for protecting them:

- An injection of varicella zoster immune globulin (VZIG) may prevent the illness if it is given within 96 hours (4 days) after contact with chicken pox. VZIG is usually reserved for those at highest risk, which includes pregnant women, newborns, and people with weakened immune systems.
- A medication called acyclovir may reduce the severity of illness if used within 24 hours after the rash appears. It may be given to anyone at increased risk for complications: in addition to the highest-risk groups above, this includes anyone over 13 years, children with chronic skin or lung disease, and children on Aspirin therapy.

Contact your doctor right away if you or your child is at increased risk and comes into contact with or develops chicken pox. To prevent illness, VZIG must be given within 96 hours (4 days) after contact with chicken pox. (If you already have symptoms, VZIG will not work.) To make chicken pox less severe, acyclovir must be given within 24 hours after the rash appears.

Prevention

Starting with children born on or after January 1, 2004, the chicken pox vaccine is now routine in BC for all children at age 12 months. The vaccine is also free for children in kindergarten or Grade 6. Babies and children who have had chicken pox do not need the vaccine.

Older teens and adults who have not had chicken pox may want to consider getting vaccinated, since the illness is often more severe in adulthood. Any adult who has not had chicken pox and has not been vaccinated should avoid exposure to children who have it and avoid exposure to people who have shingles (see page 253). Pregnant women who have never had chicken pox and have not been vaccinated should also avoid exposure, because the illness can harm the developing fetus. The vaccine cannot be given during pregnancy.

Home Treatment

- Use acetaminophen to relieve fever if your child is uncomfortable or has a very high or rapidly rising temperature. Do not give Aspirin to anyone younger than 20 who may have chicken pox, because Aspirin use is related to Reye's syndrome (see page 268).
- Control itching (see page 252). Oral Benadryl and warm baths with baking soda or Aveeno colloidal oatmeal added to the water will help. Avoid Benadryl creams because it is difficult to control the dosage when the medicine is applied to the skin.
- Cut your child's fingernails to prevent scratching. If scabs are scratched off too early, the sores may become infected.

When to Call a Health Professional

- If the child is at risk for complications from chicken pox because he or she is taking steroid medications, is receiving cancer chemotherapy, or has a weakened immune system.
- If a pregnant woman, a newborn, or a person with a weakened immune system is exposed to or develops chicken pox.
- If a teenager or adult gets chicken pox.
- If a child age 3 months to 3 years has a fever of 37.4°C or higher (taken in the armpit) for 24 hours. See Fever on page 278.
- If you notice signs of encephalitis (see page 201):
  - Fever, severe headache, and stiff neck
  - Unusual sleepiness or lethargy
  - Persistent vomiting
- If sores appear in a child's eyes.
- If bruising appears without injury.
- If severe itching cannot be controlled with home treatment.

Hand-Foot-and-Mouth Disease

Hand-foot-and-mouth disease is a viral illness that affects many children under 10 as well as young adults. It usually develops during the summer and fall months. Fever, sore throat or mouth, and loss of appetite are early symptoms. Within 2 days, blisters form in the mouth and on the tongue. In children, a blistering rash often develops on the fingers, tops of the hands, and tops and sides of the feet. Blisters sometimes form on the buttocks.

There is no treatment for hand-foot-and-mouth disease other than to give acetaminophen to reduce fever and mouth pain and to make sure the person drinks plenty of fluids. Do not give Aspirin to anyone younger than 20. Offer soft, bland foods and cool or warm (not hot) beverages. Frozen fruit pops may help relieve mouth soreness. Calamine lotion may help soothe the rash on the hands and feet.

The virus that causes hand-foot-and-mouth disease is easily spread, so a person should not go to daycare, school, or work while symptoms are present. All symptoms should go away after 7 to 10 days. The virus is spread through contact with mouth and nasal fluids and stools, so careful hand washing after blowing a runny nose or changing a diaper is important.

Colic

Colic is not a disease; it is a condition that causes otherwise healthy babies to cry inconsolably, usually in the evening and at night. Doctors aren't sure what causes colic. It is equally common among male and female babies and among breast-fed and bottle-fed babies.

All babies cry, so how do you know if your baby has colic? Colic usually follows the "rule of three": Crying starts in the first 3 weeks to 3 months after birth and continues more than 3 hours a day, more than 3 days a week, for more than 3 weeks.

Fortunately, colic goes away as the baby matures, almost always by the end of the fourth month—sooner for many babies. Although no single method always works to relieve colicky babies, there are a number of things you can try. Unfortunately, what works one time may not work the next. Be creative and persistent.

Home Treatment

- Most important: Stay calm and try to relax. If you start to lose control, take a minute to calm down. Never shake a baby; it can cause permanent brain damage and even death.
- Make sure your baby is getting enough to eat, but not too much.
- Make sure your baby isn't swallowing too much air while eating. Feed the baby slowly, holding him

or her almost upright. Burp your baby periodically. Prop your baby up for 15 minutes after feeding.

- If your baby is bottle-fed, use nipples with holes large enough to drip cold formula at least 1 drop per second. Babies will swallow more air from around the nipple if the hole is too small.
- Heat formula to body temperature. Don't overheat.
- Babies may need to suck on something for up to 2 hours a day to be satisfied. If feedings aren't enough, use a soother.
- Keep a regular routine for meals, naps, and playtime. Mealtime should be quiet and undisturbed by bright lights and loud noises.
- Make sure that your baby's diaper is clean, that he or she isn't too hot, and that he or she isn't bored.
- Don't overstimulate your baby. Some babies cry because there is too much light, noise, or activity, or too many people around them.
- Try rocking or walking your baby. Putting him or her stomach-down over your knee or forearm may be helpful.
- Calm your baby with a car ride or a walk outside. Placing your baby near the hum of a clothes dryer, dishwasher, or bubbling aquarium may have a soothing effect.
- Don't worry about spoiling a baby during the first few months; comforting a baby makes both of you feel better.
- Don't leave your baby alone for more than 5 to 10 minutes while he or she is crying. After 10 minutes, try the above suggestions again.

When to Call a Health Professional

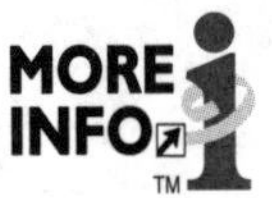

Colic generally does not require professional treatment unless it is accompanied by vomiting, diarrhea, or other signs of a more serious illness. If the baby looks healthy and acts normally between crying episodes, and if your emotions can stand the noise for the first 3 to 4 months, you have little cause for worry.

However, if colic lasts more than 4 hours a day, or if you feel like you need help, contact your doctor for advice.

In rare cases, colic may be so severe that you and your doctor may consider a medication for the baby. Ask about side effects.

Cradle Cap

Cradle cap is an oily, yellow scaling or crusting on a baby's scalp. It is caused by a buildup of normal oils on the skin.

MORE INFO For more information, see the back cover.

Home Treatment

- Wash your baby's head with baby shampoo once a day. Gently scrub the scalp with a soft-bristled brush (a soft toothbrush works well) for a few minutes to remove the scales. Rinse well.
- You can also rub mineral oil on your baby's scalp an hour before shampooing to loosen the scales.
- If the rash looks irritated and red, applying a mild hydrocortisone cream may help.

Croup

Croup is a respiratory problem that develops most often in children from 6 months to 4 years of age. Croup usually accompanies a viral infection, such as a cold. The main symptom is a harsh cough that sounds like a seal's bark and may cause the child to become very frightened. A fever up to 37.4°C (taken in the armpit) is also common. Croup may last 2 to 5 days. Symptoms usually get worse at night, but they generally improve with each passing night.

Home Treatment

- Do whatever you can to calm your child. Crying can make breathing more difficult.
- Get moisture into the air to make it easier for your child to breathe. Use a cool humidifier (do not use a hot vaporizer). Use only water in the humidifier. Set your child in your lap, and let the cool vapour blow directly into your child's face.
- If your child does not improve after several minutes, take him or her into the bathroom and turn on all the hot-water faucets to create steam. Close the door, and sit with your child while he or she breathes in the moist air for several minutes.
- If your child's breathing still does not improve, bundle him or her up and go outside into the cool night air.

When to Call a Health Professional

Call 911 or other emergency services if the child stops breathing or begins to turn blue. Give rescue breathing (see page 68) until help arrives.

Call a health professional:

- If you have been trying home treatment for 30 minutes and your child is not improving at all.
- If these signs of respiratory distress appear and persist despite home treatment:
  - Squeaky or raspy sound as the child inhales (stridor)
  - Sucking in or retraction between ribs as the child inhales
  - Flaring nostrils
- If the child is so short of breath that he or she can't walk or talk.

- If the child drools or is breathing with the chin jutting out and the mouth open.
- If the child is not calm enough to sleep after being in a room with a humidifier or breathing cold outdoor air for 20 minutes.
- If the child has a fever of 38°C or higher (taken in the armpit) or any fever that doesn't go away after 48 hours.
- If you or the child becomes hysterical and cannot calm down.
- If this is the first case of croup in your family and you need reassurance.
- If croup lasts longer than 3 nights without improving.

Diaper Rash

Diaper rash is a skin reaction, usually to the moisture and bacteria in a baby's urine and stools, to the soap used to wash diapers, or to disposable diapers. While it is uncomfortable, diaper rash is usually not dangerous.

Symptoms of the rash are a red bottom and thighs. It will be easier for you to recognize diaper rash after you have seen it the first time.

Prevention

- Change diapers as soon as possible after they have been soiled or wet. Check the diaper at least every 2 hours.
- As often as possible, leave your baby's skin open to the air for 5 to 10 minutes before applying a clean diaper.
- Wash cloth diapers with mild detergent and rinse twice. Do not use bleach or fabric softeners.
- If your baby has frequent diaper rash, avoid using plastic pants for a while. They trap moisture against the baby's skin.
- When your baby has diarrhea, protect the diaper area with zinc oxide or another cream (such as Desitin or A & D Ointment).

Home Treatment

- Change diapers frequently. Using a face cloth and water, rinse the skin in the diaper area at every diaper change. Allow the diaper area to air-dry if possible. Wash the area with a mild soap once a day.
- Stop using plastic pants when the rash appears.
- Protect healthy skin near the rash with Desitin, A & D Ointment, or zinc oxide cream. Apply cream only to dry, unbroken skin. Discontinue creams if a rash develops or they appear to slow healing.
- Try another brand of disposable diapers. Some babies tolerate one kind better than another. Unscented, non-coloured diapers may be less irritating to the skin.
- Avoid bulky or multi-layered diapers.
- Try changing detergents if the rash does not clear.

When to Call a Health Professional

- If the diaper rash becomes very red, raw, or sore-looking, or if it has blisters, pus, peeling areas, or crusty patches.
- If the rash is mainly in the skin creases, because this may indicate a yeast infection.
- If a significant rash lasts longer than 3 days.

Diarrhea and Vomiting

Diarrhea and vomiting may be caused by viral stomach flu or by eating unusual kinds or amounts of food. An infant's developing digestive system sometimes will not tolerate large amounts of juice, fruit, or even milk. Breast-fed babies are less likely to develop diarrhea.

Stomach flu often starts with vomiting that is followed in a few hours (sometimes 8 to 12 hours or longer) by diarrhea. Sometimes there is no diarrhea.

Infants and young children, especially those younger than age 1, need special attention when they have diarrhea or are vomiting, because they can quickly become dehydrated. Careful observation of the child's appearance and fluid intake can help prevent problems. For diarrhea in children age 12 and older, see Diarrhea on page 120. For vomiting in children age 4 and older, see Nausea and Vomiting on page 129.

Home Treatment

Diarrhea in babies up to 1 year:

- If your baby is breast-fed, breastfeed at more frequent intervals to replace lost fluids.
- If your baby is formula-fed, give small feedings at more frequent intervals to make up for lost fluids.
- Supplement feedings with a children's oral electrolyte solution (such as Pedialyte, Infalyte, or a store brand) only if signs of dehydration develop (see page 118). The amount of electrolyte solution your baby needs depends on his or her weight and degree of dehydration. Call your doctor if your baby shows signs of dehydration.
- You can give the oral electrolyte solution a little at a time in a dropper, spoon, or bottle. For children over 6 months of age, you can improve the taste by adding a pinch of NutraSweet or sugar-free Kool-Aid or Jell-O powder.
- Don't use sports drinks, fruit juice, or soda to treat dehydration. These drinks contain too much sugar and not enough of the minerals (electrolytes) that are being lost. Do not give your baby plain water.
- Don't use oral electrolyte solutions as the sole source of fluid for more than 12 to 24 hours.

- Offer your baby easily digestible solid foods (cereal, strained bananas, mashed potatoes) if he or she was eating them before.
- Protect the diaper area with Desitin, A & D Ointment, or zinc oxide cream. Diaper rash is common after diarrhea.

Diarrhea in children 1 year through 11 years:

- Give 120 ml to 240 ml of a children's oral electrolyte solution, half-strength orange juice, or plain water (if the child is eating food) each hour. Add NutraSweet flavourings if needed. Allow your child to drink as much as he or she wants.
- Don't give your child apple juice, chicken broth, sports drinks, soft drinks, or ginger ale. These drinks do not contain the right mixture of minerals and sugar to restore lost fluids and may make the diarrhea worse.
- Give your child frequent small meals of easily digestible foods (cooked cereal, crackers, mashed potatoes, applesauce, bananas). Avoid foods that contain a lot of sugar. Don't use an electrolyte solution as the sole source of fluids and nutrients for more than 24 hours.

As the child gets better, the stools will become smaller and less frequent. Some types of diarrhea may cause watery stools for 4 to 6 days. Watch for signs of dehydration (see page 118). You can treat the illness at home as long as the child is taking in enough fluids and nutrients, is urinating normal amounts, and seems to be improving. For home treatment of diarrhea in children 12 years and older, see page 120.

Vomiting in babies up to 6 months:

- Do not feed your baby anything for 30 to 60 minutes after he or she has vomited. Watch your baby closely for signs of dehydration.
- Do not give your baby plain water.
- If your baby is breast-fed, offer short but frequent feedings.
- If your baby is formula-fed, switch to an oral electrolyte solution (such as Pedialyte or Infalyte). Offer 15 ml every 10 minutes for the first hour. After the first hour, gradually increase the amount of fluid you offer your baby. You can return to regular feedings once 6 hours have passed without your baby vomiting.

Vomiting in children 7 months through 3 years:

- After 1 hour has passed since your child last vomited, give 30 ml of a clear liquid (not plain water) every 20 minutes for 1 hour. Increase the amount by 90 ml per hour every hour that your child does not vomit. For example, give your child 60 ml of fluid every 20 minutes during the second hour (180 ml total) and 90 ml of fluid every 20 minutes during the third hour (270 ml total). Clear liquids that are safe include children's oral rehydration solution; fruit juice mixed to half strength with water; clear broth; and gelatin dessert.

- Do not use sports drinks (such as Gatorade or Allsport), undiluted fruit juice, or soda. These drinks contain too much sugar. Do not offer plain water or diet soda, because they lack the calories and essential minerals your child needs.
- Offer your child regular foods after 6 hours with no vomiting. Avoid high-fibre foods (such as beans) and foods with a lot of sugar, such as candy or ice cream.

For home treatment of vomiting in children 4 years and older, see page 129.

When to Call a Health Professional

- If vomiting occurs with severe headache, sleepiness, lethargy, or a stiff neck. See Encephalitis and Meningitis on page 201.
- If the diarrhea is bloody, tarry, or dark red.
- If the urine becomes bloody or cola-coloured.
- If there is blood in the vomit.
- If signs of severe dehydration appear (also see page 118):
  - Sunken eyes, no tears, dry mouth and tongue
  - Sunken soft spot (fontanelle) on an infant's head
  - Little or no urine for 8 hours
  - Skin that is doughy or doesn't bounce back when pinched
  - Rapid breathing and heartbeat
  - Sleepiness, lethargy, listlessness, and extreme irritability
- If a child with diarrhea or vomiting refuses to drink or cannot take in enough liquid to replace lost fluids.
- If severe vomiting (vomiting most or all clear liquids and feedings) occurs in an infant younger than 3 months of age. For older children, call if severe vomiting continues:
  - Longer than 4 hours in an infant age 3 to 12 months.
  - 8 hours in a child age 1 to 3 years.
- If occasional vomiting occurs without other symptoms and the child is able to keep fluids down between vomiting episodes. Call if this continues longer than:
  - 1 to 2 days in an infant under 3 months of age.
  - 2 to 4 days in an infant age 3 to 6 months.
  - 1 to 2 weeks in a child age 7 months to 3 years.
- If severe diarrhea (large loose stools every 1 to 2 hours) continues for longer than:
  - 4 hours in an infant under 3 months of age.
  - 8 hours in an infant age 3 to 6 months.
  - 24 hours in a child age 7 months to 11 years.

- If mild to moderate diarrhea continues without obvious cause or other symptoms for longer than:
  - 24 hours in an infant under 3 months of age.
  - 1 to 2 days in an infant age 3 to 6 months.
  - 4 days in a child age 7 months to 11 years.
- If the child has a fever of 38.4°C or higher (taken in the armpit) or a lower fever with diarrhea for more than 12 hours.
- If the child has stomach pain that:
  - Is severe.
  - Is persistent, with frequent vomiting for more than 12 hours but little or no diarrhea.
  - Started several hours before vomiting began and seems like more than just stomach cramps.
  - Is localized to one part of the abdomen, especially the lower right section. See illustration on page 113. This may be difficult to determine in a small child.

Fever

Fever in children is usually defined as an axillary (armpit) temperature of 37.4°C or higher.

For information about taking accurate temperatures in infants and children, see page 402. **All temperatures listed in this section are axillary (armpit) temperatures. Axillary temperatures are the safest for checking for fever in a child.**

In most but not all cases, fever indicates that an illness is present. By itself, a fever is not harmful; in fact, it may help the body fight infections more effectively.

In children, viral infections, such as colds, flu, and chicken pox, can cause high fevers. Flu (see page 199) can cause a high fever for 5 days or longer. Bacterial infections, such as strep throat and ear infections, also cause fevers. Teething does not cause a fever. If a baby is teething and has a fever, other symptoms may be present that need to be evaluated. Body temperature can also rise above normal when an infant is overdressed or in a room that is too warm.

Children tend to run higher fevers than adults do. Although high fevers are uncomfortable, they do not often cause medical problems. Seizures from fever occur only occasionally. See page 280.

There is no medical evidence that fevers from infection can cause brain damage. The body limits a fever caused by infection from going above 40°C. However, heat from an external source (like sunshine on a parked car) can cause the body temperature to go above 40.6°C, and brain damage can occur rapidly.

Home Treatment

It can be hard to know when to call your doctor when your child has a fever, especially during the cold and flu season.

The height of a fever may not be related to the seriousness of the illness. The way your child looks and acts is a better guide than the thermometer is.

Most children will be less active when they have a fever. If your child is comfortable and alert, eating well, drinking enough fluids, urinating normal amounts, and seems to be improving, home treatment is all that is needed.

- Encourage the child to drink extra fluids or suck on frozen fruit pops.
- Dress the child lightly, and do not wrap him or her in blankets.

If the fever is 38°C or higher and your child is uncomfortable:

- Give acetaminophen or ibuprofen. Do not give Aspirin to anyone younger than 20, because of the risk of Reye's syndrome (see page 268).
- Keep encouraging the child to drink extra fluids, and watch for signs of dehydration (see page 118).

When to Call a Health Professional

- If fever occurs with vomiting, severe headache, sleepiness, lethargy, stiff neck, or a bulging soft spot on an infant's head. See Encephalitis and Meningitis on page 201.
- If fever is accompanied by these symptoms:
  - Rapid, difficult breathing.
  - Drooling or inability to swallow.
  - Purple rash that does not lighten when you press on it.
  - Vomiting, diarrhea, and stomach pain (see page 275).
  - Signs of dehydration (see page 118).
  - Unexplained skin rash (see page 264 for common childhood illnesses that cause rashes).
  - Ear pain (babies often pull at painful ears). See Ear Infections on page 225.
  - Pain when urinating (crying when urinating), not caused by painful diaper rash.
  - New swelling, pain, redness, or warmth in one or more joints.
  - Any unusual or severe pain.
- If an infant younger than 3 months of age has a fever of 37.4°C or higher (taken in the armpit).
- If a child age 3 months to 3 years has a fever (taken in the armpit) of:
  - 39.5°C or higher.
  - 39°C or higher that does not come down after 4 to 6 hours of home treatment.
  - 38° to 39°C for more than 12 hours.
  - 37° to 38°C for more than 24 to 48 hours.

- If the child has a fever and seems sicker than you would expect from a viral illness such as a cold or the flu.
- If the child becomes delirious or has hallucinations.
- If the child's fever began after he or she took a new medication.

For fever in children age 4 and older, see page 197.

Fever Seizures

Fever seizures are uncontrolled muscle spasms that can happen while a child's temperature is rapidly rising. Sometimes the seizure occurs before you are even aware that the child has a fever. Once a child's fever has reached a high temperature, the risk of a seizure is probably over.

A child having a fever seizure may lose consciousness. The child's muscles will stiffen, and his or her teeth will clench. Then the child's arms and legs will start to jerk. The child's eyes may roll back, and he or she may stop breathing for a few seconds. The child might also vomit, urinate, or pass stools. Seizures usually last 1 to 5 minutes.

Although frightening, fever seizures in children age 6 months to 5 years are seldom serious and do not cause harm. Four to 5 percent of children in this age group are prone to fever seizures. About 30 percent of children who have a fever seizure will have another one in the future.

Home Treatment

During a seizure:

- Try to stay calm, because that will help calm the child.
- Protect the child from injury. Ease the child to the floor, or hold a very small child face down on your lap. Do not restrain the child.
- Turn the child onto his or her side. This will help clear the mouth of any vomit or saliva and will keep the airway open so the child can breathe.
- Do not put anything in the child's mouth to prevent tongue biting, because it may injure the child.
- Time the length of the seizure, if possible.

After a seizure:

- If the child is having difficulty breathing, turn his or her head to the side and, using your finger, gently clear the mouth of any vomit or saliva so the child can breathe.
- Check for injuries.
- Give acetaminophen or ibuprofen and lukewarm sponge baths if the fever (taken in the armpit) is 38°C or higher and your child is uncomfortable. Do not give Aspirin to anyone younger than 20, because of the risk of Reye's syndrome.

- Put the child in a cool room to sleep. Drowsiness is common following a seizure. Check the child often. The child should return to his or her normal behaviour and activity level within 60 minutes after the seizure.

When to Call a Health Professional

Call 911 or other emergency services:

- If the child stops breathing for longer than 30 seconds or has difficulty breathing. Begin rescue breathing (see page 68).
- If a seizure lasts longer than 3 minutes, or if a second seizure occurs.

Call your health professional:

- If the child is younger than 6 months of age; if the child is 5 years or older; or if the seizure only affects one side of the body.
- If fever occurs with vomiting, severe headache, sleepiness, lethargy, stiff neck, or a bulging soft spot on an infant's head. See Encephalitis and Meningitis on page 201.
- If a seizure occurs without fever.
- If it is the child's first seizure, or if you haven't discussed with your doctor what to do if there is another one.

See page 279 for information on when to call a doctor because of fever.

Impetigo

Impetigo is a bacterial infection that is much more common in children than in adults. It often starts when a small cut or scratch becomes infected. Symptoms are oozing, honey-coloured, crusty sores that often appear on the face between the upper lip and nose, especially after a cold. Scratching the sores may spread impetigo to other parts of the body.

Prevention

- Wash all scratches and sores with soap and water.
- If your child has a runny nose, keep the area between the child's upper lip and nose clean to prevent infection.
- Keep your child's fingernails short and clean.

Home Treatment

Small areas of impetigo may respond well to prompt home treatment.

- Remove crusts by soaking the area in warm water (use a warm face cloth for the face) for 15 to 20 minutes; then scrub gently with a face cloth and antibacterial soap. Pat dry gently; do not rub. Repeat several times a day.
- Apply an antibiotic ointment. Cover the area with gauze taped well away from the sores. This will help keep the infection from spreading and prevent scratching.

- Adult men with impetigo should shave around the sores, not over them, and use a clean blade daily. Do not use a shaving brush.
- To prevent spreading the infection, do not share towels, face cloths, or bathwater.

When to Call a Health Professional

- If impetigo covers a total area larger than 5 cm in diameter.
- If impetigo does not improve after 3 to 4 days of home treatment, or if any new infected areas appear. Your doctor may prescribe an antibiotic.
- If there is facial swelling or tenderness, especially near the nose and lips.
- If other signs of infection develop. See page 100.

Pinworms

Pinworms are tiny, thread-like worms that infect the digestive tract. Pinworms are most common in school-age children, although anyone can become infected. The worms live in the upper end of the large intestine, near the appendix, and travel to the outside of the anus to lay their eggs.

The egg-laying almost always occurs at night and usually causes the child to scratch the anal area. When the child later sucks a thumb or licks a finger, the eggs are ingested and the cycle begins again. The eggs are very sticky and can survive on clothing and bedding for days, where they can be picked up by other family members.

Anal itching, especially at night, is the most common symptom of pinworm infection. If the infection is severe, there may also be loss of appetite, itching in the genital area, and pain when urinating. In many cases, pinworm infection does not cause any symptoms.

Prevention

Pinworms affect many families and are hard to avoid if you have young children. Teach children to wash their hands after using the toilet and before meals.

Follow the home treatment guidelines to prevent reinfection and the spread of pinworms to others.

Home Treatment

- Ask your pharmacist for a non-prescription medication for pinworms. Do not take the medication if you are pregnant and do not give it to a child under 2 years unless your health professional advises you to.
- Treat every child in the house between the ages of 2 and 10. If infection recurs, consider treating everyone in the family who is older than 2.

- On the first day of treatment, wash all underwear, nightclothes, bedding, and towels in hot water and detergent to get rid of any eggs and prevent reinfection. Sanitize toilet and sleeping areas with a strong disinfectant.
- Trim children's fingernails and keep them short.
- Require frequent hand washing, morning showers, and daily changes of pyjamas and underwear.

When to Call a Health Professional

- If a person has symptoms of pinworm infection, but you have not seen any worms. If this is the first infection, it is recommended that a health professional confirm the diagnosis.
- If the pinworm medication causes side effects, such as vomiting or pain.
- If you continue to have symptoms of pinworm infection despite using a non-prescription medication. You may need another round of treatment. Stronger prescription medications are also available.
- If a person who has a pinworm infection develops any of the following:
  - Fever or abdominal pain
  - Redness, tenderness, swelling, or itching in the genital area
  - Pain when urinating

Prickly Heat (Sweat Rash)

Prickly heat, also called heat rash, sweat rash, or miliaria, is a rash of red or pink dots that appears on an infant's head, neck, and shoulders. The dots look like tiny pimples.

Prickly heat often develops when parents dress their baby too warmly, but it can develop in any baby when the weather is hot. An infant should be dressed just as lightly as an adult and will be comfortable at the same temperature. It is normal for a baby's hands and feet to feel cold to the touch.

Prevention

Do not overdress your baby. Place your hand between the baby's shoulder blades. If the skin is hot or moist, the baby is too warm.

Home Treatment

- Dress the baby in as few clothes as possible during hot weather.
- Keep the baby's skin cool and dry.
- Keep the baby's sleeping area cool.

When to Call a Health Professional

- If the rash looks infected or lasts longer than 3 days. See Signs of Infection on page 100.
- If the infant looks sick.
- If prickly heat is accompanied by a fever of 37.4°C (taken in the armpit) in an infant younger than

3 months of age and the fever doesn't come down within 20 minutes after you remove some of the infant's clothing.

Roseola

Roseola (roseola infantum) is a mild viral illness that often starts with a sudden high fever (38.4° to 39.5°C, taken in the armpit) and irritability. The fever lasts 2 to 3 days. As the fever drops, a rosy pink rash appears on the torso, neck, and arms. The rash may last 1 to 2 days.

Since the fever is quite high and may come on quickly, fever seizures may occur (see page 280).

Roseola is most common in children from 6 months to 2 years of age. It is rare after age 4.

Home Treatment

- If the child has a fever over 38°C (taken in the armpit) and is uncomfortable, give acetaminophen or ibuprofen. Do not give Aspirin to anyone younger than 20, because of the risk of Reye's syndrome (see page 268).
- Give the child lots of liquids.
- If a fever seizure occurs, see page 280.

When to Call a Health Professional

See When to Call a Health Professional on page 279.

Fifth Disease

Another common childhood illness that causes a rash is erythema infectiosum, or "fifth disease." The main symptoms are a red rash on the face that looks like slapped cheeks and a lacy, pink rash on the backs of the arms and legs, torso, and buttocks. There may be a low fever. The rash may come and go for several weeks in response to changes in temperature and sunlight.

A child with fifth disease is most contagious the week before the rash appears. Once the rash has developed, the child is no longer contagious.

Home treatment for fifth disease consists of keeping the child comfortable and watching for signs that a more serious illness is present (fever over 38°C, taken in the armpit; child seems very sick).

Fifth disease is harmless in children, but it poses a slight risk to developing fetuses. Pregnant women should avoid exposure if possible. Contact your obstetrician if you are exposed to a child with fifth disease or develop a rash similar to the one described above while you are pregnant.

I live with the expectation that life is not fragile;
that if I push, it will not break.
Andrew Sullivan

14

Chronic Conditions

Most of the conditions described in this book are acute illnesses, which means that they get better after a short while. Chronic conditions, on the other hand, last long periods of time or come and go, often for the rest of your life. Having a chronic disease does not mean you can no longer enjoy the good things in life. Chronic diseases may not be curable, but they can often be controlled.

This chapter covers diabetes, high blood pressure, high cholesterol, and thyroid problems. Many other conditions that can be chronic—allergies, back pain, depression, headaches—are covered elsewere in the book. Use the index to find what you need.

Diabetes

During digestion the starches and sugars in the food you eat are converted to glucose, a sugar that your body uses for energy. Insulin is a hormone produced by the pancreas that helps control the amount of glucose in your blood. Without insulin, your body cannot use or store glucose, so too much sugar stays in your blood. Over a long period of time, high blood sugar levels may damage blood vessels and nerves, increasing your risk for problems that can affect the eyes, heart, kidneys, legs, and feet.

Type 1 diabetes occurs when the pancreas makes little or no insulin. Type 1 diabetes usually develops in childhood or adolescence but can develop at any age. People with type 1 diabetes must give themselves insulin shots every day.

Type 2 diabetes occurs when the pancreas cannot make enough insulin or when the body does not use insulin properly. Many people with type 2 diabetes are able to control their blood sugar by getting regular exercise; eating a healthy diet; maintaining a healthy weight; and frequently testing their blood sugar.

Some may need insulin shots or oral medications to keep their blood sugar levels within a safe range.

Risk factors for type 2 diabetes include:

- Having a family history of type 2 diabetes.
- Being age 45 or over (though the disease can develop at any age).
- Being overweight (20 percent more than your healthy weight) or having a large percentage of body fat in the abdominal area.
- Having a physically inactive lifestyle.
- Having high blood pressure (above 140/90). See page 290.
- Having a below-normal HDL cholesterol (the "good" cholesterol) level or an above-normal triglyceride level. See page 292.
- Being of African, Hispanic, Pacific Island, Asian, or First Nations and Aboriginal descent.
- Having a history of diabetes during pregnancy (gestational diabetes) or having given birth to a baby over 4 kg (9 lb).
- Having prediabetes (blood sugar levels above normal, but not as high as diabetic levels).

The symptoms of diabetes vary from person to person and are common to many conditions. A person may believe that his or her symptoms are related to an illness or to aging, not diabetes. Symptoms include:

- Dry mouth and increased thirst.
- Frequent urination (especially at night).
- Increased appetite.
- Unexplained weight loss.
- Weakness, tiredness, and dizziness.
- Frequent skin infections and slow-healing wounds.
- Recurrent vaginal yeast infections.
- Recurrent oral yeast infections, such as thrush.
- Blurry vision.
- Tingling or numbness in the hands or feet.

Your doctor needs to do a blood test to accurately diagnose diabetes.

Complications of Diabetes

Complications of diabetes are caused by the prolonged exposure of the body to high blood sugar levels. Some people develop complications early in the course of the disease; others develop them later. A person who develops complications of diabetes may have only one problem or several. By carefully controlling your blood sugar levels early in the course of the disease and practising other healthy habits, you may reduce your risk of the following complications of diabetes:

- Heart disease and problems with circulation in the feet and legs (peripheral vascular disease)
- High blood pressure
- Stroke

- Nerve damage (neuropathy), which can decrease or completely block the movement of nerve impulses or messages through organs, limbs, and other parts of the body
- Impaired ability to fight infection and heal wounds
- Foot ulcers and other foot problems
- Joint and connective tissue disease
- Kidney disease (nephropathy)
- Eye disease (retinopathy) and other eye problems
- Gum disease

Prevention

At this time, there is no known way to prevent type 1 diabetes.

The risk for developing type 2 diabetes runs in families and increases with age. However, even if you have a history of type 2 diabetes in your family, you may be able to prevent or delay its onset by maintaining a healthy body weight and exercising regularly. If you are at risk for diabetes, ask your doctor whether there are medications or lifestyle changes that can reduce your likelihood of developing the disease.

Home Treatment

- If insulin or other medications are prescribed to keep your blood sugar within a safe range, take them as directed. If you improve your diet and exercise regularly, you may need less medicine. Check with your doctor before making any changes in your medication.
- Eat a healthy diet to help keep your blood sugar within a safe range and to maintain a healthy weight. Pay special attention to eating low-fat foods, and follow the other diet recommendations in the Nutrition chapter starting on page 351. Talk to a registered dietitian if you need help.
- Get regular aerobic exercise to help regulate your blood sugar level, reduce your risk for heart disease, and control your weight. Work closely with your doctor to determine how your activity level affects your blood sugar levels and medication needs. If you have chest pain or pressure while exercising, stop exercising and call your health professional immediately.
- Check and record your blood sugar level as often as directed by your doctor. This record will help you understand how your body reacts to different foods and exercise, so you can keep your blood sugar level in the safe range. It may help you to keep your blood sugar level within the safe range if you track the following daily:
    - The time and content of each meal you eat
    - The kind and amount of exercise you get
    - How tired or energetic you feel

Diabetic Emergencies		
	Low Blood Sugar (Hypoglycemia)	**High Blood Sugar (Hyperglycemia)**
Who can be affected?	Those who inject insulin or take certain oral hypoglycemic medications	Any person who has diabetes
How does it occur?	Rapidly, over minutes or hours	Gradually, over hours or days
Blood sugar range?	Less than 4 mmol/L*	More than 10 mmol/L*
Symptoms?	Fatigue, shakiness Headache Hunger Cold, clammy skin; sweating Sudden double vision or blurred vision Pounding heart, confusion, irritability; person may appear drunk Loss of consciousness	Frequent urination Intense thirst Dry skin Blurred vision Signs of ketoacidosis: rapid breathing with fruity-smelling breath Loss of consciousness
What to do?	If the person loses consciousness, **call 911 or other emergency services**. If the person is conscious, have the person eat or drink something that contains sugar. If symptoms don't improve, call your doctor immediately.	If there are signs of ketoacidosis, call the doctor immediately. If the person loses consciousness, **call 911 or other emergency services.**
Do not give an unconscious person anything to eat or drink. If you have been taught how to give glucagon to a person who is having a diabetic emergency, do so. Always make sure the glucagon kit has not expired. If you are unsure about the cause of the diabetic emergency in a person who uses medication, have the person eat or drink something that contains sugar (glucose tablets, hard candy, honey or sugar dissolved in water, fruit juice, or a soft drink with sugar).		
**May vary for individual people. If you have diabetes, ask your doctor what your safe blood sugar range is.*		

- If you are age 30 or older, talk to your doctor about taking a low-dose Aspirin every day to help prevent heart attack, stroke, and other large blood vessel disease.
- Take good care of your feet, and check them daily for blisters, cracks, and sores. Diabetes may damage nerves and reduce blood flow to your feet, increasing your risk for infection while making you less likely to notice a problem.
- Have an eye examination every year. Eye changes caused by diabetes often have no symptoms until they are quite advanced. Diabetic eye disease can cause blindness. Early detection and treatment of diabetic eye disease may slow its progress and save your sight.
- Have regular medical checkups. Talk to your doctor about how often you need them.
- Wear a medical alert bracelet in case of an emergency.
- Attend a diabetes education program to learn more about how to take good care of yourself.

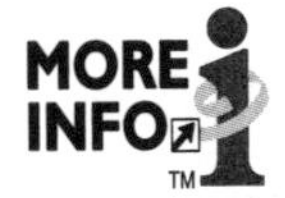

Believe that you can live a healthy life with diabetes. Controlling diabetes requires making significant, long-term lifestyle changes that may seem overwhelming at first. However, if you adopt a "take charge" attitude about your health and focus on making one change at a time, you are more likely to be successful. Work with your doctor to develop a treatment plan that fits your needs.

The Canadian Diabetes Association, 1-800-BANTING (1-800-226-8464), and the National Aboriginal Diabetes Association, 1-877-232-6232, are good resources for more information about diabetes.

When to Call a Health Professional

Call 911 or other emergency services if a person with diabetes is losing consciousness or becomes unconscious.

Call your health professional:

- If these signs of unusually high blood sugar develop in a person who has diabetes:
  - Frequent urination
  - Intense thirst
  - Blurry vision
  - Weakness, drowsiness
  - Fast breathing
  - Fruity-smelling breath
- If these signs of low blood sugar occur often or last longer than 15 minutes after a person who has diabetes has eaten something that contains sugar:
  - Sweating
  - Fatigue, weakness, shakiness, nausea

- Extreme hunger
- Blurry vision, dizziness, headache
- Rapid heartbeat, anxiousness
- Confusion, irritability, slurred speech

- If your blood sugar level continues to fall outside the range your doctor has recommended.
- If you have been diagnosed with diabetes and are sick, particularly if you are unable to eat or are vomiting.
- If you have diabetes and you suspect or know that you are pregnant.
- To get a blood sugar test if you suspect that you have diabetes but have not yet been diagnosed.

High Blood Pressure

Blood pressure is a measurement of the force of blood against the walls of the arteries. Blood pressure readings include two numbers, for example, 130/80. The first number in the reading is called the systolic pressure. It is the force that blood exerts on the artery walls as the heart contracts. The second number in the reading is the diastolic pressure. It is the force that blood exerts on the artery walls between heartbeats, when the heart is at rest.

If your blood pressure readings are consistently above 140 systolic and 90 diastolic, you have high blood pressure (hypertension). If your blood pressure readings are 120 to 139 systolic or 80 to 89 diastolic, you are more likely to develop high blood pressure. If you have high blood pressure or are at increased risk for it, treatment begins with the lifestyle changes outlined in Prevention.

Despite what a lot of people think, high blood pressure usually does not cause any symptoms. Often called the "silent killer," it increases your risk for heart attack, stroke, and kidney or eye damage. Your risk of developing these problems increases as your blood pressure rises.

Risk factors for high blood pressure and its complications include:

- Smoking.
- Being overweight.
- Having a family history of high blood pressure.
- Being of African descent.
- Having an inactive lifestyle.
- Drinking too much alcohol.
- Having too much salt or not enough potassium, calcium, or magnesium in the diet.
- Using certain medications, including steroids, decongestants, and anti-inflammatory drugs, on a regular basis.

Prevention

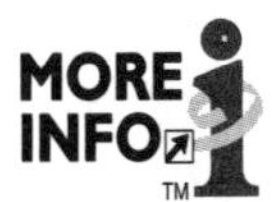

Changes in your lifestyle may help you prevent high blood pressure or help you lower your blood pressure if it's too high.

- Maintain a healthy weight. This is especially important if you tend to put on weight around the waist rather than in the hips and thighs. Losing even 4.5 kg can help you lower your blood pressure.
- Be physically active for at least 30 minutes on most days of the week. This will help you lower your blood pressure (and may also help you lose weight).
- Drink alcohol only in moderation.
- Use salt moderately. Too much salt in the diet can be a problem for some people who have high blood pressure and are also salt-sensitive.
- Make sure you get enough potassium, calcium, and magnesium in your diet. Eating plenty of fruits (such as bananas and oranges), vegetables, legumes, whole grains, and low-fat dairy products will ensure that you get enough of these minerals.
- Reduce the saturated fat in your diet. Saturated fat is found in animal products (milk, cheese, and meat). Limiting these foods will help you lose weight and also lower your risk for coronary artery disease. See page 355.
- Stop using tobacco products. Tobacco use increases your risk for heart attack and stroke. See page 25 for tips to help you quit.
- Learn how to check your blood pressure at home. See page 413.

Home Treatment

- Follow the prevention tips above even more closely if you already have high blood pressure or if your blood pressure is 120 to 139 systolic or 80 to 89 diastolic.
- Take any prescribed blood pressure medications exactly as directed, and see your doctor at least once a year. Realize that these medications help control high blood pressure but do not cure it. If you stop taking them, your blood pressure may go back up.
- If you are taking blood pressure medication, talk to your doctor before taking decongestants or anti-inflammatory drugs, because they can raise your blood pressure.

When to Call a Health Professional

- Call immediately if you have high blood pressure and:
  - Your blood pressure rises suddenly.
  - Your blood pressure is 180/110 or higher.
  - You have a sudden, severe headache.
  - You develop chest pain or discomfort.

- Call if your blood pressure is higher than 140/90 on two or more occasions (taken at home or in a community screening program). If one blood pressure reading is high, have another taken by a health professional to verify the first reading.
- Call if you develop uncomfortable or disturbing side effects from any medication taken for high blood pressure.

High Cholesterol

Cholesterol is a fat-like substance that is produced by your body and is also found in foods that come from animal sources (meat and dairy products, poultry, and fish). Your body's cells need cholesterol to function properly. However, excess cholesterol in the blood can build up inside your arteries, causing them to narrow (atherosclerosis). Atherosclerosis is the starting point for most heart and circulation problems.

Good and Bad Cholesterol

Cholesterol travels through your bloodstream attached to protein, in a combination called a lipoprotein. Two lipoproteins are the main carriers of cholesterol: low-density lipoprotein (LDL) and high-density lipoprotein (HDL). High-density lipoproteins contain more protein than fat.

- LDL ("bad cholesterol") carries cholesterol from the liver to other parts of the body. Under certain conditions, LDL cholesterol can build up on the walls of the arteries. Having a high LDL cholesterol level increases your risk for coronary artery disease (CAD), heart attack, and stroke.
- HDL ("good cholesterol") helps clear LDL cholesterol from the body by picking up cholesterol from the bloodstream and taking it back to the liver for disposal. Increasing your HDL cholesterol level may reduce your risk for heart disease, stroke, and peripheral vascular disease.

Triglycerides are another type of fat that can be found in the bloodstream. A high triglyceride level may increase your risk of coronary artery disease and stroke.

Cholesterol Screening

You and your doctor can determine the screening schedule that is best for you based on your risk factors for coronary artery disease. Most healthy adults who are not at high risk should have their cholesterol tested every 5 years. Another recommendation is to start cholesterol screening at age 35 for men and age 45 for women.

If your total cholesterol is high, or if you have any of the following **risk factors for coronary artery disease**, you may want to have your cholesterol checked more often:

- Having a family history of early heart attack (before age 55 in father or brother; before age 65 in mother or sister)

- Being a cigarette smoker
- Having high blood pressure (over 140/90) or taking high blood pressure medication
- Having diabetes
- Having a below-normal HDL level or an above-normal triglyceride level in a previous cholesterol test

If your total cholesterol is over 4.14 mmol/L and you don't know what your HDL and LDL levels are, more extensive testing can help you better estimate your actual risk.

How to Reduce Your Cholesterol

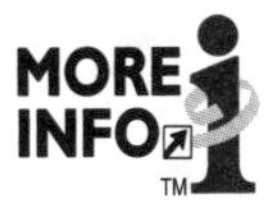

For most people, regular exercise and a diet low in saturated fat are enough to lower cholesterol. People who have very high cholesterol, diabetes, or coronary artery disease (or who are at very high risk for CAD) may need medication as well as exercise and a low-fat diet to lower their cholesterol.

What Do the Numbers Mean?

There are guidelines doctors rely on to evaluate your cholesterol numbers and assess your risk for heart disease. The importance of the numbers varies from person to person, depending on whether a person has additional risk factors for heart disease or actually has heart disease. The following ranges apply to people who are at average risk for heart disease. The numbers are given in mmol/L.

Total cholesterol

Desirable: Less than 4.14

Borderline high: 4.15 to 6.19

High: 6.20 and above

HDL cholesterol

High (desirable): 1.55 and above

Acceptable: 1.04 to 1.54

Low (not desirable): Less than 1.04

LDL cholesterol

Optimal: 2.5 and below

Near optimal: 2.6 to 3.5

Borderline high: 3.6 to 4.0

High: 4.1 to 4.9

Very high: 5.0 and above

Triglycerides

Normal: Less than 1.7

Moderately high: 1.7 to 6.0

Very high: Above 6.0

To reduce your cholesterol:

- Eat less total fat, especially saturated fat. Follow the guidelines for eating less fat on page 355.
- Attend a nutrition workshop or consult a registered dietitian to learn ways to lower your saturated fat intake to 7 percent or less of total calories and your dietary cholesterol to less than 300 mg per day. Your total fat intake can be up to 30 percent of total calories, as long as most of it is unsaturated fat.
- Eat at least 5 servings of fruits and vegetables each day.
- Eat 2 to 3 servings (113 to 170 g) of baked or broiled fish per week. The safety and value of fish oil supplements is not yet known.
- Eat more soluble fibre (fruit, dry beans and peas, cereal grains). See page 354.
- Exercise more. Exercise increases your HDL cholesterol level and may lower your LDL level.
- Quit smoking. Smoking increases the risk of heart attack and stroke, even in people with low cholesterol.
- Lose weight. Losing even 2.5 to 4.5 kg can lower triglyceride levels and raise HDL levels. In some people, LDL levels may fall as well.

Thyroid Problems

The thyroid is a butterfly-shaped gland that wraps around the windpipe. It functions as a kind of "throttle" for the body, regulating your metabolism. As the thyroid gland releases more hormones, the body runs faster. As thyroid hormone levels decrease, the body slows down. The pituitary gland in the brain controls the thyroid and usually keeps the level of thyroid hormones fairly constant. The pituitary gland is in turn controlled by the hypothalamus, another area of the brain.

Thyroid problems are most common among older people but can occur at any age. The symptoms may develop so slowly that they go unnoticed.

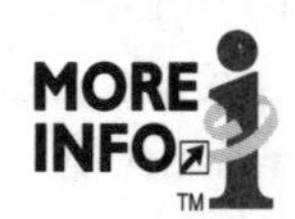

Thyroid hormone tests can detect changes in the amount of thyroid hormone in your body, even before you have noticed symptoms. If you have a family history of thyroid problems or have been exposed to radiation, either at work or as part of medical treatment, ask your doctor whether you need a thyroid test.

The thyroid gland can cause problems in two ways: by producing too much thyroid hormone or by producing too little of it. Symptoms of too much thyroid hormone, or **hyperthyroidism**, include:

- Weight loss with or without loss of appetite.
- Increased discomfort in warm temperatures.
- Soft stools or diarrhea.
- Itchy, irritated, and puffy eyes.
- Hair loss.
- Rapid, pounding, or irregular heart rhythm.
- Shortness of breath, even when resting.
- Night sweats.
- Difficulty sleeping.
- Chronic fatigue and lack of energy.
- Progressive muscle weakness, especially in the large muscles of the legs.
- Difficulty concentrating, mood swings, or nervousness.
- An enlarged thyroid gland, or goiter, which looks like a swollen area in the throat.

These symptoms are often confused with those caused by other diseases. Graves' disease, the most common cause of hyperthyroidism, occurs when the immune system makes the thyroid gland overactive. When drug treatment for hyperthyroidism is complete, thyroid function may return to normal. However, some people require radioactive iodine treatment to destroy part of the thyroid gland in order to cure hyperthyroidism. In rare cases, surgery to remove part or all of the thyroid gland may be necessary.

Symptoms of too little thyroid hormone, or **hypothyroidism**, include:

- Chronic fatigue, sluggishness, and weakness.
- Memory loss, difficulty concentrating, or depression.
- Inability to tolerate cold temperatures.
- Dry skin, brittle nails, and dry, coarse hair; hair loss.
- Constipation.
- Unexplained weight gain.
- Slowed heartbeat and reflexes.
- An enlarged thyroid gland, or goiter.
- Swelling of the arms, hands, legs, and feet, and facial puffiness, particularly around the eyes.
- Hoarseness.

Treatment of hypothyroidism is quite simple. Your doctor can prescribe a medication that acts like natural thyroid hormone in your body. You will probably have to take the medication for the rest of your life. You will need regular blood tests (usually once a year) to make sure your medication does not need to be adjusted.

Home Treatment

If you have a prescription for daily thyroid medications, take them every day.

When to Call a Health Professional

- If a person with **hyperthyroidism** develops any of the following symptoms:
  - Fever.
  - Extreme weakness or fatigue.
  - Rapid or irregular heartbeat.
  - Heavy sweating or inability to tolerate warm temperatures.
  - Restlessness, agitation, or delirium.
  - Abnormally high or low blood pressure.
  - Unexpected weight loss.
- If the following symptoms develop and persist, especially in a person who has been diagnosed with **hypothyroidism**:
  - Extreme intolerance of cold temperatures.
  - Weakness and fatigue.
  - Dry skin, brittle nails, or hair loss.
  - Constipation.
  - Memory problems, depression, or difficulty concentrating.
- If you suspect that you have a thyroid function problem.
- If you have a family history of thyroid problems or a history of radiation exposure, especially in the head or neck area.

Amyotrophic Lateral Sclerosis (ALS)

Also known as Lou Gehrig's disease, ALS is a progressive wasting away of certain nerve cells of the brain and spinal column. These cells, called motor neurons, control the muscles that allow movement.

ALS is a disabling, usually fatal disease. It may progress over a period of months or years. As muscles throughout the body weaken, walking, speaking, eating, swallowing, breathing, and other basic functions become more difficult. These problems can lead to injury, illness, and other complications, such as pneumonia or heart failure.

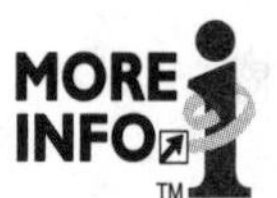

Treatment can help maintain strength and independence, manage symptoms, and avoid complications for as long as possible. How aggressively to treat the problems caused by ALS is a personal decision. Regardless of your choices, your comfort can be maintained. It is important to discuss treatment options and share any concerns with your doctor.

Behind every successful woman is herself.
New American proverb

15

Women's Health

This chapter focuses on health problems that are unique to women. If you are looking for general guidelines for making healthy lifestyle choices to prevent illness and injury, see Living a Healthy Life starting on page 15. Specific tips for developing a fitness plan, eating a healthy diet, maintaining a healthy body weight, managing stress, and preventing sexually transmitted diseases are included in other chapters. Use the index to find the information you need.

Breast Health

Breast cancer is the second leading cause of cancer deaths in women. The good news is that breast cancer can often be cured if it is detected early. There are three methods of early detection: mammography, clinical breast examination, and breast self-examination.

One of the most important risk factors for breast cancer is age. The risk goes up significantly after age 50. Women younger than 50 are at lower risk for breast cancer. However, if your mother or a sister had breast cancer before menopause, talk with your doctor about starting mammography and other screenings before age 40.

Mammography

A mammogram is a breast X-ray that can reveal breast tumours that are too small to be detected by breast self-examination or a clinical breast examination.

Studies have shown that mammograms save lives. In women over 50, mammograms reduce breast cancer death rates by up to one-third. Mammograms reduce breast cancer deaths in women under 50 as well, but the total number of deaths prevented is small because breast cancer is rare before age 50.

Breast Pain

Breast pain is common and, fortunately, is rarely a serious problem. Many women's breasts become achy, heavy, or sore a week or so before their menstrual periods start. This is called cyclic pain. It is caused by hormonal changes that occur during the menstrual cycle. The symptoms usually go away at the end of a woman's period. Cyclic breast pain usually ends after a woman completes menopause.

Non-cyclic breast pain, which is not associated with a woman's periods, is usually described as sharp or burning. This pain usually occurs on one side only; it may go up toward the armpit; and it may come and go. Pain in one spot that does not go away should be checked by a health professional.

Stress, estrogen therapy, and the use of certain medications can make breast pain worse. Sore breasts can also be a sign of pregnancy.

If breast pain occurs with other premenstrual symptoms (such as bloating and weight gain), avoid salty foods before your period starts, and try taking 400 mg of magnesium daily. There is some evidence that taking evening primrose oil reduces breast pain. Wearing a more supportive bra, especially when exercising, may also help.

If pain or any other changes in your breasts concern you, talk to your health professional. If you are over 40 or have a family history of breast cancer, discuss breast cancer screening with your doctor.

Your doctor may tell you how often he or she would like you to get a mammogram. The following intervals are recommended for women in BC who are not at increased risk for breast cancer:

- Younger than 40: mammograms not usually done for routine screening.
- Age 40 to 49: mammograms every 1 to 2 years or according to a schedule agreed upon by the woman and her doctor.
- Age 50 and older: mammograms every 1 to 2 years.

Yearly mammograms are recommended for any woman who has had cancer in one breast. If you have a female relative (especially your mother or a sister) who had breast cancer before menopause, talk to your doctor about when to start and how often to have mammograms.

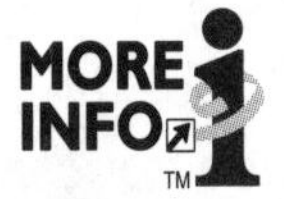

Getting all the facts and thinking about your own needs and values will help you make a wise decision about mammography. Always see your health professional if you find a lump or change in your breast.

To schedule an appointment for a routine mammogram, call the Screening Mammography Program of BC at 1-800-663-9203.

Preparing for a Mammogram

- Arrange to have your mammogram 1 to 2 weeks after your period ends.

MORE INFO For more information, see the back cover.

- Do not wear deodorant, perfume, powder, or lotion, because they can affect the quality of the X-ray.
- Wear clothing that allows you to easily undress from the waist up.
- If you had a previous mammogram at a different facility, have it sent before your test or bring it with you on the day of your mammogram.

Clinical Breast Examination

During a clinical breast examination, a doctor or nurse looks at your breasts and gently feels them for lumps or other unusual changes. During the examination, the doctor or nurse can also teach you how to examine your breasts yourself.

A clinical breast examination is recommended every 1 to 2 years after age 40. A clinical breast examination is also done whenever a woman has symptoms indicating that there may be a problem with her breasts.

Breast Self-Examination

The breast self-examination is a simple way for you to learn what is normal for your breasts and how to notice changes in them. It is useful for finding lumps (most of which are not cancerous), cysts, and other noncancerous problems. Once you know what your breasts normally look and feel like, you will be better able to recognize any changes in your breasts and know when to get help early instead of waiting until your next checkup. A self-examination is not a substitute for a mammogram or a clinical breast examination by a health professional.

Few women have breasts that match exactly. It is normal for one breast to be slightly larger than the other. Most women's breasts have some lumpiness or places where the tissue feels thicker. If the lumpiness is the same in both breasts, it is probably normal. If you find a lump that feels different or much harder than the rest of your breast tissue, or if you find anything else that worries you, have it checked by your health professional.

Establish a regular time each month to examine your breasts. A good time is a few days after your period ends, when your breasts are less likely to be swollen or sore. Women who do not menstruate can examine their breasts at any time of the month.

The breast self-examination takes place in two stages. Ask your health professional for help in learning the technique.

Stage 1: In front of the mirror

Stand in front of a well-lighted mirror and examine your breasts carefully: first with your arms at your sides; then with your hands pushing firmly on your hips to tighten your chest muscles; then with your arms raised overhead; and finally while bending forward (arms at sides).

Look for changes in the shape of your breasts (indentations, flattening, or puckering of the skin) as you move your arms. Both breasts should change in the same way. Also check to see if either nipple appears to be turning inward when it never did before, and look for changes in the skin of the nipple. Squeeze each nipple carefully between your thumb and index finger to feel for lumps. A milky discharge that happens only when you squeeze your breast or nipple is usually normal.

Stage 2: Lying down

To examine your right breast, place a pillow or folded towel under your right shoulder. Put your right arm under your head and use your left hand to examine your breast. Using the pads of your fingers (not just the fingertips), move your fingers in coin-sized circles over your skin, and push down gently to feel for lumps, thickening, or changes of any kind. Be sure to feel all of your breast, including the nipple, as well as your breastbone, the area under the breast, and the armpit.

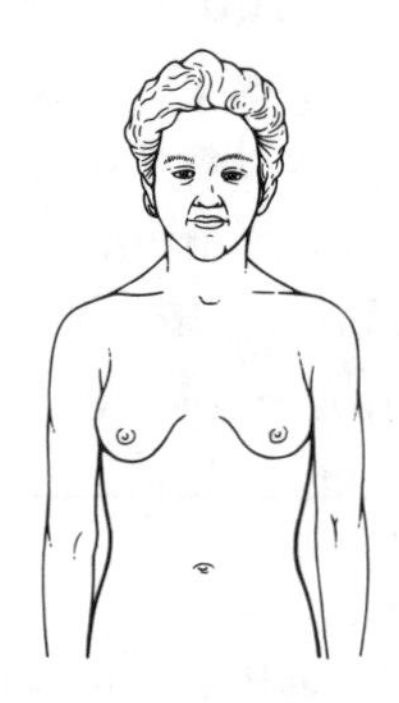

Look at your breasts in a mirror.

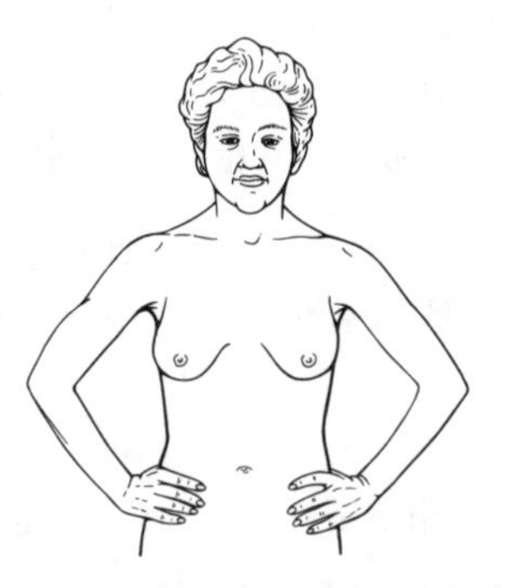

Put your hands on your hips.

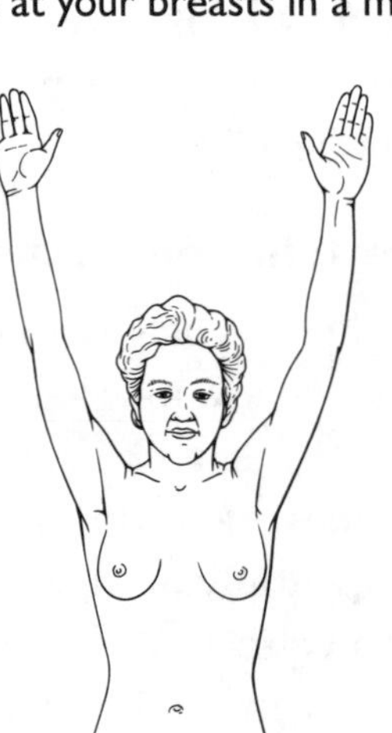

Raise your arms.

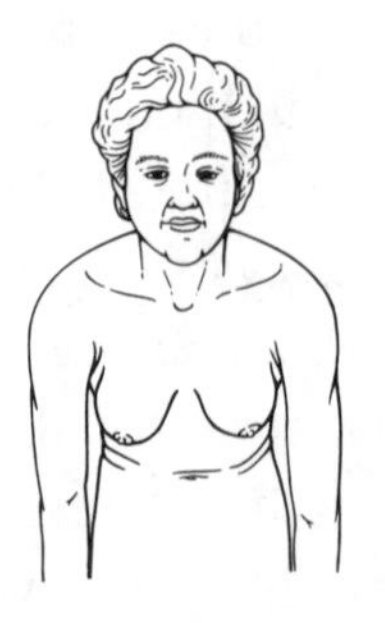

Bend forward, still looking in the mirror.

Move the pillow or towel to the left shoulder. Use your right hand to examine your left breast.

Instead of lying down, some women like to do the second stage of the examination while standing in the shower. If your skin is wet and soapy, it may be easier to feel your breast tissue. Stand with one arm raised (hand behind your head) and feel the breast with your other hand.

Prevention and Early Detection of Breast Cancer

- Limit alcohol to 1 drink per day. Moderate to heavy drinking increases your risk for breast cancer.
- Eat a low-fat diet. Although it has not been proven that a diet low in fat will prevent cancer, women in populations that consume a high-fat diet are more likely to die of breast cancer than those in populations that consume a low-fat diet. Cut down on fried foods and high-fat meats and dairy products. Choose lean meats and low-fat dairy products instead, and eat plenty of fruits and vegetables.
- Have a clinical breast examination every 1 to 2 years after age 40.
- If you are age 40 to 49, discuss an appropriate mammogram schedule with your doctor (or see page 298). If you are age 50 or older, have a mammogram every 1 to 2 years.
- If you have a strong family history of breast cancer, talk with your doctor about approaches that may lower your risk.

When to Call a Health Professional

- If you find a lump in your breast or armpit that concerns you, particularly if it is hard and unlike other tissue in your breasts.
- If you find a breast lump and you are past menopause.
- If you have a bloody or greenish discharge from a nipple, or a watery or milky discharge that occurs without pressing on the nipple or breast.
- If one of your breasts changes shape, or if it seems to pucker or "pull" when you raise your arms.
- If the skin of one breast becomes dimpled like an orange peel.
- If you notice a change in the colour or feel of the skin of a breast or the darker area (areola) around a nipple.
- If you have a new pain in one breast, not caused by an injury, that lasts longer than 1 or 2 weeks.
- If you have any signs of infection in a breast. See page 100.
- If you are a man and you find a lump in your chest area.

Gynecological Health

Regular pelvic examinations and Pap tests are vital components of women's health. These examinations can give you early indications of any abnormalities in your reproductive organs. It is better to catch any disease in its early stages, when it may be easier to treat.

Self-Examination

Self-examinations will help you better understand your own body and what is normal for you. Periodically examine your entire genital area for any sores, warts, red swollen areas, or unusual discharge. A normal vaginal discharge may be white to yellowish white and smell slightly like vinegar. It can be either thick or thin and may vary in amount throughout your menstrual cycle; every woman is different. During ovulation (the midpoint between periods), there is often a large amount of clear, slippery mucus. If your discharge seems unusual in amount, smell, or texture, see Vaginitis on page 316.

There should be no pain or straining when you urinate, and the urine should come out in a fairly steady stream. The urine should be pale yellow, and it should not have a strong ammonia smell. If you experience pain or burning when you urinate, see Urinary Tract Infections on page 138 or Vaginitis on page 316.

If you have problems with bladder control, see Urinary Incontinence on page 137.

Pelvic Examination and Pap Test

A pelvic examination given by a health professional will generally include an external genital examination, a Pap test, and a manual examination.

The Pap test is the screening examination for cancer of the cervix (the opening of the uterus). When done regularly, the Pap test detects 90 to 95 percent of cervical cancers, making it a reliable and important test. To do the test, your health professional will insert an instrument (speculum) into your vagina to spread apart the vaginal walls. Then, using a cotton swab, small brush, or wooden or plastic spatula, your health professional will gather several samples of cells from your cervix. The cells are then sent to a lab for classification. Your health professional should let you know the results of your Pap test when they return from the lab. Ask for an explanation of your results if you don't understand them.

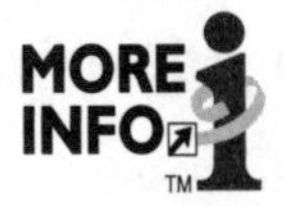

If your Pap test results are abnormal, you will be asked to return for more testing. You may have another Pap test, or your health professional may use a special magnifying device (colposcope) to try to find the area in your cervix that contains abnormal cells.

To do a manual examination, your health professional will insert two gloved and lubricated fingers into your vagina and press on your lower abdomen with his or her other hand to feel for any abnormalities in the shape or size of your ovaries and uterus.

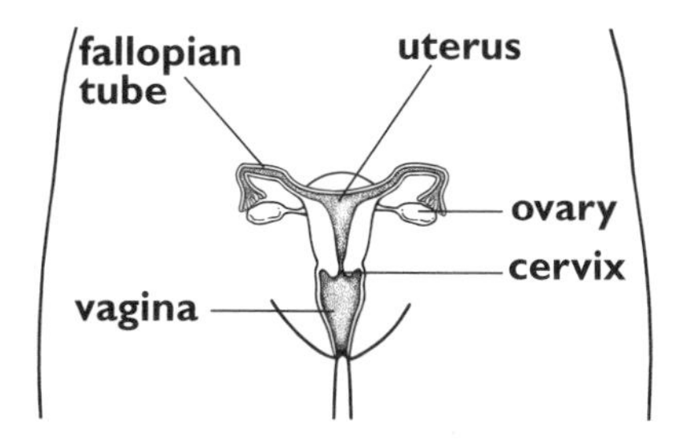

Female pelvic organs

Scheduling a Pelvic Examination

It is recommended that you have your first Pap test when you become sexually active or at age 18. After that, a Pap test should be done every year for 3 years. If the results of these 3 tests are normal, Pap tests are recommended every 1 to 3 years, depending on whether you have risk factors for cervical cancer. You may not need annual Pap tests if:

- You have had 3 or more normal Pap tests in a row (done annually).
- You have only one sex partner.
- You do not smoke.
- You do not have a history of abnormal Pap tests, cervical cancer, a sexually transmitted disease such as genital warts or HIV infection, or exposure to the drug diethylstilbestrol (DES).
- You have had a hysterectomy for a reason other than cancer.
- You are older than 65 and have had normal Pap tests over the past 10 years.

If you do have risk factors for cervical cancer or a history of abnormal Pap tests, it is recommended that you have a Pap test each year. Talk to your doctor about the best schedule for you.

Arrange to have the test 1 to 2 weeks after your period ends. Do not douche, have sexual intercourse, or use feminine hygiene products for at least 24 hours before a Pap test, because doing any of these things can alter the test results.

Pregnancy: How to Make a Healthy Baby

You can increase the chances that your baby will be healthy. The following guidelines will help.

Before Conception

Your health before conception and during the first weeks after is particularly important for your baby's health. Start helping your baby even before you become pregnant:

- Get a thorough physical checkup. If any problems or needs are found, deal with them early. Have a blood test to check your rubella immunity. If you test negative, you will need an immunization. After being vaccinated, wait at least 3 months before you get pregnant. Exposure to rubella during early pregnancy can harm your baby.

Dangers of Alcohol During Pregnancy

Do not drink alcohol while you are pregnant. When a pregnant woman drinks alcohol, the alcohol passes from her blood to the developing baby. Alcohol can hurt your baby. No amount of alcohol is safe. There is no time during pregnancy that is known to be safe to drink alcohol.

Alcohol use while you are pregnant can cause a child to have growth retardation, abnormal facial features, birth defects, mental retardation, or behaviour and learning problems. It can also lead to miscarriage, early delivery, or stillbirth.

Health Canada recommends that pregnant women and women who are planning to become pregnant do not drink alcohol. If you are affected by problematic substance use and plan to get pregnant, get help to stop drinking before you try to get pregnant. Use birth control until you have stopped drinking alcohol completely.

- During your checkup, you may want to ask for a "pre-pregnancy examination," which can help determine any risks to you or your children from pregnancy. Knowing the possible risks may help you decide whether you wish to see a general practitioner, a registered midwife, or an obstetrician for care during your pregnancy. It may also help you decide what tests you want to have done during pregnancy.
- You and your partner may want to be screened for potential genetic problems, such as sickle cell anemia if you are of African descent, or Tay-Sachs disease if you are of Jewish-European or French-Canadian descent.
- If you have diabetes, high blood pressure, seizure disorders, or any inherited diseases, talk with your doctor before getting pregnant. Your doctor may want to modify your treatment and may be able to prescribe medicine that is safer for the developing baby.
- See your dentist and have any necessary fillings or other work done before you get pregnant.
- If you have symptoms of a sexually transmitted disease or are unsure of your partner's sexual history, arrange for an examination and testing. See Sexually Transmitted Diseases on page 332.

- Eat well. Make sure your diet includes plenty of green, leafy vegetables and legumes.
- Take a multivitamin supplement that contains 0.4 mg of folate (folic acid). Folic acid helps prevent certain birth defects such as spina bifida. Other good sources of folic acid include fortified cereal and whole wheat bread.
- Exercise and control your weight as advised by your doctor.
- Stop smoking, and cut down on caffeinated drinks such as coffee, tea, and cola.
- Stop drinking alcoholic beverages, including beer, wine, and hard liquor. See Dangers of Alcohol During Pregnancy on page 304.
- Stop all illegal drug use and eliminate any medications that are not absolutely essential.
- If you are anxious or depressed, get help. See pages 370 and 372.
- Get your free copy of *Baby's Best Chance*. Ask your public health unit how to get a copy.

Early Pregnancy (Weeks 1 to 14)

- Continue to avoid smoking, alcohol, and drugs.
- Make the first visit to your health professional in the first 10 to 12 weeks of your pregnancy.
- Get tested for HIV infection.

Morning Sickness

Many women experience nausea and vomiting during the first few months of pregnancy. Morning sickness, which can occur at any time of day, is a normal result of the body's adjustment to pregnancy. The following home treatment can help.

- Eat five or six small meals a day to avoid having an empty stomach. Include some protein in each of the meals.
- Eat crackers or dry toast as soon as you get up in the morning.
- Increase your intake of vitamin B_6 by eating more whole grains and cereals, wheat germ, nuts, seeds, and legumes. Talk with your health professional before taking vitamin supplements during early pregnancy.
- Avoid foods or smells that make you nauseous.
- Get plenty of rest.

Call your health professional if your symptoms are so severe that you cannot hold down food or liquids, if you are vomiting more than 3 times a day, or if you are losing weight.

- Continue to improve your nutrition.
- Continue taking a multivitamin supplement containing 0.4 mg of folate.
- Avoid touching cat feces and litter boxes. Also, wash your hands after handling raw meat and cook all meat well before you eat it. Cat feces and raw or undercooked meat can carry toxoplasmosis, an infection that can cause a miscarriage or brain damage in the fetus.
- Avoid all chemical vapours, paint fumes, and poisons.
- If you drink coffee or soda with caffeine, cut back to 240 ml or less per day.

Middle Pregnancy (Weeks 15 to 28)

- Continue with the guidelines described above.
- Reduce your risk for injury and falls:
  - Wear sensible shoes.
  - Continue moderate levels of your regular exercises, but do not become exhausted or significantly short of breath.
  - Avoid sports with a high risk for falls or impact, such as skiing or horseback riding.
- Increase your calcium intake by drinking more milk (1 litre of skim or low-fat milk per day) or through other sources of calcium. See page 359.

Late Pregnancy (Weeks 29 to 40)

- Follow all the guidelines listed above.
- Get plenty of rest.
- Take childbirth classes with your partner or designated coach.
- Educate yourself about early signs of labour.
- Have your other children take a class to help them adjust to the new baby.
- Practise relaxation exercises (see page 386). They will be helpful during labour.
- Develop a written birth plan with your health professional that outlines your wishes and expectations throughout the labour and delivery.
- Maintain a good sense of humour.

Caesarean Deliveries

Most babies are delivered vaginally, just as nature intended. However, when the health of the baby or mother is at risk, doctors can deliver the baby through an incision in the mother's abdomen. This is called a Caesarean delivery or a C-section.

There are three main concerns with Caesarean deliveries:

- More risk. Many mothers who have C-sections develop infection or bleeding that requires additional medications or treatment. A C-section is a major surgery, which always carries risks.
- Longer recovery. You can usually go home within 1 day after a vaginal delivery. The hospital stay after a Caesarean delivery may be 2 to 4 days. After a C-section, you must limit your activity over the next 4 to 6 weeks to allow the incision to heal.
- Less involvement. Caesarean delivery is a surgery, which limits family involvement. The mother and other family members can be more involved with a vaginal delivery.

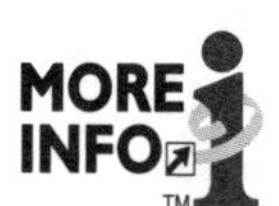

C-sections are a good idea when either the baby or the mother is in danger. A Caesarean delivery should not be done just because it is easier to schedule. If you previously had a C-section delivery, you may still be able to have a vaginal delivery with your next pregnancy. Ask your health professional to discuss this option with you.

Breast-Feeding

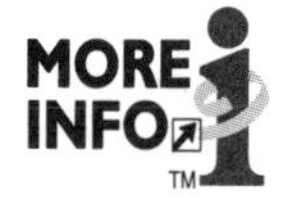

Breast milk is the ideal food for your new baby. Consider taking a breast-feeding class before your baby is born. See page 265.

A nursing mother needs to consume 500 more calories per day than she did before becoming pregnant. Although you don't need to drink milk to make milk, extra calcium and protein are important, and your doctor may prescribe a vitamin supplement. Avoid smoking and do not drink alcohol; limit caffeine to one or two beverages per day. Do not take any medication while breast-feeding before discussing it with your health professional.

Abortion Services in BC

Abortions are available in BC and, for BC residents who have current coverage, are paid for by the Medical Services Plan. Several clinics, doctors, and hospitals throughout the province offer these services. Counselling about pregnancy options, the procedure itself, birth control, and other topics are available at most of the clinics and through either of these toll-free information lines:

- Pregnancy Options Referral Service: 1-888-875-3163. This service provides information and referral for all abortion services, including counselling, available to BC residents.
- Facts of Life Line: 1-800-739-7367, or, from the Lower Mainland, 604-731-7803. This service offers general sexual and reproductive health information as well as referral to resources throughout BC.

Women may self-refer to any of the abortion clinics in BC or may call the Pregnancy Options Referral Service (see above) for referral to a doctor in their area.

Abortion is safest when done as early as possible in the pregnancy. Medical abortion, which uses medication to cause the abortion, can be done up to 7 weeks after the last menstrual period. This procedure can be done in a doctor's office. For more information about the availability of medical abortion in your area, talk to your health care provider or call one of the numbers above.

Surgical abortion can be done from the 5th week after the last menstrual period up to the 20th week of pregnancy. With a referral to the United States, it can be done up to the 24th week or later, if there is a problem with the fetus. The surgery is safest when done in the first 12 weeks of pregnancy. After 12 weeks, a 2-day procedure is usually needed. Access to abortion between 12 and 20 weeks from your last period is limited to a small number of facilities that provide this service. The Pregnancy Options Referral Service can refer you to a facility.

Birth Control Failure

If you have recently had unprotected sex—a condom broke, you skipped a birth control pill, you did not use birth control—and you do not want to get pregnant, see a health professional or pharmacist immediately. Emergency contraception (the "morning-after pill") can help prevent pregnancy and should be taken within 72 hours (3 days) of unprotected sex. It may be effective if taken up to 5 days after sex, but the sooner you take it, the more effective it will be. See page 332.

Bleeding Between Periods

Many women experience bleeding or spotting between periods. It does not necessarily mean a serious condition is present. Use of an intrauterine device (IUD) may increase your chances of spotting. Some minor bleeding is common during ovulation and during the first few months of using birth control pills. Other hormonal birth control methods, such as Depo-Provera injections, can cause bleeding between periods. Women who are breast-feeding often have irregular vaginal bleeding or spotting. Stress and hormonal imbalances are other common causes of irregular bleeding. In all these situations, if the bleeding is not heavy and occurs only occasionally, there is probably no cause for concern. Avoid Aspirin, which may prolong the bleeding.

There are other, less common causes of bleeding between periods that may be more serious:

- In a woman who is pregnant, bleeding may indicate a problem with the pregnancy.
- A woman who is having a miscarriage will usually have cramping, lower abdominal pain, and vaginal bleeding.
- Ectopic pregnancy (when a fertilized egg attaches somewhere other than the uterus; also called tubal pregnancy) usually causes lower abdominal pain, and there may be vaginal bleeding.
- Non-cancerous uterine growths (uterine fibroids) can cause spotting or bleeding between periods in some women.
- Rarely, irregular bleeding can be caused by uterine cancer.
- A pelvic infection may cause bleeding between periods. Fever, cramping pain, painful sexual intercourse, and a bad-smelling vaginal discharge are other symptoms.
- If the opening of the uterus (cervix) is inflamed or has an abnormal growth on it, there may be bleeding, especially after sexual intercourse or douching.
- A woman who has gone through menopause and is not on hormone replacement therapy should not have any vaginal bleeding. If she does, she may have an abnormal growth in her uterus and should see a health professional. Women taking hormones may have some post-menopausal bleeding, which they should discuss with their health professional.

When to Call a Health Professional

Call 911 or other emergency services if you have severe vaginal bleeding (soaking more than 8 pads or super tampons in 8 hours) and signs of shock (see page 103).

Call a health professional:

- If you are pregnant and have any vaginal bleeding.
- If you have new lower abdominal pain with unexpected vaginal bleeding.
- If the bleeding is severe.
- If you have irregular vaginal bleeding and a fever of 37.7°C or higher.
- If bleeding between periods lasts longer than 1 week or occurs 3 months in a row.
- If bleeding occurs after sexual intercourse or douching.
- If you are over 35 and have any bleeding between periods or prolonged bleeding with periods.
- If you are using a hormonal method of birth control and your periods are different from what your doctor told you to expect.
- If bleeding occurs after you have gone through menopause.

Menopause

For most women, menopause occurs between the ages of 45 and 55, when the production of female hormones (estrogen and progesterone) begins to decline. These hormonal changes may cause irregular menstrual periods before periods stop altogether. You may also experience hot flashes, vaginal dryness, or mood changes. Every woman is unique and will experience menopause differently. Menopause can also occur as the result of having a hysterectomy.

Osteoporosis is directly linked to the decrease in estrogen that comes with menopause. See Osteoporosis on page 172.

Most women can expect to live one-third of their lives after menopause, so it is important to manage any problems related to menopause.

Irregular periods. The hormonal changes that occur during menopause may cause you to have irregular periods before your periods stop altogether. This may mean that your menstrual flow will be lighter or heavier than usual; that the intervals between your periods will be shorter or longer; or that you will have spotting between periods. Some women have regular periods until their periods stop suddenly, and others have irregular periods for a long time until menopause.

Birth control. Although you may be less fertile during the years just before the onset of menopause, you continue to release eggs (ovulate) and could become pregnant. If you do not wish to become pregnant, continue to use birth control until your doctor confirms that you have reached menopause or until you have not had a menstrual period for 12 months.

Hot flashes. Hot flashes are sudden periods of intense heat, sweating, and flushing. A hot flash usually begins in the chest and spreads out to the neck, face, and arms. Seventy-five to eighty percent of women going through menopause will have hot flashes. Hot flashes may occur as frequently as once an hour and can last from a few minutes to an hour. If they occur at night, they may disrupt your sleep patterns. Disrupted sleep can lead to insomnia, fatigue, irritability, or inability to concentrate.

Hot flashes usually stop within 1 or 2 years but may persist for several years. They are rarely noticed by others.

Vaginal changes. Vaginal changes that occur during menopause include vaginal dryness caused by the loss of lubrication and moisture in the vagina; thinning of the vaginal walls and loss of elasticity in them; and shrinkage of the outer lips (labia) of the vagina. These vaginal changes can lead to soreness during and after sexual intercourse and may also increase your risk for vaginal infections and urinary incontinence. See Vaginitis on page 316 and Urinary Incontinence on page 137.

Mood changes. The hormonal and physical changes of menopause can cause mood changes. Symptoms such as nervousness, lack of energy, insomnia, moodiness, or depression are common.

Many women think that menopause means emotional upset and the loss of sexuality. Other women feel positive about the changes that occur with menopause, such as freedom from menstruation and the need for birth control. Understanding what is happening to you and having a plan for dealing with symptoms will help you through menopause.

Home Treatment

Irregular periods

Keep a written record of your periods in case you need to discuss them with a health professional.

Hot flashes

Hot flashes usually improve after 1 to 2 years. In the meantime:

- Keep your home and workplace cool, or use a fan.
- Wear layers of loose clothing that can be easily removed. Wear natural fibres such as cotton and silk.
- Drink cold beverages rather than hot ones, and limit your intake of caffeine and alcohol.
- Eat smaller, more frequent meals to avoid the heat generated by digesting large amounts of food.
- Try the relaxation tips on page 386.

Vaginal dryness

Use a water-soluble vaginal lubricant, such as Astroglide or Replens, to ease discomfort during sexual intercourse. Vegetable oil will also work. Do not use Vaseline or other petroleum-based products.

Mood changes

The best thing you can do for yourself is realize that you are not alone. Discuss your symptoms with other women. Give yourself, and ask others for, abundant amounts of love, caring, and understanding. Try to develop a relaxed attitude about menopause. Tension and anxiety may make your symptoms worse. Exercise regularly to relieve stress.

Hormone therapy may improve hot flashes, vaginal dryness, and mood changes, in addition to protecting you from osteoporosis, but it also has side effects and risks. See page 312. Certain antidepressants can also help with hot flashes and mood swings.

When to Call a Health Professional

- If your menstrual periods are unusually heavy, irregular, or prolonged (1½ to 2 times longer than usual).

- If bleeding occurs between periods when your periods have been regular.
- If bleeding recurs after periods have stopped for 6 months.
- If vaginal dryness is not relieved with a vaginal lubricant. Your doctor may prescribe a vaginal cream or suppository that contains estrogen.
- If your symptoms are interfering with your life and home treatment does not help.
- If you are considering hormone therapy or other medical treatment.
- If you have unexplained bleeding (different from what your health professional told you to expect) while you are taking hormones.

Hormone Therapy

During and after menopause, a woman's body produces much less of the hormones estrogen and progesterone. Hormone therapy may be prescribed to treat symptoms of menopause. There are two types of hormone therapy:

- Estrogen replacement therapy (ERT). ERT is estrogen alone. Because ERT may increase the risk of endometrial (uterine) cancer, it is usually prescribed only for women who have had a hysterectomy.
- Hormone replacement therapy (HRT). HRT combines estrogen with progestin, another female hormone. Progestin reduces the effect of estrogen on the uterine lining and protects against endometrial cancer.

Hormone pills are taken every day. Some forms of hormone therapy are available as skin patches, vaginal creams, or vaginal rings.

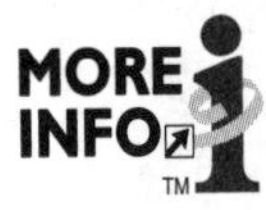

Hormone therapy reduces the discomfort of menopausal symptoms such as hot flashes and vaginal dryness and helps maintain bone density. It can also have unpleasant side effects such as bloating, breast tenderness, and irregular vaginal bleeding. Hormone therapy appears to have significant risks, including an increased risk of breast cancer, stroke, and heart conditions. For some women, however, the short-term benefit of reducing menopausal symptoms may outweigh the risks. Talk with your doctor about whether starting or continuing hormone therapy is a good idea for you.

Hormone therapy usually is not recommended for women who have had breast cancer, endometrial cancer, problems with blood clots, heart attack, stroke, liver disease, or undiagnosed uterine bleeding.

MORE INFO For more information, see the back cover.

Menstrual Cramps

Many women suffer from painful menstruation (dysmenorrhea). Symptoms include mild to severe cramping in the lower abdomen, back, or thighs; headaches; diarrhea or constipation; nausea; dizziness; and fainting. During the menstrual cycle, the lining of the uterus produces a hormone called prostaglandin. This hormone causes the uterus to contract, often painfully. Women who get severe cramps may produce higher-than-normal amounts of prostaglandin or may be more sensitive to its effects.

A copper intrauterine device (IUD) can cause increased cramping during your period for the first few months of use. If menstrual cramping persists or gets worse, you may need to consider having the IUD removed and choosing another birth control method. A levonorgestrel IUD or birth control pills can reduce menstrual cramping. Pain caused by endometriosis (a condition in which cells from the lining of the uterus become implanted on other pelvic organs) usually occurs 1 to 2 days before menstrual bleeding begins and continues through the period. Pelvic infections may cause pain at any time, but the pain often occurs after menstrual bleeding has begun. Some women who have non-cancerous uterine growths (uterine fibroids) have severe menstrual cramps.

Home Treatment

- Ibuprofen and naproxen sodium generally help ease cramps better than Aspirin and acetaminophen do. Take either ibuprofen or naproxen sodium the day before your period starts, or at the first sign of pain. Take these products with milk or food. Otherwise, they may upset your stomach.
- Exercise. Regular workouts decrease the severity of cramps. See Fitness starting on page 343.
- Use heat (hot water bottles, heating pads, or hot baths) to relax tense muscles and relieve cramping.
- Herbal teas (such as camomile, mint, raspberry, and blackberry) may help soothe tense muscles and anxious moods.
- If symptoms other than cramping (such as weight gain, headache, and tension) occur before your period begins, see Premenstrual Syndrome on page 315.

When to Call a Health Professional

- If sudden, severe pelvic pain occurs, with or without menstrual bleeding.
- If your menstrual cramps have become worse.
- If pelvic pain seems unrelated to your menstrual cycle.
- If you have cramps and a fever of 37.7°C or higher.

- If cramps begin 5 to 7 days before your period starts or continue after your period stops.
- If cramps do not respond to home treatment for 3 cycles, or if they interfere with your normal activities.
- If you suspect that your copper intrauterine device (IUD) is causing cramps, and the pain is more than you can stand or worse than what your doctor told you to expect.

Missed or Irregular Periods

Missed or irregular periods have many possible causes. Pregnancy is usually the first cause to be considered, but other common causes include:

- Stress; weight loss or weight gain; increased exercise (missed periods are common in endurance athletes); and travel.
- Use of hormonal birth control methods, such as birth control pills or Depo-Provera injections, which may cause lighter, less frequent, or skipped periods.
- Menopause.
- Menarche (the start of menstrual periods). For the first few years of menstruation, periods may be irregular.
- Medications, including steroids, tranquilizers, and diet pills, or recreational drugs.
- Hormonal imbalance or problems in the pelvic organs.
- Breast-feeding.
- Untreated thyroid disease.

If you've skipped a period, try to relax. Restoring your life to emotional and physical balance may help. Many women miss periods now and then. Unless you are pregnant, chances are your cycle will return to normal next month. If you could be pregnant, treat yourself as if you are until you know for sure.

Home Treatment

- If you had sex during the previous month, do a home pregnancy test. See page 414.
- Avoid fad diets that greatly restrict calories and food variety, and avoid rapid weight loss. To maintain a healthy weight, focus on eating a variety of low-fat foods. See Nutrition starting on page 351.
- Increase exercise gradually. If you are an endurance athlete, cut back on training and talk with a doctor about hormone and calcium supplements to protect against bone loss.
- Learn and practise relaxation techniques to reduce and cope with stress. See page 386.
- If you are age 45 or older, you may be starting menopause. See page 310.

When to Call a Health Professional

- Call your doctor immediately if it is possible that you may be pregnant and you are having lower abdominal pain.
- If a home pregnancy test indicates you are pregnant, see a doctor to confirm the test and begin pregnancy counselling.
- Call a health professional if you have missed 2 regular periods and there is no obvious cause such as those listed previously.
- If you miss 2 or 3 periods while taking birth control pills, and you have not skipped any pills.
- If you have not started having menstrual periods by age 16.

Premenstrual Syndrome

Many women have mild symptoms related to menstruation, such as cramps and breast tenderness. These symptoms are considered a normal part of the menstrual cycle. A diagnosis of premenstrual syndrome (PMS) is reserved for symptoms that occur during the 2 weeks before a woman's period begins and that are severe enough to disrupt her life.

About 40 percent of women are affected by PMS at some time in their lives. PMS occurs most often in women in their 20s and 30s and is rare in teenagers.

Many physical and psychological symptoms have been attributed to PMS. Symptoms vary greatly from woman to woman. They can include physical changes such as breast swelling, water retention, bloating, weight gain, and acne; mood and behaviour changes such as irritability, depression, difficulty concentrating, decreased sex drive, and aggression; painful symptoms such as headaches, breast tenderness, and muscle aches; and other symptoms such as food cravings, lack of energy, and sleep disturbances.

If you suspect that you have PMS, keep a menstrual diary in which you record:

- Your symptoms and how severe they are.
- Dates when symptoms occur.
- Days when you have your period.

If symptoms consistently appear shortly before your period and end shortly after your period, you may want to follow the home treatment recommendations. Many women find that making small changes in their lives significantly improves their PMS symptoms.

Home Treatment

- Eat small meals every 3 to 4 hours. Include plenty of whole grains, fruit, and vegetables. Limit fats and sweets, and reduce salt to help limit bloating.

- Eliminate tobacco, alcohol, and caffeine. This may help relieve some symptoms.
- Exercise regularly to help minimize PMS symptoms.
- Try a non-prescription PMS medication such as Midol or Pamprin. Many products contain a combination of drugs to help relieve cramps, bloating, and headache.
- Be good to yourself. Reduce your stress level as much as possible. Try yoga (see page 397) or other relaxation techniques (see page 386).
- Create a support system. Talk with your family, friends, and any others who may be affected by your symptoms. Join a support group for women who have PMS.
- Try taking calcium (1,200 mg daily), magnesium (400 mg daily), or vitamin B_6 (no more than 100 mg daily). These may improve your mood, reduce fluid retention and pain, and help with other PMS symptoms.

When to Call a Health Professional

- If PMS symptoms regularly disrupt your life and keep you from doing your regular activities.
- If you feel out of control because of PMS symptoms.
- If PMS symptoms do not end within a few days after your menstrual bleeding starts.

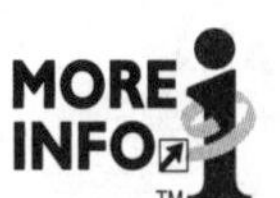

If PMS symptoms are severely disrupting your life, make an appointment with your doctor. He or she may prescribe medication to reduce these symptoms.

Vaginitis

Vaginitis is any vaginal infection, inflammation, or irritation that causes a change in normal vaginal discharge. General symptoms include a change in the amount, colour, odour, or texture of vaginal discharge; itching; painful urination; and pain during sexual intercourse. Common causes of vaginitis include yeast infection (see page 319), bacterial vaginosis, and trichomoniasis, which is caused by a parasite spread through sexual contact (see page 336). Some other sexually spread diseases can cause unusual vaginal discharge or vaginal irritation. See page 332. Douching frequently, wearing tight clothing, or using strong soaps, perfumed feminine hygiene products, or spermicides may also contribute to vaginal irritation or infection.

If you have burning and pain when you urinate and feel the need to urinate often, see Urinary Tract Infections on page 138.

Symptoms of bacterial vaginosis often include a thin, greyish white, fishy-smelling vaginal discharge. The odour is often worse after sex. Bacterial vaginosis is commonly associated with having multiple sex partners, using an intrauterine device (IUD) or diaphragm, exposure to a sexually transmitted disease (STD), or frequent douching. However, it may also occur in women who don't have these risk factors.

Symptoms of trichomoniasis may include a large amount of frothy, foamy, white, yellow, green, or grey vaginal discharge; vaginal redness, irritation, and swelling; and vaginal odour. See page 336.

Prevention

- Limit the number of your sex partners and use condoms during sexual intercourse. Having multiple sex partners may increase your risk for vaginitis by changing the normal environment of your vagina.
- If you think frequent vaginal infections may be related to use of a diaphragm or IUD, spermicidal foams or jellies, or condoms, discuss other birth control options with your health professional.
- Wipe from front to back after using the toilet to avoid spreading bacteria from your anus to your vagina.
- Wash your vaginal area once a day with plain water. Rinse well and pat dry. Do not douche unless your health professional advises you to do so.

Hysterectomy Guidelines

Hysterectomy is the surgical removal of the uterus. It is generally done to treat disease. However, there are times when other treatments may work as well with fewer risks.

Hysterectomy is often the best treatment for:

- Uterine, ovarian, or cervical cancer.
- Severe uterine bleeding.
- Severe endometriosis.
- Large, non-cancerous tumours (fibroids) that cause severe bleeding and pain or press on the bladder.
- Severe uterine prolapse (uterus falls into the opening of the vagina).

Conditions that may respond to non-surgical treatments include:

- Abnormal uterine bleeding.
- Fibroids that cause mild symptoms.
- Mild to moderate uterine prolapse.
- Pelvic pain or mild endometriosis.
- Pelvic inflammatory disease.

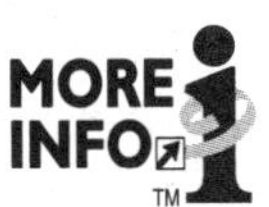

Getting all the facts and thinking about your own needs and values will help you make the best decision about hysterectomy.

- Do not use feminine deodorant sprays and other perfumed products. They irritate and dry tender skin.
- During your period, change tampons at least 3 times a day, or alternate tampons with pads. Remember to remove the last tampon used during your period.
- Antibiotic medications can kill the healthy bacteria that grow in your vagina. If you are taking an antibiotic, drink acidophilus milk or eat yogourt that contains live *Lactobacillus* cultures to help prevent vaginitis.
- Do not wear panty hose or tight nylon underwear, which limit air circulation to your vaginal area.
- Consider using a vaginal lubricant during sex if you have a problem with dryness.

Home Treatment

A vaginal infection may clear up without treatment in 3 or 4 days. If your symptoms do not improve, call your doctor.

- Follow the prevention guidelines.
- Avoid sexual intercourse to give irritated vaginal tissues time to heal.
- Do not scratch. Relieve itching with a cold-water compress or cool bath.
- Make sure the cause of vaginitis is not a forgotten tampon or another foreign object.
- If you think you may be pregnant, do a home pregnancy test. See page 414. Bacterial vaginosis can be more serious if it occurs during pregnancy.
- If itching is the most bothersome symptom, try a non-prescription vaginal cream or suppositories for yeast infections. See Yeast Infections on page 319. If you are pregnant, talk with your doctor before using a non-prescription treatment.

When to Call a Health Professional

- If you have pelvic or lower abdominal pain, fever, and unusual vaginal discharge.
- If you have pain or bleeding after sexual intercourse (and the pain is not eased by using a vaginal lubricant such as Astroglide).
- If you have an unusual or foul-smelling vaginal discharge.
- If you have vaginal itching that does not go away after you use a non-prescription medication for yeast infections.
- If you think you've been exposed to a sexually transmitted disease (see page 332). Your sex partner may need to be treated too.

If you plan to see a health professional, do not douche, use vaginal creams, or have sexual intercourse for 48 hours before your appointment. Doing these things may make your problem more difficult to diagnose.

Yeast Infections

A vaginal yeast infection (candidiasis) is caused by an excess growth of yeast organisms in the vagina. Yeast infections are common in women of child-bearing age. They can cause severe discomfort but rarely cause serious problems.

Common symptoms of yeast infection include vaginal itching (often severe); white, curdy, usually odourless vaginal discharge; and pain when urinating and during sexual intercourse. The skin around the vagina (labia) may be red and irritated. If you have burning and pain when urinating and feel the need to urinate often, see Urinary Tract Infections on page 138.

Yeast infections are commonly associated with antibiotic or steroid use, pregnancy, diabetes, and illnesses that weaken the immune system. In addition, douching frequently, wearing tight clothing, or using strong soaps or perfumed feminine hygiene products may contribute to vaginal irritation or infection. Yeast infections are not spread by sexual contact.

Prevention

- Drink acidophilus milk or eat yogourt that contains live *Lactobacillus* organisms. Some studies suggest that yogourt may help prevent vaginal yeast infections.
- Wear cotton or cotton-lined underwear. Avoid tight-fitting pants and undergarments. They increase heat and moisture in the vaginal area, which may allow yeast to grow more easily in your vagina.
- Avoid feminine sprays, talcs, or perfumes in your vaginal area, because they may affect the balance among the micro-organisms in your vagina. Do not douche unless your health professional advises you to do so.
- Wipe your vaginal area from front to back after using the toilet and when bathing.
- Eat a well-balanced diet. This helps maintain a normal balance in your vagina.
- If you have diabetes, keep your blood sugar level within the range recommended by your doctor.

Home Treatment

Left untreated, vaginal yeast infections often clear up on their own, usually when your period begins. Be sure you have a yeast infection before you try self-treatment. If you are pregnant, talk to your doctor first.

- Follow the prevention guidelines above.
- Use a non-prescription antifungal medication for yeast infections (such as Monistat, Canesten, or a store brand) as directed.

- Avoid excessive cleaning of your vaginal area. Wash once a day with plain water or a mild, non-perfumed soap.
- Don't use tampons while using topical cream or vaginal suppositories for a vaginal yeast infection. The tampons can absorb the medication. Use sanitary pads instead.
- If sexual intercourse causes discomfort, avoid it until your symptoms go away.

When to Call a Health Professional

- If you develop lower abdominal pain or a fever higher than 37.7°C along with symptoms of a vaginal yeast infection.
- If you think this is the first time you've had a yeast infection, or if you aren't sure whether your symptoms are being caused by a yeast infection.
- If home treatment with a non-prescription antifungal product fails to clear up a yeast infection within 3 or 4 days, or if you are using antifungal creams repeatedly.
- If you have symptoms of a urinary tract infection. See page 138.
- If you are or may be pregnant and you have symptoms of a vaginal infection.
- If symptoms of a yeast infection return within 2 months and you have not been taking antibiotics.

If you plan to see a health professional, do not douche, use vaginal creams, or have sexual intercourse for 48 hours before your appointment. Doing these things may make your problem more difficult to diagnose.

The man who says it cannot be done should not interrupt the man doing it.
Old Chinese proverb

16

Men's Health

This chapter focuses on health problems that are unique to men. If you are looking for general guidelines for making healthy lifestyle choices to prevent illness and injury, see Living a Healthy Life starting on page 15. Specific tips for developing a fitness plan, eating a healthy diet, maintaining a healthy body weight, managing stress, and preventing sexually transmitted diseases are included in other chapters. Use the index to find the information you need.

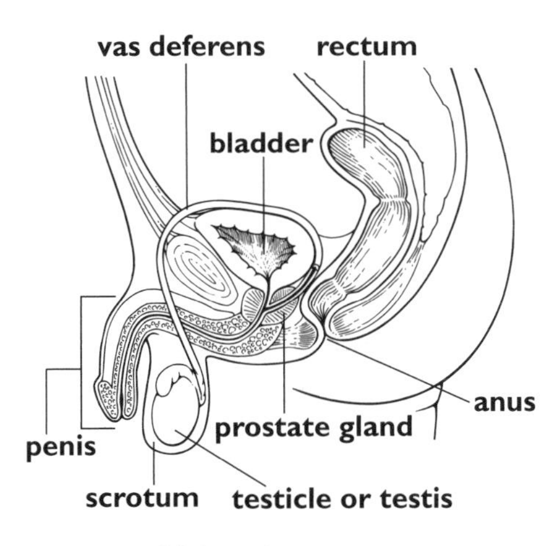

Male pelvic organs

Genital Health

Daily cleansing of the penis, particularly under the foreskin of an uncircumcised penis, can prevent bacterial infection and reduces the already low risk of penile cancer. Boys should be taught by age 3 or 4 to start to gently pull back (retract) the foreskin and wash beneath it. The foreskin may not be fully retractable until puberty. Do not forcibly retract a child's foreskin if it is painful or difficult to do so.

Erection Problems

Erection problems are common and can often be solved with self-care. By definition, an erection problem is difficulty in getting or maintaining an erection capable of intercourse.

Erection problems are often caused by stress, tension in relationships, depression, fatigue, lack of privacy, physical injury, or side effects of medications. These causes are generally temporary and will usually resolve with home treatment. Less reversible causes include diabetes, a long history of smoking, nerve damage, and vascular disease.

The ease of gaining and sustaining erections generally decreases with age. However, with the right foreplay and environment, healthy men can have erections at any age.

Prevention

Most erection problems can be prevented or resolved by taking a more relaxed approach to lovemaking and watching for possible side effects from medications or illnesses.

Home Treatment

- Rule out medications first. Many drugs, especially blood pressure medicines, water pills (diuretics), and mood-altering drugs, can cause erection problems. Ask your doctor or pharmacist to check your medications for possible effects on sexual function, or look it up yourself. Do not stop taking any medication without talking to your doctor first.
- Avoid alcohol and smoking, which can make erection problems worse.
- Cope with stress (see page 384). Tension in your life can distract you and make getting erections difficult. Regular exercise and other stress-relieving activities may help ease tension.
- Talk to your partner about your concerns, and take time for more foreplay. Let your partner know that you would enjoy some stroking. Slow down; then slow down some more.
- Make sure you're ready. If you have recently experienced a loss or change in a relationship, you may not yet be emotionally ready for erections. Generally, your stress will subside and your erection problem will disappear over time. Do what you can to relax.
- Find out if you can have erections at other times. If you can have an erection during masturbation or on awakening, the problem is probably stress-related or may be caused by an emotional problem.

When to Call a Health Professional

- If an erection lasts longer than 4 hours after you use an erection-producing medication.
- If you have taken an erection-producing medication (such as Viagra, Levitra, or Cialis) in the past 24 hours and you are having chest pain. Do not take nitroglycerine if you have taken Viagra, Levitra, or Cialis in the past 24 hours.
- If you think that a medication may be causing the problem. Your doctor may be able to prescribe a different medication for you.
- If you are unable to have an erection at all, or think that your problem may be a physical one.

- If you have other symptoms such as urinary problems, pain in the lower abdomen or lower back, or fever.
- If your symptoms developed after a recent injury.

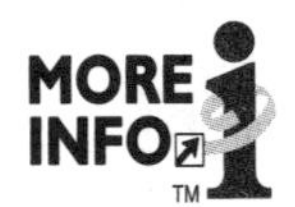

If you have tried home treatment for a few months but your symptoms have not improved, you may wish to talk with your doctor about erection-producing medications or injections, a vacuum device, or a penile implant. Getting all the facts and thinking about your own (and your partner's) needs and values will help you make a wise decision about treatment for erection problems.

Prostate Infection (Prostatitis)

The prostate is a small gland that lies under the bladder, about halfway between the rectum and the base of the penis. It encircles the urethra, the tube that carries urine from the bladder out through the penis. The prostate produces some of the fluid that transports sperm during ejaculation.

Prostatitis is a painful condition of the prostate gland. Types of prostatitis include acute and chronic bacterial prostatitis, inflammatory chronic pelvic pain, and non-inflammatory chronic pelvic pain. With the exception of acute bacterial prostatitis (in which the symptoms are severe, come on suddenly, and may include fever and chills), it is difficult to determine the kind of prostatitis a man has based on symptoms alone.

In general, symptoms may include:

- A frequent urge to urinate, with only small amounts of urine being passed.
- A burning sensation when urinating.
- An inability to empty the bladder completely.
- Difficulty starting urination; interrupted or weaker-than-normal urine flow; and dribbling after urinating.
- Urinating excessively at night.
- Pain or discomfort in the lower back; the scrotum; the area between the scrotum and the anus; the lower abdomen; the upper thighs; or above the pubic area.
- Pain or vague discomfort during or after ejaculation.

Bacterial prostate infections usually respond well to self-care and antibiotics. If the infection recurs, long-term antibiotic treatment may be needed. Pelvic pain and prostate inflammation that are not caused by bacteria usually respond to home treatment.

Prevention

- Practise good hygiene, and wash your penis daily.

- Drink enough water and other fluids so that you urinate regularly.
- If you develop symptoms of a urinary tract infection, seek treatment early. See Urinary Tract Infections on page 138.
- If your doctor prescribes an antibiotic for bacterial prostatitis, take the full amount prescribed. This can reduce your risk of having another infection in the future.

Home Treatment

- Avoid alcohol, caffeine, and spicy foods, especially if they make your symptoms worse.
- Take hot baths to help soothe pain and reduce stress.
- Eat plenty of high-fibre foods, and drink enough water to avoid constipation. Straining to pass stools can be very painful when your prostate is inflamed.
- Take Aspirin, ibuprofen, or acetaminophen to help relieve pain. Do not give Aspirin to anyone younger than 20.

When to Call a Health Professional

- If urinary symptoms occur with fever, chills, vomiting, or pain in the back or abdomen.
- If your urine is bloody, red, or pink and there is no dietary reason for this (see page 136).
- If symptoms continue for 5 days despite home treatment.
- If your symptoms suddenly change or get worse.
- If you have pain during urination, ejaculation, or bowel movements. If there is also an unusual discharge from your penis, see pages 332 to 336.
- If you have urinary symptoms such as trouble starting to urinate, inability to empty your bladder completely, or frequent urination (especially at night), and they are not related to drinking more fluids.

Prostate Enlargement

As a man ages, the prostate may enlarge (benign prostatic hyperplasia or hypertrophy). This seems to be a natural process and is not really a disease. However, as the gland gets bigger, it may squeeze or partially block the urethra and cause urinary problems, such as:

- Difficulty getting the urine stream started and completely stopped (dribbling).
- Frequent urge to urinate, or being awakened by the urge to urinate.
- Decreased force of the urine stream.
- Having the sense that the bladder is not completely empty after urinating.

An enlarged prostate gland is not a serious problem unless urination becomes difficult or backed-up urine causes bladder infections or kidney damage. Some dribbling after urination is very common and not necessarily a sign of prostate problems.

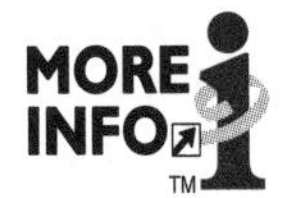

Surgery is usually not necessary for prostate enlargement. Many men find that their symptoms are stable, and sometimes symptoms even clear up on their own. In these cases, the best treatment may be no treatment at all. Drugs are available that may help improve symptoms in many men. Your doctor can advise you about the various treatment options.

Home Treatment

- Avoid antihistamines, decongestants, and nasal sprays, which can make urinary problems worse.
- If you are bothered by a frequent urge to urinate at night, cut down on beverages before bedtime, especially those that contain alcohol or caffeine. Drink at least 8 glasses of water and other fluids during the day.
- Don't postpone urinating, and take plenty of time. Try sitting on the toilet instead of standing.
- Also see Urinary Incontinence on page 137.

When to Call a Health Professional

- If you are unable to urinate, or if you feel as if you cannot empty your bladder completely.
- If you develop fever, back or abdominal pain, or chills.
- If there is blood or pus in your urine.
- Water pills (diuretics), tranquilizers, antihistamines, decongestants, and some antidepressants can aggravate urinary problems. If you take any of these drugs, ask your doctor if there are other medications you could use that do not cause these urinary side effects.

Prostate Cancer

Prostate cancer is the second leading cause of cancer deaths in men. When detected early, before it has spread to other organs, prostate cancer may be curable. Most cases develop in men over 65. Prostate cancer sometimes runs in families and tends to be more common in men who eat a high-fat diet.

Because prostate cancer tends to develop late in life and usually grows slowly, it does not usually shorten a man's life. However, the younger you are and the larger or more advanced the cancer is, the more serious the disease may be.

There are no specific symptoms of prostate cancer. Most men have no symptoms at all. In a few cases, it can cause urinary symptoms very similar to those of prostate enlargement (see page 324). Other symptoms, such as pain, may develop if the cancer spreads to other organs or to the bones.

Prostate cancer treatment is tailored to each individual. Work with your doctor to be sure that you will receive the long-term benefits from the treatment you choose.

Learn all you can about the available treatment options, which may include watchful waiting, so that you and your doctor can select the one best suited for you. Your age, overall health, and other medical conditions, as well as the characteristics of the cancer, are all important factors to consider when you make treatment decisions.

Prevention

There is no known way to prevent prostate cancer. However, you may reduce your risk of developing prostate cancer by:

- Eating a low-fat diet that includes plenty of fruits and vegetables.
- Adding foods that contain tomato or tomato sauce to your diet.
- Increasing your intake of soy products.

Talk to your health professional about whether you should take dietary supplements. Researchers are studying the possibility that vitamins D and E, selenium, and green tea may help prevent prostate cancer.

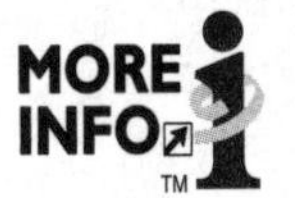

Early detection may be the most important part of prevention, but there is controversy about the value of using digital rectal examinations and the prostate-specific antigen (PSA) blood test to screen all men for prostate cancer. Detecting early prostate cancer may not improve quality of life or prolong life, especially in men who are older or have other serious health problems. Therefore, many experts are uncertain whether routine screening is appropriate for all men. Talk with your doctor for more information about prostate cancer screening.

When to Call a Health Professional

- If you have blood or pus in your urine.
- If any urinary symptoms (see Prostate Enlargement on page 324) come on quickly, are bothersome enough that you want help, or last longer than 2 months.

Testicular Problems

The testicles produce sperm and male hormones. Males normally have two testicles, located behind the penis inside a sac of skin called the scrotum. It is normal for one testicle to be slightly larger than the other.

Each testicle is suspended at the end of a spermatic cord, which consists of blood vessels, nerves, and a tube called the vas deferens. Sperm cells leave the testicle through the epididymis (a coiled tube located at the top and back of the testicle). They are stored in the epididymis. At the time of ejaculation, they are propelled through the vas deferens and prostate, into the urethra. Sperm mix with fluids produced by the seminal vesicles and the prostate to create semen, which exits the body through the penis during sexual activity.

The location of the testicles makes them prone to injury, especially during contact sports. Pain caused by a testicular injury should go away within an hour or so.

Testicular torsion occurs when one of the testicles rotates, twisting the spermatic cord and cutting off blood flow to the testicle. Testicular torsion can occur at any age, but it is most common in teenage boys. It may occur after strenuous physical activity or after an injury, but it often has no specific cause and may occur while a boy is sleeping.

Symptoms of testicular torsion include sudden, severe pain in one testicle that may spread to the lower abdomen; swelling high in the scrotum; nausea and vomiting; and fever.

Testicular torsion is a medical emergency. Surgery is often needed to restore blood flow to the testicle. If the procedure is not done within a few hours after the onset of symptoms, the testicle can be permanently damaged and may have to be removed.

Epididymitis is inflammation of the epididymis. It can be caused by a bacterial infection (including chlamydia, which is spread through sexual contact; see page 333) or by irritation resulting from a bladder infection or injury. Epididymitis causes pain and swelling in the scrotum; the pain and swelling develop gradually, over hours or days, and can become severe. The scrotum may feel hot and be tender to the touch, and the person may have a fever. Bacterial epididymitis is usually treated with antibiotics.

Orchitis is inflammation of the testicle. It may be caused by a bacterial infection or by a virus, most often the mumps. Orchitis can also occur with epididymitis or a prostate infection (prostatitis). Symptoms include scrotal pain, swelling (usually on one side of the scrotum), and a feeling of heaviness in the scrotum. If it is not treated, orchitis can cause infertility.

Testicular cancer is rare and most often affects males between the ages of 15 and 35. Those at highest risk include males whose testicles have not descended or did not descend until after age 6 and males with a family history of testicular cancer. Testicular cancer usually affects only one testicle and responds well to treatment if detected early. Symptoms of testicular cancer may include a painless lump or swelling or a feeling of heaviness in one testicle.

Prevention

- Prevent testicular injury by wearing a protective athletic cup when you play sports.

- Prevent bacterial infections that are spread through sexual contact by following the safer sex guidelines on pages 336 and 337.
- Make sure your child has completed the measles, mumps, and rubella (MMR) vaccination series. See page 18.

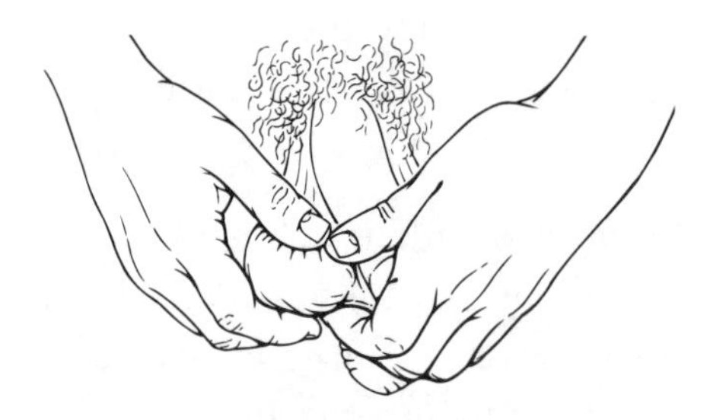

Gently feel each testicle for hard lumps or a change in size.

- Teenage boys and men should do a testicular self-examination once a month. After taking a warm bath or shower:
  - Stand and place your right leg on an elevated surface such as the side of the bathtub or the toilet seat.
  - Examine the surface of your right testicle by gently rolling it between the thumb and fingers of both hands. Feel for any hard lumps or nodules. The testicle should feel round and smooth.
  - Feel for any enlargement of the testicle or a change in its consistency. It is normal for one testicle to be slightly larger than the other. Report any major size differences or any changes in feeling or appearance to a health professional.
  - Repeat the examination on your left testicle.

Home Treatment

- Elevating the scrotum with a pillow and applying ice may help relieve pain caused by an injury.
- Wearing a jockstrap daily may relieve scrotal pain.
- Take Aspirin or acetaminophen to relieve pain caused by orchitis. Do not give Aspirin to anyone younger than 20. Warm baths may also help relieve pain.

When to Call a Health Professional

- If pain in a testicle or the scrotum comes on suddenly and is severe. This may be a sign of testicular torsion, which requires immediate treatment.
- If you find a lump in a testicle.
- If you notice any enlargement in a testicle or a change in its consistency.
- If pain or swelling in a testicle or the scrotum worsens over a period of several hours or days or does not lessen after a few days.
- If pain or swelling in a testicle or the scrotum is accompanied by fever.
- If pain or swelling in the scrotum develops after exposure to the mumps virus.
- If you have a feeling of heaviness in one testicle.

I wasn't kissing her, I was whispering in her mouth.
Groucho Marx

17 Sexual Health

This chapter covers specific health issues of concern to people who are sexually active, from birth control to sexually transmitted diseases (STDs), including infection with the human immunodeficiency virus (HIV), which causes AIDS. It also addresses sexual issues unique to older adults.

Birth Control

Birth control can help prevent unplanned pregnancies. However, no birth control method (except abstinence) is 100 percent effective and without risks. The text that follows and the chart on page 330 briefly describe the most common birth control methods.

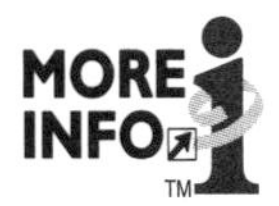

Review each of the birth control methods presented in this chapter before deciding which one meets your needs. Your health professional can help you better understand the effectiveness and risks of each method.

Use all birth control methods exactly as your doctor or the package instructions recommend. Proper use helps ensure effectiveness.

Hormonal methods of birth control for women either prevent the ovaries from releasing an egg each month (ovulation) or thicken the mucus at the opening of the uterus so sperm can't get to the uterus to fertilize an egg. Almost all hormonal birth control methods require a doctor's prescription. Hormonal methods of birth control do not protect against STDs.

Oral contraceptives (the Pill) are taken daily. Depo-Provera is a hormone injection given by a health professional once every 3 months. The transdermal patch (Ortho Evra) is a newer form of hormonal contraception.

Birth Control		
Method	**Pregnancies***	**Comments**
Sterilization		Consider it permanent.
Tubal ligation (women)	Fewer than 1	
Vasectomy (men)	1 to 2	
Hormonal Methods		
Oral contraceptives (the Pill)	80	Increased risk of circulatory disorders and high blood pressure in women who smoke.
Depo-Provera (shot)	30	Depo-Provera may cause irregular menstrual bleeding.
Intrauterine Device (IUD)		May be expelled without being noticed. Copper IUD may cause bleeding and cramping. LNg IUD reduces bleeding and cramping and has reduced risk of pelvic infection.
Levonorgestrel (LNg) IUD	1	
Copper IUD	8	
Barrier Methods		
Condom (male)	150	For maximum protection against STDs, use latex or polyurethane condoms every time you have sex.
Condom (female)	210	
Diaphragm (with spermicide)	160	
Cervical cap (with spermicide)	160 to 320	Higher failure rate (320 per 1,000) is for women who have given birth vaginally.
Spermicides (alone)	290	Use with a condom for best protection.
Jelly, cream, foam, suppositories		
Periodic abstinence	200 to 250	
(natural family planning: basal body temperature, mucus, or rhythm/calendar method)		Natural family planning can be used either to plan or to avoid a pregnancy.
Withdrawal	270	
No method (chance)	850	

*Typical number of accidental pregnancies per 1,000 women in 1 year. When birth control methods are used exactly as directed, pregnancy rates are lower. Adapted from: Trussell J, Kowal D. The essentials of contraception. In: R. Hatcher et al., *Contraceptive Technology*, 18th ed., 2004.

The intrauterine device (IUD) is a plastic or metal device that is inserted into the uterus by a doctor. The levonorgestrel (LNg) IUD releases a hormone to prevent conception; it also reduces menstrual cramping and bleeding. Other IUDs are made of copper, which causes changes in the uterus that kill sperm and prevent implantation of a fertilized egg. IUDs do not provide any protection against STDs.

Barrier methods of birth control keep sperm from entering the uterus and reaching the egg. They are often used with spermicides, which kill sperm. Barrier methods work best when two methods are combined (for example, male condoms used with spermicidal foam).

The male condom is a thin, flexible tube of latex rubber, polyurethane, or animal skin that is placed over the man's erect penis before sexual intercourse to catch ejaculated semen. There are also condoms for women that fit inside the vagina. Latex or polyurethane condoms provide the most reliable, but not total, protection against STDs, including HIV. Lambskin condoms are not effective in preventing STDs. Condoms are available without a doctor's prescription. Condoms can be used with other birth control methods for added protection against STDs.

Spermicides are foams, jellies, and suppositories that contain chemicals which kill sperm. Many condoms are lubricated with a spermicide. Spermicides are available without a doctor's prescription. Most spermicides contain nonoxynol-9. Some people are allergic to nonoxynol-9 and may develop sores in the vagina or on the penis after coming in contact with it. Sometimes the allergic reaction is triggered by other chemicals in the spermicide, and switching to a different product solves the problem.

The diaphragm and cervical cap are small rubber caps that are filled with spermicide and inserted into the vagina to cover the opening of the uterus (cervix) before sexual intercourse begins. They are left in place for 6 hours or longer after sexual intercourse. When used alone, these barrier methods provide minimal protection against STDs.

Surgical methods are the most effective forms of birth control. During a vasectomy, the tubes (vas deferens) that carry a man's sperm from his testes are clamped or cut off, thus preventing sperm from being ejaculated in semen. Tubal ligation procedures close off or cut the tubes (fallopian tubes) that carry a woman's eggs from her ovaries to her uterus. This prevents eggs from being fertilized or implanting in the uterus. Both vasectomy and tubal ligation should be considered permanent, but in some cases they can be successfully reversed with surgery. Surgical methods of birth control do not protect you against STDs.

Emergency Contraception

Emergency contraception either prevents the release of an egg from a woman's ovaries (ovulation) or prevents a fertilized egg from implanting in the uterus. It can be very effective for preventing unwanted pregnancy if you use it soon after you have unprotected sex.

Sometimes called the "morning-after pill," emergency contraceptive pills (usually a high-dose form of regular birth control pills) should be taken within 72 hours (3 days) after unprotected sex but may be effective up to 5 days after sex. Inserting a copper intrauterine device (IUD) within 5 days after ovulation (up to 8 days after unprotected sex, in some cases) is another method of emergency contraception.

Regardless of method, the sooner you use emergency contraception, the more effective it is in preventing pregnancy.

If you have sex and are concerned about a possible pregnancy because you did not use birth control or because your birth control may have failed (for instance, if a condom or diaphragm tore), call your health professional or pharmacist immediately for information about emergency contraception. In BC, emergency contraception may be prescribed by a doctor or a pharmacist.

Natural family planning (fertility awareness) methods help a couple estimate when the woman is most likely to become pregnant (before and during ovulation) so they can avoid sexual intercourse during that time or have intercourse to get pregnant. To estimate when ovulation occurs, a woman records her temperature, examines her vaginal mucus discharge, and tracks her menstrual periods. You can also buy urine test strips that help estimate when ovulation occurs. Like any birth control method, natural family planning is most effective when used correctly. Couples who do not receive or follow proper instruction in using the method have a much higher rate of accidental pregnancy. Natural family planning does not provide protection against STDs.

Sexually Transmitted Diseases

Sexually transmitted diseases (STDs) or venereal diseases (VD) are infections passed from person to person through sexual intercourse, genital contact, or contact with fluids such as semen, vaginal fluids, and blood (including menstrual blood). Many of these diseases can also be spread by sharing needles and other items that may be contaminated with infected blood or body fluids.

Chlamydia, genital herpes, genital warts, gonorrhea, hepatitis B,

HIV (which causes AIDS), syphilis, and trichomoniasis are among the most common STDs. If you think you might have symptoms of any of the STDs as described below, call your doctor, your public health unit, or the BC NurseLine for advice.

Chlamydia, gonorrhea, hepatitis B, herpes simplex virus, HIV, and syphilis can be spread from an infected mother to her unborn baby or infant. Treatment during pregnancy can prevent the spread of many of these diseases from mother to child. If you are infected with any of these diseases, talk to your doctor about how you can protect your baby before and after it is born.

Chlamydia

Chlamydia is a bacterial infection that affects millions of men and women. It may be difficult to detect chlamydia; about 80 percent of women and 50 percent of men with the disease have no symptoms, but they can still infect their sex partners. If symptoms do show up, they occur 1 to 3 weeks after exposure to the bacteria. In women, symptoms may include vaginal discharge or irregular menstrual bleeding, pain or burning when urinating, or lower abdominal pain. In men, there may be a discharge from the penis and pain or burning when urinating.

Chlamydia is easily treated with antibiotics. If undetected and untreated, chlamydia can cause pelvic inflammatory disease (infection in the ovaries and fallopian tubes), which may lead to sterility (inability to conceive a child). Both partners need to be treated.

Genital herpes

Genital herpes is caused by the herpes simplex virus, which also causes cold sores (see page 250).

Genital herpes is easily spread through sexual contact and any other direct contact with genital herpes sores.

Symptoms of the first genital herpes outbreak occur 2 to 7 days after contact with an infected person. It is also possible to be infected with genital herpes and have no symptoms.

The first outbreak of genital herpes may be quite severe, with many painful sores or blisters. Fever, swollen lymph nodes, and headache or muscle aches may also occur. If the sores develop inside the urethra (the tube that carries urine out of the body) or the vagina, there may be pain when urinating or vaginal discharge. The sores crust over and disappear in 2 to 3 weeks.

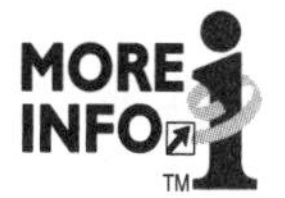

There is no known cure for genital herpes, although medication can reduce pain and speed healing of sores during an outbreak. Most people with genital herpes have recurrent outbreaks. Having 4 outbreaks per year is typical. Outbreaks tend to become less frequent and less severe over time. Itching, burning, or tingling may occur at the place where the sores will later appear.

If you have frequent or severe outbreaks, taking medication every day can help reduce how often outbreaks occur and how long they last.

Genital warts

Genital warts are caused by the human papillomavirus (HPV), which is spread through sexual contact. The warts generally look like small, fleshy bumps or flat, white patches on the lips around the vagina (labia), inside the vagina, on the penis or scrotum, or around the anus. A person infected with HPV may never develop genital warts, or the warts may be too small to be seen. Certain types of HPV increase the risk of cervical cancer in women. A Pap test can occasionally detect the virus.

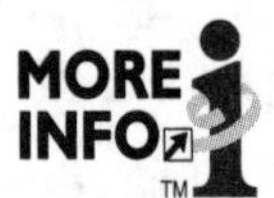

If genital warts are bothersome or develop on the cervix, they can be treated by a health professional. However, treatment does not cure HPV infection, and the warts may persist or recur. There does not appear to be an effective cure for HPV infection at this time. However, in many people the infection goes away by itself and does not cause further problems.

Gonorrhea

Gonorrhea is a bacterial infection that is spread through sexual contact. Symptoms, which appear 2 days to 2 weeks after infection, may include pain or burning when urinating, vaginal discharge, irregular menstrual bleeding, or a thick discharge from the penis. Many people who are infected have no symptoms.

Untreated gonorrhea can lead to pelvic inflammatory disease and sterility in women; it can lead to prostate infection (see page 323) in men. Gonorrhea sometimes spreads to a person's joints, causing arthritis. Antibiotic treatment cures the infection. Both sex partners need to be treated to keep from passing the infection back and forth.

Hepatitis B

Hepatitis B is a viral infection that is spread through contact with infected blood, semen, or vaginal fluid (see page 122). The hepatitis B virus (HBV) is very contagious and may be spread to household contacts (other than sex partners) by sharing such things as razors and toothbrushes. Most people with hepatitis B recover completely after 4 to 8 weeks, but a small percentage of adults remain infected for months or years. Chronic infection can lead to life-threatening liver damage or cancer. Drug treatment for chronic HBV infection is not very effective.

In British Columbia, you can get a free hepatitis B vaccine if:

- You are a sexual partner of someone who has hepatitis B.
- You are a male who has sexual contact with other males.
- You inject illegal drugs or are a sexual partner of someone who does.

- You have many sexual partners or have a recent history of a sexually transmitted disease.
- You have hepatitis C.

See page 19 for more information about the vaccine.

Human immunodeficiency virus (HIV)

Human immunodeficiency virus (HIV) is spread when blood, semen, or vaginal fluids from an infected person enter someone else's body. Once a person becomes infected, the virus attacks and gradually weakens his or her immune system. AIDS (acquired immunodeficiency syndrome) is the last phase in HIV disease, when the body is no longer able to fight infection or disease. Without treatment, AIDS develops in most people 12 to 13 years after they first become infected with HIV. With treatment, AIDS may be delayed for many more years.

A person is said to be HIV-positive if antibodies to the virus are detected in his or her blood. It may take up to 6 months after infection for the antibodies to appear. However, the virus can be spread to others before antibodies or symptoms are apparent.

The specific behaviours that spread HIV include:

- Having more than one sex partner.
- Having unprotected sex, especially unprotected sex between men (unless both sex partners have sex only with each other and neither is infected).
- Sharing needles, syringes, or other "drug works" with someone who is HIV-positive.
- Having a sex partner with any of the above risk factors.

Babies born to or breast-fed by women who are HIV-positive are also at high risk for becoming infected with the virus.

Because all donated blood has been tested for HIV since 1985, the risk of getting the virus from transfused blood or blood products is extremely low.

HIV is not spread by mosquitoes; toilet seats; being coughed on by an infected person; casual contact with someone who is HIV-positive or who has AIDS; or by donating blood. Being touched, hugged, or lightly kissed by someone who is HIV-positive will not transfer the virus to you.

A simple, confidential blood test can determine if you are HIV-positive. Call your health care provider to arrange for a test. If you engage in activities that put you at risk for HIV infection, have an HIV test every 6 months. Early diagnosis and treatment of HIV are important even before symptoms develop. If you think you have been exposed to HIV, but you test negative, you should be tested again 6 months after your last known exposure to HIV.

If you are pregnant and have any reason to believe that you may ever have been exposed to HIV, getting tested is the most important thing you can do for your baby. If you are HIV-positive, drug treatment during pregnancy can greatly reduce the likelihood that you will pass the infection on to your baby.

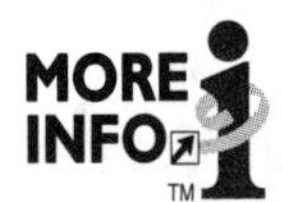

People who educate themselves about HIV infection learn how to prevent the spread of the virus and seek treatments that may improve their chances for staying healthy longer.

Syphilis

Syphilis is a bacterial infection spread through sexual contact, through sharing needles contaminated with an infected person's blood, or from an infected mother to her unborn baby. When syphilis is spread through sexual contact, symptoms appear about 3 weeks after infection occurs. The first symptom is a red, painless sore that appears on the genitals, rectal area, or mouth. The sore may go unnoticed. Swollen lymph nodes near the sore are another possible symptom.

If syphilis is not treated, it can proceed to a second phase after about 2 months. Symptoms of the second phase include a rash, patchy hair loss, fever, swollen lymph nodes, and flu-like symptoms that are easily confused with other illnesses.

Syphilis can be cured with antibiotics. If untreated, syphilis may cause serious health problems and death. Both partners need to be treated.

Trichomoniasis

Trichomoniasis is a bacterial infection that is spread through sexual contact. In women, the bacteria usually infect the vagina or urethra. In men, infections can develop in the urethra or under the foreskin of the penis.

Up to 50 percent of women who have trichomoniasis have no symptoms, and symptoms in infected men are rare. If symptoms do occur, they appear 4 to 28 days after infection. Symptoms in women may include vaginal discharge, itching, and irritation and pain during sexual intercourse and when urinating. In men there may be a discharge from the penis and pain when urinating.

Trichomoniasis usually does not lead to serious illness. However, the infected person and his or her sex partner need to be treated with antibiotics to keep from passing the infection back and forth. Condoms should be used until treatment is completed.

Prevention

Preventing a sexually transmitted disease is easier than treating an infection once it occurs. Only monogamy (you and your partner have sex only with each other) between uninfected partners or sexual abstinence completely eliminates the risk of HIV infection and other sexually transmitted diseases. The following safer sex guidelines will help you reduce your risk.

- If you are beginning a new sexual relationship:
  - Take time before having sex to talk about HIV and other STDs. Find out if your partner has ever been exposed to or infected with an STD or if your partner's behaviour puts him or her at risk for HIV infection. Tell your partner if you've ever engaged in high-risk behaviour. Remember that it is possible to be infected with an STD without knowing it.
  - Use latex condoms every time you have sex (vaginal, anal, or oral) until you are certain that you and your partner are free of STDs and you both agree not to have unprotected sexual contact with anyone else while your relationship lasts.
  - If you plan to use HIV testing to decide whether it is safe to have unprotected sex, have the test done 6 months after the last time you engaged in high-risk behaviour. In the meantime, use condoms every time you have sexual contact.
- Avoid unprotected sexual contact with anyone who has symptoms of or who has been exposed to an STD, or whose behaviour puts him or her at risk for HIV infection. Keep in mind that a person may still be able to transmit STDs even if no symptoms are present.
- Avoid unprotected vaginal, anal, or oral sex with anyone whose sexual history may not be risk-free or who has sores on the genitals or mouth. Use latex condoms from the beginning to the end of sexual contact to reduce your risk. "Natural" or lambskin condoms do not protect against HIV infection or other STDs.
- Avoid sexual contact while you or your partner is being treated for an STD.
- If you or your partner has genital herpes, avoid sexual contact when a blister or an open sore is present or when tingling or pain occurs in the genital area, which may signal an outbreak. At other times, use latex condoms to help reduce the spread of the virus. A person can transmit genital herpes even when no sores are present.
- Do not rely on spermicides or a diaphragm to protect against STDs. If spermicide irritates the skin or tissues in your genital area, it may increase your risk of infection. Except for abstinence, latex condoms provide the best protection against STDs, including HIV.

In addition to the guidelines above, taking the following precautions will reduce your risk of getting HIV and hepatitis B:

- Avoid activities that may spread HIV (see page 335). Safer activities include closed-mouth kissing, hugging, massage, and other pleasurable touching.
- Never share needles, syringes, razors, or other personal items that could be contaminated with blood.

If your job or behaviour puts you at risk for HIV infection, or if you come in contact with HIV-infected blood (for example, an accidental needle prick), contact a health professional immediately. In some cases, medications may prevent HIV infection if they are started within a few hours after you are exposed to the virus. Have a blood test 6 months after any activity or accident that puts you at risk for HIV infection.

For more information, check the phone directory for the HIV/AIDS hotline in your area.

When to Call a Health Professional

All STDs need to be diagnosed and treated by a health professional. Call your doctor, public health nurse, or the BC NurseLine for confidential help. Your sex partner may also need to be treated, even if he or she has no symptoms. Otherwise, your partner may reinfect you or develop serious complications.

Call a health professional:

- If you suspect that you have been exposed to an STD.
- If you notice any unusual discharge from the vagina or penis, burning during urination, or any sores, redness, or growths on the genitals.
- If your behaviour puts you at risk for exposure to HIV, or if your sex partner has high-risk behaviour or is HIV-positive.
- If you are pregnant and have any reason to believe that you may have been exposed to an STD, especially HIV.
- If you have symptoms such as fatigue, weight loss, fever, diarrhea, cough, or swollen glands that do not go away after a short period of time and do not seem to be related to any illness.
- If you are HIV-positive and you develop any of the following:
  - Fever higher than 39.4°C.
  - Fever higher than 38.3°C that lasts 3 days or longer.
  - Increased outbreaks of cold sores or any unusual skin or mouth sores.
  - Severe numbness or pain in the hands and feet.
  - Unexplained weight loss.
  - Unexplained fever and night sweats.
  - Severe fatigue.
  - Diarrhea or other bowel changes.
  - Shortness of breath and a persistent dry cough.
  - Swollen lymph nodes in the neck, armpits, or groin.
  - Personality changes, difficulty concentrating, confusion, or severe headache.

Sexuality and Aging

FOR SENIORS

Sex and sexuality communicate a great deal: affection, love, esteem, warmth, sharing, and bonding. These gifts are as much the birthright of those in their 80s and 90s as of those who are much younger.

In most healthy adults, pleasure and interest in sex do not diminish with age. Age alone is no reason to change the sexual practices that you have enjoyed throughout your life. However, you may have to make a few minor adjustments to accommodate any physical limitations you may have or the effects of certain illnesses or medications.

Common Physical Changes in Men

- A man's sexual response begins to slow down after age 50. However, a man's sexual drive is more likely to be affected by his health and his attitude about sex and intimacy than by his age.
- It may take longer for a man to get an erection, and more time needs to pass between erections.
- Erections will be less firm. However, a man who has good blood flow to his penis will be able to have erections that are firm enough for sexual intercourse throughout his entire life. For information about erection problems, see page 321.
- Older men are able to delay ejaculation for a longer time.

Common Physical Changes in Women

Most physical changes take place after menopause and are the result of decreased estrogen levels. These changes can be altered if a woman is taking hormone therapy.

- It may take longer for a woman to become sexually excited.
- A woman's skin may feel more sensitive and irritable, making caressing and skin-to-skin contact less pleasurable.
- The walls of the vagina become thinner and drier and are more easily irritated during sexual intercourse. Use a water-based vaginal lubricant to reduce the irritation. Do not use petroleum jelly. A doctor can also prescribe a vaginal cream containing estrogen, which will help reverse the changes in the vaginal tissues.
- Orgasms may be somewhat shorter than they used to be, and the contractions experienced during orgasm can be uncomfortable.

Not all women experience these problems. Those who do can experiment to find ways to enjoy sex despite these physical changes.

Sexuality and Cultural and Psychological Changes

In addition to physical changes, there are cultural and psychological factors that affect sexuality in later years. For example, in our society, sexuality is equated with youthful looks and youthful vigor. Too many people seem to think that as a person ages, he or she becomes less desirable and less of a sexual being. Older adults may accept this stereotype and buy into the notion that they are not permitted or expected to be sexual.

Joy in sex and loving knows no age barriers. Almost everyone has the capacity to find lifelong pleasure in sex. To believe in the myth that older people have no interest in sex is to miss out on wonderful possibilities.

Being single through choice, divorce, or widowhood can present a problem as well. As you get older, you may not have as many people in your age group to choose from for partners. Women and men who are single may not know how to deal with their sexual feelings. Generally speaking, it is better to express your desires than to suppress them until you are no longer aware that they exist.

Physical and emotional needs change with time and circumstance. Intimacy and sexuality may or may not be important to you. The issue here is one of choice. If you freely decide that sex is no longer right for you, then that is the correct decision. However, if you choose to continue enjoying your sexuality, you deserve support and encouragement.

Use It or Lose It: Staying Sexual

Just as exercise is the key to maintaining fitness and health, having sex on a regular basis is the best way to maintain sexual capacity.

And just as it's never too late to start an exercise program, it's never too late to start having sex. Many older people who have been celibate for years develop satisfying sexual practices within new loving relationships. For others, self-stimulation is common and poses no health risks or side effects.

Here are some additional considerations:

- To enhance sexual response, use more foreplay and direct contact with sex organs.
- The mind is an erogenous zone. Fantasy and imagination help arouse some people. Try setting the mood with candlelight and soft music, or whatever else "turns you on."
- Many medications, especially high blood pressure medications, tranquilizers, and some heart medications, inhibit sexual response. Ask your doctor about

these side effects. Your doctor may be able to reduce your dosage or prescribe different medications. Do not stop taking prescription medications without consulting your doctor first.

- Colostomies, mastectomies, and other procedures that involve changes in physical appearance need not put an end to sexual pleasure. Communicating openly about your fears and expectations can bring you and your partner closer together and help you overcome barriers. If necessary, a little counselling for both of you can help you adjust.
- People who have heart conditions can enjoy full, satisfying sex lives. Most doctors recommend that you abstain from sex for only a brief time following a heart attack. If you have angina, ask your doctor about taking nitroglycerin before you have sex. Do not take Viagra, Levitra, or Cialis if you are using nitroglycerin.
- If arthritis keeps you from enjoying sex, experiment with different positions. Try placing cushions under your hips. Also try home treatment for arthritis pain. See page 158.
- Use lubricants if vaginal dryness or irritation is a problem.
- Drink alcohol only in moderation. Small amounts of alcohol may heighten your sexual responsiveness by reducing your inhibitions. Larger amounts of alcohol may increase your sexual desire, but they decrease sexual performance.
- Prescription medications that can enhance the sexual response—such as sildenafil citrate (Viagra) for men and testosterone for women—are available. Some people find that herbs such as ginkgo biloba and ginseng enhance their sexual function. Both prescription drugs and herbal remedies carry the risk of side effects. Your health professional can help you decide whether these options are right for you.

Other Aspects of Sexuality

Sexuality goes far beyond the physical act itself. It is part of who we are. It involves our needs for touch, affection, and intimacy.

Touch

Touch is a wonderful and needed sensation. Babies who are not touched do not thrive. Children who are not touched develop emotional problems. Touch is important to older adults as well. Touch helps us feel connected with others and enhances our sexuality.

- Get a massage. Professional massages are wonderful, but simple shoulder and neck rubs feel great too. Find a friend who will trade shoulder rubs with you.
- Look for hugs. Everybody needs them. Some people are a little shy about hugs, but it's okay to ask, "Would you like a hug?"

- Consider getting a pet. Caring for a pet can help meet your needs for touch. Some studies have shown that older people who have pets to care for live longer.

Affection

To give and receive affection is a wonderful feeling. If you like someone, be sure to let them know. If someone seems to like you, appreciate it. It is never too late to make new friends and strengthen bonds with longtime companions.

Intimacy

Intimacy is the capacity for a close physical or emotional connection with another person. Intimacy is a great protector against depression.

Talking with a confidant can help ease life's problems. When you lose a loved one, intimacy may be what you miss most. You may not find someone to fully replace a loved one who died, but you can begin to rebuild intimacy in your life in the following ways:

- Turn to your children, siblings, or old and new friends.
- Look for another person who is in the same situation as you are. One of the richest benefits of support groups is that members often find intimacy with one another.
- Be available to others. Just as you need people, there are people who need you too.

If exercise could be packed into a pill, it would be the single most widely prescribed, and beneficial, medicine in the nation.
Robert Butler, MD

18

Fitness

Do you want to feel less stressed? Less tired? More in control of your weight and appearance? More healthy? Do you want to reduce your risk of heart disease, diabetes, and many other health problems? Believe it or not, there is one thing that can help you do all of this, and it doesn't come in a bottle. It's regular physical activity.

If just thinking about exercise makes you sweat, you may be pleasantly surprised by the information in this chapter. If you have already made physical activity a routine part of your life, you may find new reasons to keep your body moving.

Your Personal Fitness Plan

No one can prescribe the perfect fitness plan for you. You have to figure it out based on what you enjoy doing and what you will continue to do. The next few pages can be a big help.

Consistency is the most important, the most basic, and the most often neglected part of people's efforts to become more fit. No matter which activities you choose to do, you need to do them consistently in order to get the most benefit.

Don't forget the important role that nutrition plays in your healthy lifestyle. A balanced diet and regular physical activity go hand in hand to help you maintain a healthy weight. To learn how active people can get adequate nutrition, see Nutrition starting on page 351.

A good fitness plan has three parts: aerobic fitness, muscle strengthening, and flexibility. Many physical activities stress two or all three of these aspects of fitness. Read the sections that follow to learn about each aspect of fitness; then see Setting Your Fitness Goals on page 350.

FOR SENIORS

Benefits of Exercise for Older Adults

Exercise is one of your best defenses against many problems that are associated with aging.

Problem	How Exercise Helps
Arthritis	Improves flexibility and range of motion; improves muscle strength; helps protect joints.
Chronic obstructive pulmonary disease (COPD)	Improves endurance and feeling of well-being.
Constipation	Regular activity keeps waste moving through your bowels.
Depression and confusion	Improves mood; increases energy level; improves thinking; improves self-image.
Diabetes (type 2)	Helps the body use blood sugar more efficiently; helps control weight; helps you live longer.
Heart disease	Helps lower cholesterol; improves the heart's ability to pump blood; helps you live longer.
High blood pressure	Lowers blood pressure; improves heart and lung health.
Insomnia	Reduces stress and promotes relaxation; may improve sleep.
Obesity	Reduces weight by burning calories; helps maintain a healthy body weight.
Osteoporosis	Weight-bearing exercise (walking, lifting weights) helps maintain bone strength.

Aerobic Fitness

Aerobic conditioning improves the ability of your heart and lungs to deliver oxygen to your muscles. Aerobic fitness allows you to do more with less fatigue.

Generally speaking, anything that raises your heart rate can be considered aerobic exercise. Some of the more common aerobic exercises include brisk walking, running, bicycling, swimming, and dancing.

You don't have to go out of your way to improve your aerobic fitness. Many activities that you do each day will help you become more fit if you do them regularly and at least at a moderate intensity. The following ordinary activities all count as aerobic activity:

- Sweeping or mopping floors (perhaps to fast-paced music)
- Raking leaves, shovelling snow, or pushing a lawn mower
- Walking the dog
- Taking the stairs to your office instead of taking the elevator
- Walking to a nearby restaurant for lunch instead of driving there

How Hard Should I Exercise?

In order to benefit from aerobic exercise, you need to work hard enough to increase your heart rate. Work hard enough to feel the effort, but not so hard that you become out of breath. Above all, listen to your body. If the exercise feels too hard, slow down. You will reduce your risk of injury and enjoy the exercise much more.

Try the "talk-sing test" to determine your ideal exercise pace:

- If you can't talk and exercise at the same time, you are going too fast.
- If you can talk while you exercise, you are doing fine.
- If you can sing while you exercise, it would be safe to increase your pace a little.

Target Heart Rate

Age	10-second heart rate (multiply by 6 for heart rate per minute)
20	20–27
25	20–26
30	19–25
35	19–25
40	18–24
45	18–23
50	17–23
55	17–22
60	16–21
65	16–21
70	15–20

Target heart rate is 60 percent to 80 percent of maximum heart rate. (Maximum heart rate per minute = 220 minus your age.)

Target Heart Rate

Another way to see how hard you are exercising is to check your heart rate. You get the most benefit from aerobic exercise when your exercising heart rate is 60 percent to 80 percent of your maximum heart rate (220 minus your age). After exercising for about 10 minutes, stop and take your pulse for 10 seconds (see page 103). Compare the number to the chart on page 345. Adjust the intensity of your exercise so that your heart rate stays between the two numbers. Remember, the target heart rate is only a guide. Everyone's body is different, so pay attention to how you feel.

How Often and How Long Should I Exercise?

The three factors that you need to consider when planning a fitness routine are:

1. Frequency (how often you exercise).

2. Duration (how long you exercise).

3. Intensity (how hard you exercise).

Achieving a balance between these three factors will give you better results than if you take any one of them to an extreme. You may choose to do a vigorously paced physical activity (such as swimming, fast dancing, or cycling) 3 times a week for 30 minutes per session. Or you may choose to exercise at a moderate intensity (by walking or doing yard work) 5 to 6 times a week for 30 minutes per session. You can also mix shorter, more intense exercise sessions with longer, less strenuous sessions.

In general, try to get at least 30 minutes of moderate physical activity most days of the week. Children should be even more active (at least 60 minutes a day).

Warm Up and Cool Down

For the first 5 or 10 minutes of your activity routine, go slowly and easily, gradually increasing your pace, so your muscles have a chance to warm up. After a few minutes of warm-up, do some stretches to prepare your muscles for the workout.

End your activity with a cool-down period of about 8 to 10 minutes. Gradually slow your pace for about 5 minutes; then do a few stretches (see page 348) to improve flexibility.

Drink water before, during, and after the activity.

Making Progress

As you build aerobic endurance, your heart rate will not rise as high as it once did during the same activity. You will need to do the activity longer, harder, or more often to get the same benefits from it. You can use your target heart rate to decide how much harder your workout needs to be. You can also add some new element of difficulty or variety to your current workout, such as increasing your pace, alternating between an aerobic activity and a strength-training activity (cross-training), or trying a new aerobic activity that is slightly harder for you.

Be careful to progress slowly. Overdoing it can lead to injury or burnout.

Muscle Strengthening

Strengthening your muscles enables you to do more work and to work longer before you become exhausted. Strong muscles also help protect your joints.

Muscles become stronger through a three-step process:

1. Stress
2. Recovery (rest)
3. Repeated stress

A program for increasing your muscle strength can be as formal or informal as you'd like it to be. You may choose to do resistance training with free weights, weight-training equipment, inexpensive rubber tubing, or even canned goods.

Other simple, safe, and effective strengthening exercises include bent-knee curl-ups, chin-ups, push-ups, side leg-lifts, and other exercises that improve abdominal, neck, arm, shoulder, and leg strength.

As your muscles grow stronger, you will notice that you can work longer without tiring. If a muscle-strengthening activity starts to feel too easy, gradually add more resistance. Remember to work slowly, and move your muscles through their full range of motion.

Flexibility

Flexibility comes from stretching. Stretching is a simple and relaxing activity that has a variety of health benefits. Stretching regularly gives you flexible muscles and joints, which helps prevent injury and improves your range of motion. Being flexible also helps you have a better sense of balance.

Stretching is particularly important during the cool-down phase of exercise, when your muscles are warm. Your muscles are repeatedly shortened when they are used, especially during exercise. See the stretches on page 348.

- Stretch slowly and gradually. Don't bounce. Maintain a continuous tension on the muscle.
- Relax and hold each stretch for a count of 10.
- Exhale as you stretch to further relax your muscles. If stretching hurts, you have gone too far or you are doing something incorrectly.

Try to stretch a little every day. Take a stretch break instead of a coffee break, or take dance, martial arts, or yoga classes, which may appeal to your sense of fun and adventure as well as improve your flexibility.

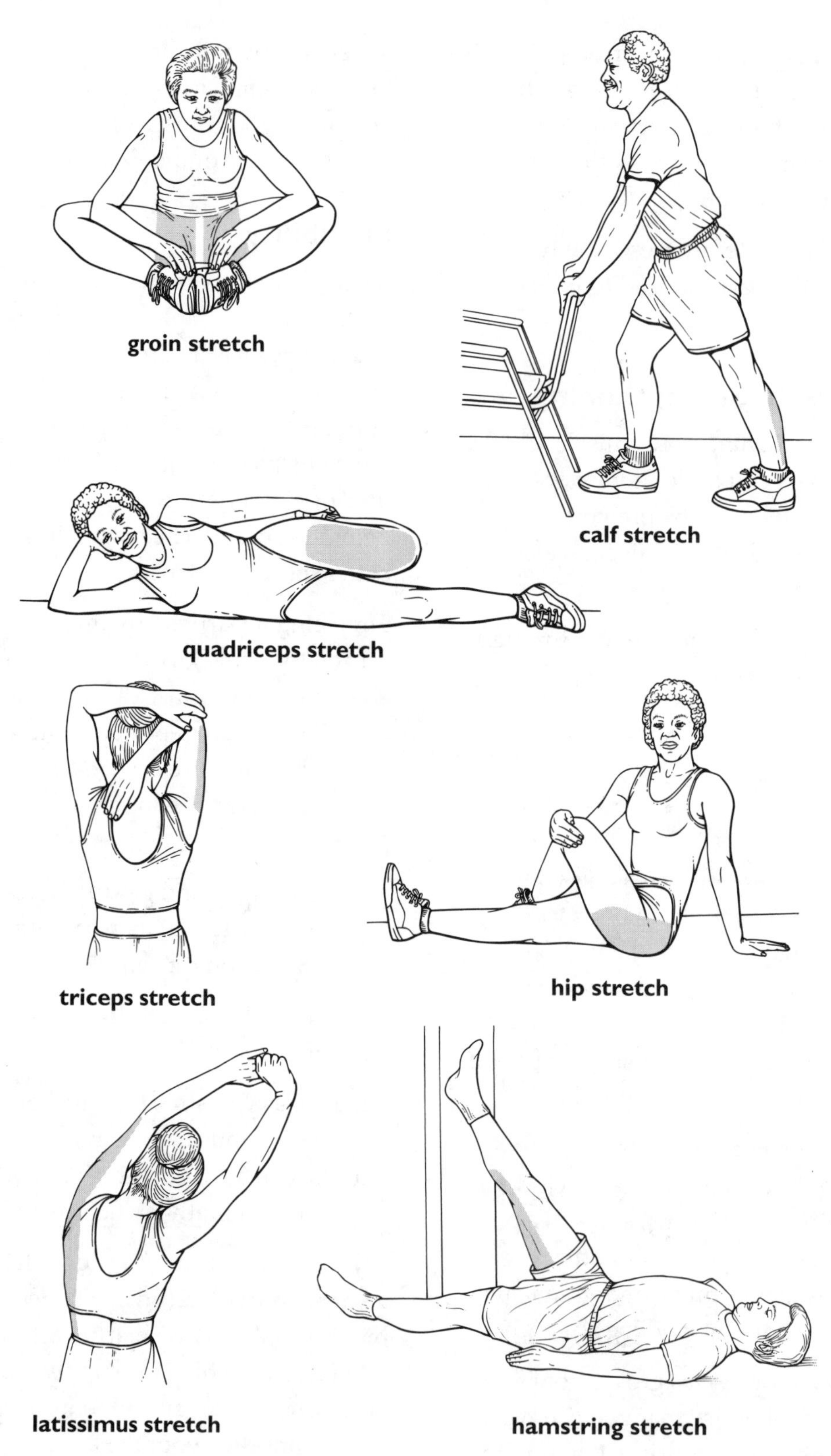

Stretching exercises. Shaded areas show where stretches are felt.

Exercise Cautions

Moderate exercise is safe for most people. However, if you answer yes to any of the following questions, talk with your doctor before starting an exercise program.

- Do you have heart trouble?
- Do you often have pains in your heart or chest?
- Do you have high blood pressure?
- Do you often feel faint or have dizzy spells?
- Do you have arthritis or other bone or joint problems that might be made worse by exercise?
- Do you have diabetes? (Increased exercise affects your insulin needs.)
- Are you over age 40 with 2 or more risk factors for heart disease*?
- Are you over age 40 and planning to do hard exercise?

*Cholesterol over 5.17 mmol/L; blood pressure over 140/90; smoking; diabetes; obesity; family history of heart disease before age 50.

Overcoming Barriers to Exercise

There are many barriers to getting regular physical activity, some of which are easier to overcome than others. Here are a few common barriers and some suggestions for getting past them.

1. No time? Try shorter periods of activity spread throughout the day, such as walking 3 times a day for 10 minutes each time.

2. Too tired? It's often lack of exercise that makes you tired. Exercise gives you energy. Try it.

3. Embarrassed? Many people are, especially at first. Be proud that you're taking care of your body.

4. No partner? Yes, it's more fun to exercise with a friend. If your regular exercise partner quits, find another one.

5. Bad weather? Too hot, too cold, too wet, too windy—it never seems right for exercise. Lots of people exercise come rain or shine. You can too; just dress properly. Try a variety of indoor and outdoor activities.

6. Too costly? You had to let the fitness club membership expire. You can't afford fancy exercise equipment. You panic at the price of running shoes. It all costs money. But can you afford not to exercise? Try a low-cost option, such as walking, riding a bicycle, or dancing.

7. Not the athletic type? Physical activity doesn't require any special athletic skill. Everyone's body is made to move.

Setting Your Fitness Goals

Are you as strong, flexible, and physically fit as you would like to be? If you are, good for you. You can use this chapter to reaffirm your commitment to physical fitness and stay motivated. However, if you want to make some improvements, here's one piece of advice: Try to take it one step at a time.

- Pick one aspect of fitness (aerobic, strength, flexibility) that you want to improve first.
- Pick an activity that you enjoy. You're more likely to keep doing something you like.
- Set a 1-week goal that you think you can reach. For example, plan to walk for 10 minutes at lunch 3 days a week or to stretch for 5 minutes each morning.
- Start today. Keep a record of what you do.
- When you reach your first goal, reward yourself! Then set a new goal. Once you get used to meeting weekly goals, try setting monthly goals.
- If you haven't met your goal, think about what changes you need to make to be successful, and try again.

Consistency brings success. Small successes can quickly add up to a level of physical fitness that will make a big difference in your life.

Maintaining the Lifestyle

Staying motivated is essential to making physical activity a long-term lifestyle commitment. If you choose activities wisely, your body will let you know how enjoyable becoming more fit can be.

If you're just starting out with a fitness plan, reaching one goal and then striving for another may be enough to keep you going. Before long, you'll start to notice changes in your endurance, strength, flexibility, energy level, and appearance that will probably encourage you to continue your efforts.

People who are moderately active or very active may become bored with their usual activities and need to find new ways to stay motivated. Vary your activity, or vary when or where you exercise. If you don't already do so, try working out with a partner. Continue to set goals for yourself. You might want to train for a competitive event related to your activity. Another great way to stay motivated is to help someone else who is just starting a fitness program. You will be a role model for that person, you'll have another reason for staying consistently active, and you'll probably learn ways to vary your routine.

Never eat more than you can lift.
Miss Piggy

19

Nutrition

This chapter gives some guidelines for good eating and some hints on how to help your children establish healthy eating habits. Children learn best by example, so practise good eating habits along with them.

Simple Guidelines for Eating Well

The guidelines below are aimed at improving health and reducing the risk of disease, especially high blood pressure, heart disease, stroke, type 2 diabetes, osteoporosis, and certain types of cancer. The guidelines recommend the following ways to build a base for good health:

1. Aim for a healthy weight. Healthy bodies come in many shapes and sizes. Work toward achieving and maintaining the weight that is best for you by choosing a variety of healthy foods and getting regular physical activity.

2. Be physically active every day. Regular physical activity that is vigorous enough to raise your heart rate has many benefits. When combined with a healthy diet, it is the best way to maintain a healthy body weight.

3. Use the Food Guide to make your choices. Canada's Food Guide to Healthy Eating on pages 356 and 357 is a simple, flexible guide designed to help you follow a balanced diet. It encourages eating a variety of foods in balance with one another so that your body gets the nutrients it needs every day.

4. Choose a variety of grains daily, especially whole grains. Foods made from grains are the foundation of good nutrition. They provide vitamins, minerals, fibre, and carbohydrates and are often low in fat. Whole grains may help protect against heart disease and high blood pressure.

5. Choose a variety of fruits and vegetables daily. These foods are key parts of your daily diet, but most people eat fewer than the recommended minimum of 5 servings. Fruits and vegetables taste great, are easy to prepare, and may help prevent some types of cancer.

6. Keep food safe to eat. Prevent food poisoning by keeping hot foods hot and cold foods cold. See Stomach Flu and Food Poisoning on page 133 for more information on how to store, handle, and prepare food safely.

7. Choose a diet low in saturated fat and cholesterol and moderate in total fat to reduce your risk for heart disease, cancer, and high blood pressure. Choosing more grains, fruits, and vegetables can help you reduce the amount of total fat in your diet.

8. Choose beverages and foods that limit your sugar intake. Added sugars have no other nutrients, and when consumed in excess, they crowd healthier foods out of your diet.

9. Choose and prepare foods with less salt to help reduce your risk of high blood pressure. Reducing your salt intake can also help lower your blood pressure if it is already high. See High Blood Pressure on page 290.

10. If you drink alcoholic beverages, do so in moderation. Alcohol supplies calories but few nutrients. Drinking alcohol is the cause of many health problems and accidents and can lead to addiction. Moderate alcohol consumption is defined as no more than 2 drinks a day for men and no more than 1 drink a day for women and older adults. Women who are pregnant or trying to become pregnant should avoid alcoholic beverages altogether.

Tips for People Who Are Underweight

If you have trouble gaining weight or maintaining your minimum healthy weight, try the following:

- Eat 3 meals plus 3 snacks a day. Don't skip meals.
- Use liquid supplements, such as Ensure, between meals to add calories.
- Choose the higher-calorie items from each food group (for example, whole milk instead of skim milk).
- Eat the highest-calorie items first in a meal.
- Add extra fat to the foods you prepare.

Eating Alone?

FOR SENIORS

Many older adults live and eat alone. This can affect your nutritional status, since you may not eat as well alone as you would when dining with others. You may not take the time to make balanced meals, or you may skip meals.

If you often eat alone, consider the following:

- Plan your meals for the week, and shop from a list. You are more likely to eat meals for which you have planned and have all the ingredients.
- Take turns with friends preparing meals and eating together.
- Make a big pot of hearty stew or soup that you can enjoy for several meals. Freeze leftover portions.
- Visit the deli section of your local store, and buy single servings.
- Contact your local health authority to find out about community meal programs in your area. They provide low-cost, nutritious meals and opportunities to be with other people.
- Find out if your community has a Meals on Wheels program. If you are temporarily or permanently homebound, this service will deliver a hot, nutritious, and inexpensive meal once a day.

Eating Well: A Basic Plan

Eat a variety of foods from Canada's Food Guide to Healthy Eating on pages 356 and 357 each day. Most people who follow the diet outlined by the Food Guide will get all the vitamins, minerals, and other nutrients their bodies need and may have less trouble controlling their weight.

Grain Products

Grains are the foundation of a healthy diet. Try to eat 5 to 12 servings from this group each day, and choose foods made from whole grains as often as possible. Whole grains, such as whole wheat breads and pastas, oats, and brown rice, contain large amounts of vitamins, minerals, fibre, and complex carbohydrates. Carbohydrates are the body's fuel and should provide 45 to 65 percent of total calories for most people.

Fruits and Vegetables

Fruits and vegetables are another important part of the Food Guide. Notice that the "plant-based" foods in this group and the grain group represent about two-thirds of what you should eat each day. Aim to eat 5 to 10 daily servings of fruits and vegetables.

Fruits and vegetables provide vitamins, minerals, fibre, and carbohydrates. They also contain compounds that appear to protect against heart disease, high blood pressure, and some types of cancer. These compounds include antioxidants, such as vitamin C, vitamin A (beta-carotene), and other carotenoids, as well as non-nutrient compounds called phytochemicals (see page 361).

To make the most of the nutrients and healthy compounds in fruits and vegetables:

- When shopping for fruits and vegetables, avoid damaged and wilted produce. Choose produce that is in season and locally grown, if possible. Frozen or canned fruits and vegetables are also good choices.
- Store fruits and vegetables in the crisper drawer of your refrigerator. If they need to ripen, leave them at room temperature until ripe; then refrigerate them.
- Before eating fruits or vegetables, rinse them well but don't soak them. Chop vegetables into large pieces just before cooking. Microwave, steam, stir-fry, or sauté vegetables in a small amount of water or oil until they are just tender.

Fibre

Fibre is the indigestible part of plants. It is not absorbed into the bloodstream like other nutrients.

However, by providing "bulk," it plays an important role in keeping your digestive tract healthy.

There are two types of fibre found in foods: insoluble fibre and soluble fibre.

Insoluble fibre, which can be found in whole-grain products such as whole wheat flour, provides bulk for your diet. Together with fluids, insoluble fibre stimulates your colon to keep waste moving out of your bowels. Without fibre, waste moves too slowly, increasing your risk for constipation, diverticulosis, and possibly colon cancer.

Soluble fibre, which is found in fruit, legumes (dry beans and peas), and oats, helps lower blood cholesterol, reducing your risk for heart disease. Soluble fibre, especially the fibre in legumes, can also help regulate your blood sugar level.

Do you need more fibre in your diet? If your stools are soft and easy to pass, you probably get plenty of fibre. If they are hard and difficult to pass, more fibre and water may help. See page 116 for more information about constipation.

To increase fibre in your diet:

- Eat 5 to 10 servings of fruits and vegetables a day (see the Food Guide on pages 356 and 357). Eat fruits with edible skins and seeds: kiwifruit, figs, blueberries, apples, and raspberries. Eat more raw or lightly cooked vegetables.
- Switch to whole-grain and whole wheat breads, pasta, tortillas, and cereals. The first ingredient listed should be whole wheat flour.
- Eat more cooked dry beans, dry peas, and lentils. These high-fibre, high-protein foods can replace some of the high-fat, no-fibre meats in your diet.

- Popcorn is a good high-fibre snack. However, avoid added oil, butter, and salt. Use an air or microwave popcorn popper to eliminate oil, and add flavour with salt substitute or herb mixtures.

Sugar

In moderation, sugar does little harm. However, if too many of your calories come from sugar, you may gain weight and may not get enough of the other nutrients you need. Sugar also contributes to dental cavities.

To reduce sugar in your diet:

- Be aware that all sugars are basically alike. Honey and brown or raw sugar have no advantage over other sugars. Corn syrup is another commonly used form of sugar.
- Processed foods and drinks can be full of sugar. Flavoured yogourt, breakfast cereals, and canned fruits often have sugar added. Look for breakfast cereals that have 6 g or less of added sugar per serving.
- Limit foods and drinks that list sugar among the first few ingredients.
- You can reduce the amount of sugar added to homemade baked goods by up to one-half without affecting the texture. Try using more sweet spices, such as cinnamon and nutmeg, in your recipes.
- Make it a habit to eat a sweet piece of fruit instead of a sugary dessert most of the time.
- Drink water, sparkling water, or milk instead of soft drinks or sweetened fruit drinks.

Fats in Foods

It is recommended that 20 to 35 percent of your total calorie intake come from fat. No more than 10 percent of total calories should come from saturated fats. Reducing dietary fat to 30 percent will slow the development of heart disease, reduce your cancer risk, and improve your overall diet.

The Food Guide is designed to help you eat a low-fat diet. If you need help reducing fat in your diet, a registered dietitian can create a menu plan that will help you meet your goal. In BC, you can call Dial-A-Dietitian at 1-800-667-3438 for professional, friendly, and reliable nutrition advice. Check their Web site at www.dialadietitian.org.

Simple Ways to Reduce Harmful Fats

When eating meat:

- Keep serving sizes at 57 to 85 g (about the size of a deck of cards), and don't eat second helpings. If you eat red meat, choose the leanest cuts, such as tenderloin, flank steak, chuck, or top and bottom round.
- Eat more poultry (without skin) and fish. They contain less saturated fat than red meat does.

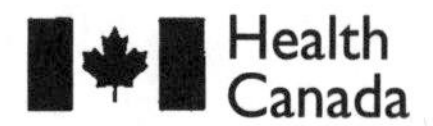
Health
Canada
Santé
Canada

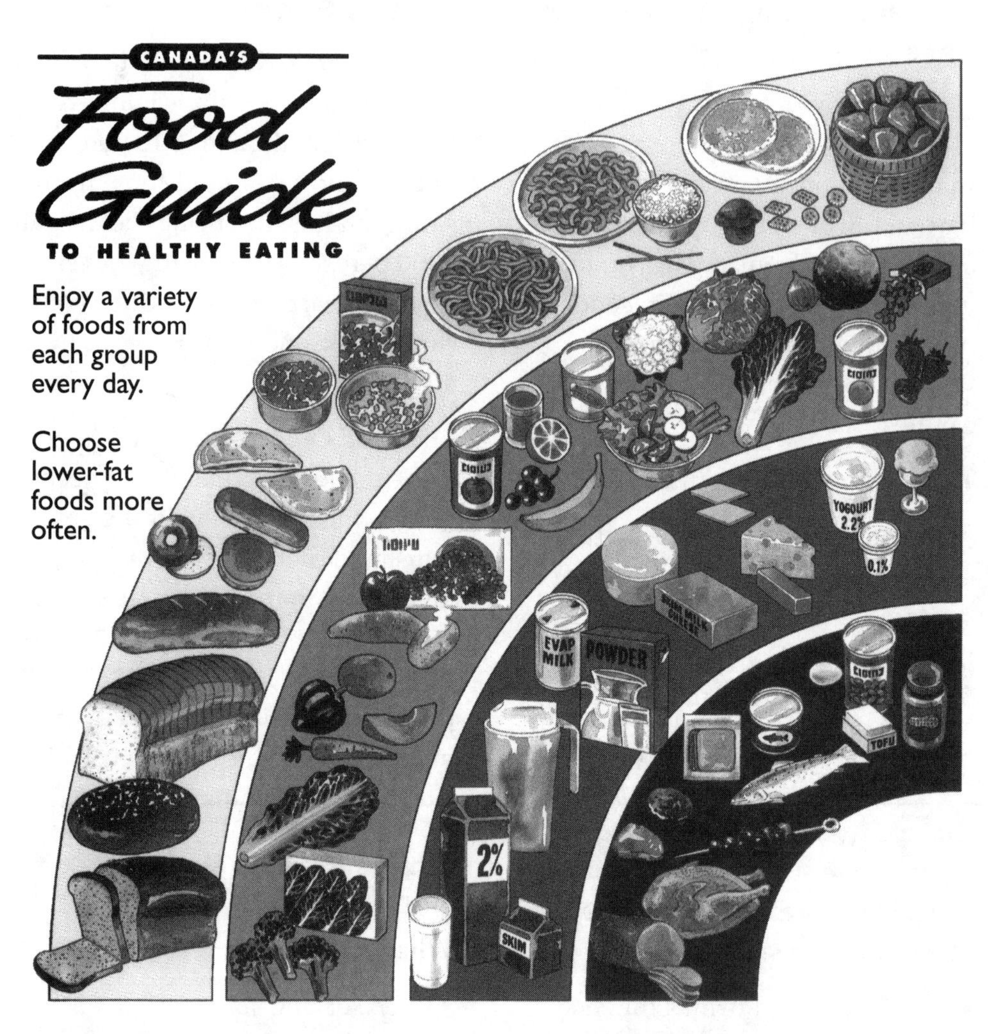
CANADA'S
Food Guide
TO HEALTHY EATING
Enjoy a variety of foods from each group every day.
Choose lower-fat foods more often.
YOGOURT
2.2%
0.1%
EVAP
MILK
POWDER
2%
SKIM
TOFU

Grain Products

Choose whole grain and enriched products more often.

Vegetables & Fruit

Choose dark green and orange vegetables and orange fruit more often.

Milk Products

Choose lower-fat milk products more often.

Meat & Alternatives

Choose leaner meats poultry and fish, as well as dried peas, beans and lentils more often.

Canada

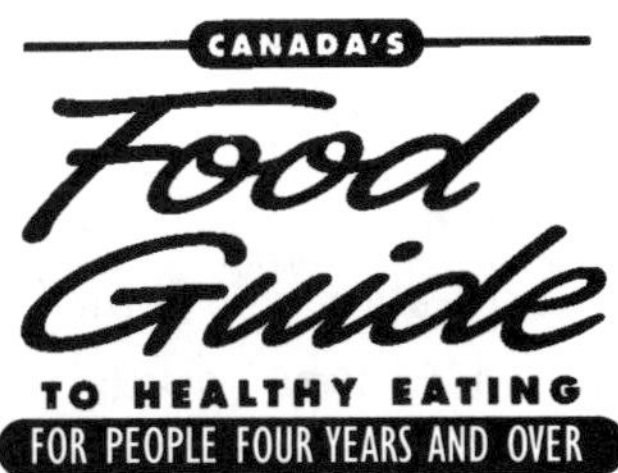
CANADA'S
Food Guide
TO HEALTHY EATING
FOR PEOPLE FOUR YEARS AND OVER

Different People Need Different Amounts of Food

The amount of food you need every day from the 4 food groups and other foods depends on your age, body size, activity level, whether you are male or female and if you are pregnant or breast-feeding. That's why the Food Guide gives a lower and higher number of servings for each food group. For example, young children can choose the lower number of servings, while male teenagers can go to the higher number. Most other people can choose servings somewhere in between.

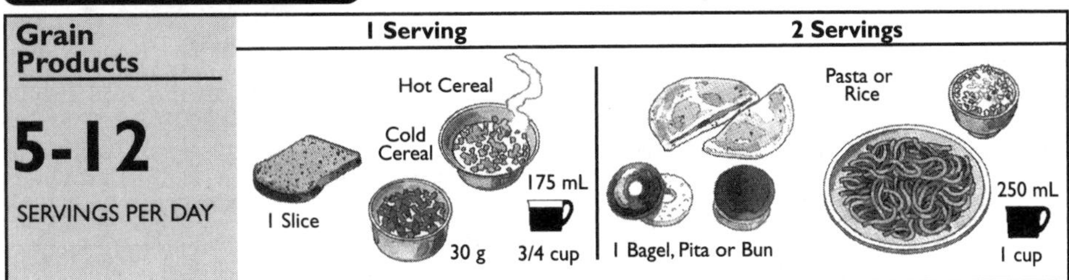

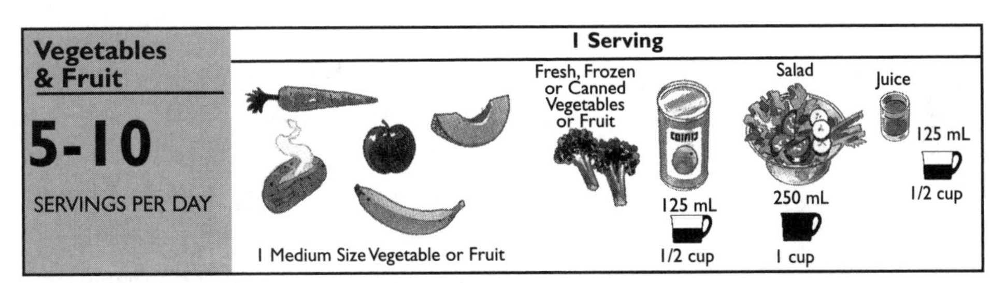

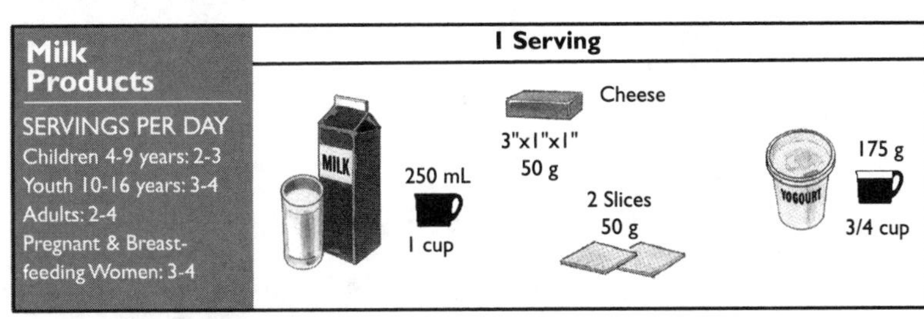

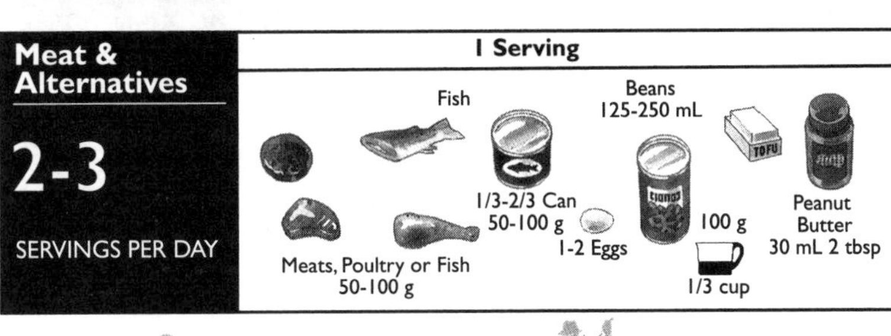

Other Foods

Taste and enjoyment can also come from other foods and beverages that are not part of the 4 food groups. Some of these foods are higher in fat or Calories, so use these foods in moderation.

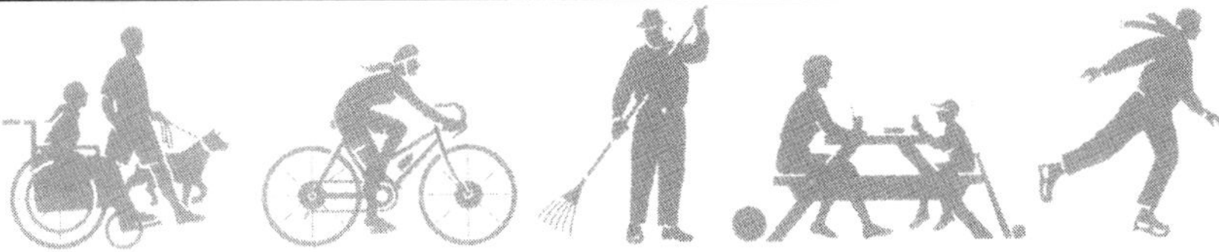

Enjoy eating well, being active and feeling good about yourself. That's 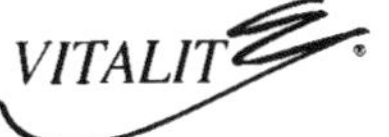

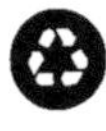

 ISBN 0-662-19648-1

- Remove all visible fat from meat, poultry, and fish before cooking. Remove poultry skin either before or after cooking.
- Bake, broil, or sauté meats, poultry, and fish instead of frying in butter or fat.
- A couple of times a week, serve a combination of legumes (dry beans, peas, lentils) and grains in place of a meat entree.

When using dairy products:

- Use skim, ½%, or 1% milk.
- Choose cheeses made with skim or part skim milk, or look for cheeses that have no more than 5 g of fat per ounce (read the label).
- Try low-fat cottage cheese or yogourt in place of cream and sour cream; or use fat-free sour cream and fat-free cream cheese.

When cooking:

- Steam vegetables. If you choose to sauté them, use a mono-unsaturated oil (olive, canola, or peanut oil), or try using other liquids such as wine, defatted broth, or cooking sherry.
- Use non-stick pans, or add a small amount of oil to a preheated pan (less oil goes farther this way).
- Season vegetables with herbs and spices instead of butter and sauces. Dress salads with olive or canola oil-based dressing, lemon juice, fat-free mayonnaise, or fat-free dressing.
- Use a cooking oil that is mono-unsaturated, such as canola, olive, or peanut oil.
- Experiment with using less oil than is called for in recipes. You may need to increase other liquids. Use applesauce, prune puree, or mashed bananas to replace some of the fat in baked goods.

Cholesterol

For many people, a diet high in saturated fat raises the amount of cholesterol in the blood, which increases the risk of heart attack and stroke. (See page 292.) Review the tips for reducing fat in your diet starting on page 355. Mono-unsaturated fats, such as olive, canola, and peanut oil, improve cholesterol levels, so choose these over saturated fats whenever possible.

Protein

Protein is important for maintaining healthy muscles, tendons, bones, skin, hair, blood, and internal organs. It should provide 10 to 35 percent of your total calories each day. Most adults in North America get all the protein they need in their diets. If you eat animal products (milk, cheese, eggs, fish, meat), your diet will contain plenty of protein. However, if you eat little meat, poultry, or fish and use no dairy products, your diet will require careful planning in order for you to get all the protein and other nutrients you need.

Vitamins

Vitamins are tiny elements of food that have no calories but are essential to good health. Vitamins A, D, E, and K are fat-soluble and can be stored in the liver or in fat tissue for a relatively long time. Other vitamins, including all the B vitamins and vitamin C, are water-soluble. Your body can only retain them for a short time, so it is important that you consume them often.

Most people who eat a variety of foods from the Food Guide (see pages 356 and 357) get all the necessary vitamins. However, if you typically eat fewer than 1,500 calories per day, you may want to consider taking a vitamin-mineral supplement. Unless your doctor prescribes a specific supplement, choose a balanced, multivitamin-mineral supplement rather than a specific vitamin or mineral. Avoid taking much more than 100 percent of the dietary reference intake (DRI) of any vitamin or mineral unless it is prescribed by a doctor.

Certain vitamins found in foods have been shown to prevent some diseases. However, researchers are still trying to determine whether those vitamins have the same preventive effects when taken as supplements. If possible, add more variety and balance to your diet rather than trying to make up for a poor diet by taking supplements.

Minerals

Minerals have many important roles in the structure and function of your body. You need minerals to build and maintain healthy teeth and bones; to carry nerve signals to and from your brain; to carry oxygen to your cells; to regulate blood sugar levels; and to maintain a healthy immune system.

More than 20 minerals have been determined to be essential to health, and many more have been discovered in the human body. Eating a variety of foods is the best way to get all the minerals you need.

Calcium

Calcium is the primary mineral needed for building and maintaining strong bones. Calcium is especially important for growing children and for women, especially in the peak bone-building years between the teens and early 30s. Calcium also helps women prevent osteoporosis, which can occur after menopause. See Osteoporosis on page 172.

Children from 1 to 3 years of age need 500 mg of calcium per day; those from 4 to 8 years of age need 800 mg per day; and those from 9 to 18 years of age need 1,300 mg per day. Adults between 19 and 50 years of age need 1,000 mg per day. Adults age 51 and older need 1,200 mg per day.

Lactose Intolerance

People whose bodies produce too little of the enzyme lactase have trouble digesting the lactose (sugar) in milk. Symptoms of lactose intolerance include gas, bloating, cramps, and diarrhea after drinking milk or eating milk products.

If you have mild to moderate lactose intolerance:

- Eat small amounts of milk products at any one time.
- Try eating cheese. Most of the lactose in cheese is removed during processing.
- Eat yogourts made with active cultures, which provide their own enzymes that digest the lactose in milk.
- Drink milk with reduced lactose, or try enzyme tablets (such as Lactaid), which will digest the lactose for you.
- You may be able to tolerate milk if you drink it with snacks or meals.

If you have severe lactose intolerance:

- Read labels to avoid any form of lactose in foods.
- Be sure to include non-dairy sources of calcium in your diet (see page 359). Ask your doctor or a dietitian if you need to take a calcium supplement.
- Plan your diet so it gives you the nutrients that milk products would normally provide.

Fat-free or low-fat milk products are the best source of dietary calcium. Each serving provides about 300 mg of calcium. Milk products provide other nutrients in addition to calcium, such as protein and vitamin D. Other foods, such as tofu, fortified soy milk, broccoli, certain greens, and calcium-fortified orange juice, provide calcium in varying amounts and can help meet your body's calcium needs.

While dietary calcium is preferred, low-dose calcium supplements (such as Tums) can also help keep bones strong. If you are not sure you are getting enough calcium in your diet, talk to your health professional about whether a calcium supplement would be helpful.

Salt

Most people get far more salt (sodium) than they need. For some people, excess salt causes high blood pressure. See page 290.

In general, processed foods contain the most salt, while unprocessed foods, such as fresh fruits and vegetables, have the least. If you want to cut back on the salt in your diet:

- Read the Nutrition Facts labels on foods for sodium content. Choose foods that contain less sodium.
- Limit ready-mixed sauces and seasonings, frozen dinners, and canned or dehydrated soups. These foods usually contain large amounts of salt. Products labelled "low sodium" contain less than 140 mg of sodium per serving.

- Eat lots of fresh or frozen fruits and vegetables. These foods contain very little sodium.
- Don't put the salt shaker on the table, or get a salt shaker that allows very little salt to come out. Use salt substitute or "lite salt" sparingly.
- Always measure the salt in recipes, and use half of what is called for.
- Avoid fast foods, which are usually very high in salt. In a restaurant, ask the chef not to salt food during cooking.

Iron

Your body needs small amounts of iron to make hemoglobin, which carries oxygen in your blood. Adult men need 8 mg of iron per day; adult women need 18 mg per day. Infants and young children have higher iron needs relative to their size than other age groups. People who have increased blood loss caused by ulcers or heavy menstrual periods or who take arthritis medications (such as Aspirin) are at high risk for iron deficiency anemia. Symptoms of iron deficiency anemia include paleness and fatigue. A blood test is needed to confirm the diagnosis, and further testing may be needed to determine the cause of the blood loss.

To get more iron in your blood:

- Eat foods with vitamin C along with iron-rich foods. Vitamin C helps you absorb more iron from food. To get the most iron from a bowl of iron-enriched cereal, drink a glass of orange or other citrus juice when you eat the cereal, or add berries to your cereal. High-iron cereals have at least 25 percent of the dietary reference intake (DRI) of iron.
- Eat meat with vegetables or grains. The iron in animal tissues (heme iron) improves absorption of the iron in these other foods.
- Avoid caffeinated tea with meals. It interferes with iron absorption.

Iron Supplements

Women who menstruate and who eat fewer than 1,500 calories per day may wish to consider taking a multivitamin-mineral supplement that contains iron. (Men are much less likely to need iron supplements.) A low-dose ferrous-form iron supplement or iron chelate containing no more than 60 mg is safe for most women to take daily. However, too much iron can cause a number of serious medical problems or mask the development of others. Iron supplements are best absorbed when taken between meals, at bedtime, or on an empty stomach. Keep iron supplements away from children.

Non-nutrients in Foods

In addition to essential nutrients, foods contain non-nutrient compounds that have important functions in the body. These include phytochemicals (found in plants), many of which protect against cancer and heart disease.

Some foods contain compounds that have medicinal effects, such as the compound found in cranberries that may flush bacteria from the urinary tract and prevent urinary tract infections.

The non-nutrients in foods are of great interest today, and many of them are just being discovered. Foods are made up of hundreds of chemicals that cannot be duplicated in a supplement. Taking a supplement cannot provide "insurance" against a poor or inadequate diet. If you think that your diet is poor, the best advice is to improve your food choices.

Nutrition for Older Adults

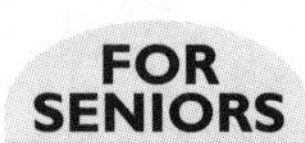

As you age, certain things can happen that may change both what you need and what you choose to eat.

- Your metabolism slows down, so you don't need to take in as many calories as you did when you were younger. However, your nutrition needs do not change—your body still needs the same balance of healthy foods.
- Physical changes may make different foods more attractive to you. For example, soft foods may be more appealing if you have dental problems. Sweet or salty foods may appeal to you if your senses of taste and smell have changed.
- Constipation can be a problem for many seniors, brought on by a low-fibre diet, not enough fluids, medication side effects, and decreased physical activity. You may find it helpful to increase the amount of fibre and fluid in your diet.
- Your lifestyle may change. You may eat alone more often, which may make you less inclined to prepare complete meals. Arthritis and other health problems may make shopping and meal preparation difficult.

Although your body needs fewer calories, it still needs plenty of vitamins, minerals, protein, and fibre to stay healthy. That's why planning a nutritious diet becomes even more important as you get older.

Nutrition for Children

Your whole family can follow the diet outlined in the Food Guide (pages 356 and 357). Offer nutritious foods as well-planned, pleasant meals and snacks. Then sit back and let your child decide how much to eat (or even if he or she wants to eat at all). This is a good division of responsibility that allows children to tune in to their own appetites and takes the pressure off the parents.

Child-Sized Environment

Imagine yourself eating at a giant's table. That's how a child can feel eating at an adult-sized table in an adult-sized chair.

- Provide a booster seat and child-sized utensils. However, fingers are fine until a child can hold utensils easily.
- Give children smaller plates and smaller servings (15 g per year of age is a good serving size guide). If the child is hungry for seconds, he or she will ask for them.

Healthy Snacks

Young children have small stomachs and high energy needs, so they need frequent snacks to supplement meals. Plan between-meal snacks as part of the day's total food intake. Snacks should provide good nutrition, not just empty calories.

- Fruits and fruit juices are good snacks. Other good choices are raw vegetable sticks with low-fat dip, cereal, yogourt, cheese, peanut butter on bread or crackers, or soup.
- Serve meals and snacks on a regular schedule. Do not serve snacks so close to a meal that they interfere with the child's appetite.
- Choose desserts that are low in fat and high in nutrients. Fruit, yogourt, and other foods found in the Food Guide are good choices.

The 80-20 Rule

If you are generally healthy, you don't need to worry about maintaining a perfect diet. If you make healthy eating choices 80 percent of the time, occasionally eating high-fat or high-calorie foods the remaining 20 percent of the time won't be a problem.

He who laughs, lasts.
Mary Pettibone Poole

20

Mental Health, Addictions, and Mind-Body Wellness

This chapter is organized in two sections. The first section covers some common mental and emotional health problems and describes what you can do to treat them at home and when you should seek professional help. The second section describes the relationship between your mental health and your physical health.

This chapter does not address all mental health and problematic substance use concerns. If you have symptoms that are not described here, contact a health professional or visit the Mental Health and Addictions Web site at www.healthservices.gov.bc.ca/mhd.

Mental Health and Problematic Substance Use

Mental health and problematic substance use concerns are similar to other health problems: some can be prevented; others will go away on their own with home treatment; and some need professional attention. Many problems begin when physical stress (such as an illness or injury) or emotional stress (such as the loss of a family member or friend) triggers chemical changes in the brain. The goal of treatment for these concerns—including self-care and professional treatment—is to reduce stress and restore the normal chemical processes in the brain.

In general, it is a good idea to seek professional help when:

- A symptom becomes severe or disruptive.
- A symptom becomes a continuous or permanent pattern of behaviour and does not respond to self-care.
- Symptoms become numerous, affect all areas of your life, and do not respond to self-care or communication efforts.
- You are thinking about hurting yourself or someone else.

For more information, call the BC Mental Health Information Line at 1-800-661-2121 or visit the Web site at www.heretohelp.bc.ca.

Alcohol and Drug Problems

The overuse or abuse of alcohol or other drugs is called problematic substance use. It is common, costly, and associated with many medical problems.

Alcohol Problems

A person has problematic substance use if he or she continues to drink even though alcohol is interfering with his or her health or daily living. Alcoholism is defined as a physical or psychological dependence on alcohol.

Problematic substance use patterns vary. Some people get drunk every day. Some drink large amounts of alcohol at specific times, such as weekends. Others may be sober for long periods and then go on drinking binges that last for weeks or months.

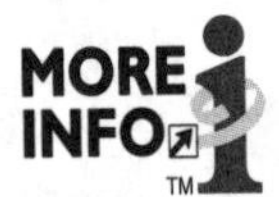

Long-term heavy drinking causes liver, nerve, heart, and brain damage; high blood pressure; depression; stomach problems; sexual problems; and cancer. Problematic alcohol use can also lead to violence, accidents, social isolation, and difficulties at work, at home, or with the law.

Are You a Problem User?

Answer the following questions honestly. They refer to your use of alcohol and drugs, including prescribed and illegal drugs.

- Have you ever felt that you ought to cut down on your drinking or drug use?
- Do you get annoyed when others criticize your drinking or drug use?
- Do you ever feel guilty about your drinking or drug use?
- Do you ever take an early-morning drink or use drugs first thing in the morning to get the day started or to eliminate "the shakes"?

A person who answers yes to any of these questions may have a problem with alcohol or drugs. Call a health professional to arrange for other tests to diagnose alcohol or drug dependence.

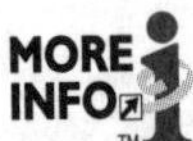

For more information, see the back cover.

Signs that a person is dependent on alcohol include not remembering what happened while he or she was drinking (blackouts), drinking more and more for the same effect, and being uncomfortable in situations where alcohol isn't served. A person with alcoholism may gulp or sneak drinks, drink alone or early in the morning, and suffer from "the shakes."

A person whose body is dependent on alcohol may suffer serious withdrawal symptoms (such as trembling, delusions, hallucinations, sweating, and seizures) if he or she stops drinking suddenly or tries to reduce his or her alcohol intake. Once alcohol dependency develops, it is very difficult for a person to stop drinking without outside help. Medical detoxification may be needed.

Problematic Substance Use

Problematic substance use includes the use of marijuana, cocaine, heroin, or other "street drugs," and the misuse of legal prescription drugs. Tranquilizers, sedatives, painkillers, and amphetamines are misused most often, sometimes unintentionally. Some people turn to drugs as a way to get a high or to deal with stress or emotional problems.

Drug dependence (addiction) occurs when a person develops a physical or psychological need for a drug. A person may not be aware that he or she has become dependent on a drug until he or she tries to suddenly stop taking it. Withdrawing from the drug can cause uncomfortable symptoms such as muscle aches, diarrhea, or depression. Your doctor can help you set up a plan to stop using the drug and to manage withdrawal effects.

Prevention

- Look for signs of mental stress. Try to understand and resolve sources of depression, anxiety, or loneliness. Don't use alcohol or drugs to deal with these problems.
- Educate your children about the effects of alcohol and drugs. Children are less likely to use alcohol or other drugs if their parents teach them early (during the elementary school years) about their effects.

Signs of Problematic Substance Use

- Chronic red eyes, sore throat, dry cough, and fatigue (in the absence of allergies)
- Major changes in sleeping or eating habits
- Moodiness, hostility, or abusive behaviour
- Work or school problems, absenteeism
- Loss of interest in favourite activities
- Social withdrawal or changes in friends
- Stealing, lying, and poor family relationships

- If you drink, do so in moderation: not more than 2 drinks a day for men and not more than 1 drink a day for women and older adults. One drink is 360 ml (12 fl oz) of beer, 150 ml (5 fl oz) of wine, or 44 ml (1.5 fl oz) of hard liquor.
- Don't drink alcohol or use drugs if you are pregnant or trying to become pregnant. Doing either can seriously harm your baby. See Dangers of Alcohol During Pregnancy on page 304.
- Ask your pharmacist or doctor if any of your current medications could potentially lead to misuse or dependence. Be especially cautious when taking painkillers, tranquilizers, sedatives, or sleeping pills. Follow the instructions carefully, and do not exceed the recommended dose.
- Do not suddenly stop taking any medication without your doctor's supervision.
- Avoid alcohol when you are taking medications. Alcohol can react with many drugs and cause serious complications.

Home Treatment

- Recognize early signs that alcohol or drug use is becoming a problem. See Are You a Problem User? on page 366.
- Attend an Alcoholics Anonymous or Narcotics Anonymous meeting. These are self-help groups devoted to helping members get sober and stay sober.
- If you are concerned about another person's alcohol or drug use:
  - Never ignore the problem. Discuss it as a medical problem.
  - Build up the person's self-esteem and reaffirm his or her value as a person. Help the person see that he or she can be successful without alcohol or drugs. Let the person know you will support his or her efforts to change.
  - Ask if the person will accept help. Don't give up if you get a negative response; keep asking periodically. If the person eventually agrees, act that very day to arrange for help. Call a health professional, Alcoholics Anonymous, or Narcotics Anonymous for an immediate appointment.
  - Attend a few meetings of Al-Anon, a support group for family members and friends of alcoholics. Read some 12-step program information.

When to Call a Health Professional

Call 911 or other emergency services:

- If a person loses consciousness after drinking alcohol or taking drugs.
- If a person who has been drinking alcohol or using drugs threatens to commit suicide or harm someone else.

- If a person who suddenly stops using alcohol has withdrawal symptoms (trembling, hallucinations, seizures).

Call a health professional:

- If you answer yes to any of the questions under Are You a Problem User? on page 366.
- If you recognize an alcohol or drug problem in yourself and are ready to accept help. Both outpatient and in-patient treatment programs are available. Call the BC NurseLine for confidential advice.

Anger and Hostility

Anger signals your body to prepare for a fight. When you get angry, adrenaline and other hormones are released into your bloodstream. Your blood pressure, pulse, and respiration rate all go up.

Anger can be a normal response to daily events. It is the appropriate response to any situation that poses a threat. Anger can be directed to become a positive, driving force behind your actions.

Hostility is being ready for a fight all the time. Continual hostility keeps your blood pressure high and may increase your risk for heart attack and other illnesses. Being hostile also isolates you from other people.

Home Treatment

- Try to understand the real reason why you are angry. Is it the current situation that is making you angry or something that happened earlier in the day?
- Notice when you start to become angry, and take steps to deal with your anger in a positive way. Don't ignore your anger until you "blow up." Express your anger in healthy ways:
  - Count to 10 or practise some other form of mental relaxation (see page 386). When you have calmed down, you will be better able to discuss the conflict rationally.
  - Try screaming or yelling in a private place, not at other people.
  - Go for a short walk or jog.
  - Talk with a friend about your anger.
  - Draw or paint to release the anger, or write about it in a journal.
- Use "I" statements, not "you" statements, to discuss your anger. Say "I feel angry when my needs are not being met" instead of "You make me mad when you are so inconsiderate."
- If you are angry with someone, listen to what the other person has to say. Try to understand his or her point of view.

- Forgive and forget. Forgiving helps lower blood pressure and ease muscle tension so you can feel more relaxed.
- Read books about anger and how to handle it. See page 379 for additional information about anger and violent behaviour.

When to Call a Health Professional

- If anger has led or could lead to violence or harm to you or someone else.
- If anger or hostility interferes with your work, family life, or friendships.

Anxiety and Panic Disorder

Feeling worried, anxious, and nervous is a normal part of everyday life. Everyone frets or feels anxious from time to time.

Anxiety can cause both physical and emotional symptoms. A specific situation or fear can cause some or all of these symptoms for a short time. When the situation passes, the symptoms go away.

Physical symptoms of anxiety include:

- Trembling, twitching, or shaking.
- Light-headedness or dizziness.
- A feeling of fullness in the throat or chest.
- Muscle tension, aches, or soreness.
- Restlessness.
- Fatigue.
- Insomnia.
- Breathlessness or rapid heartbeat.
- Sweating or cold, clammy hands.

Emotional symptoms of anxiety include:

- Feeling keyed up and on edge.
- Excessive worrying.
- Fearing that something bad is going to happen.
- Poor concentration.
- Irritability or agitation.
- Constant sadness.

Many people, including children and teens, develop anxiety disorders in which these symptoms occur for no identifiable or rational reason. This type of anxiety can become overwhelming and is not normal. People with an anxiety disorder may develop irrational and involuntary fears (phobias) of common places, objects, or situations.

Panic disorder is a common anxiety-related disorder. People with panic disorder have periods of sudden, intense fear and anxiety when there is no clear cause or danger. These panic attacks can cause frightening (but not life-threatening) symptoms, such as a pounding heart, shortness of breath, a feeling of choking or suffocation, and a sense that you are about to lose control or die. People who have had panic attacks may try to avoid any situations or behaviours that might trigger another attack. This often results in a higher level of anxiety.

Self-care, often combined with counselling and medication, can be effective in managing anxiety and panic disorder.

Home Treatment

The following home treatment tips can relieve simple anxiety and can also help if you are receiving medical treatment for anxiety or panic disorder.

- Recognize and accept your anxiety about specific fears or situations. Then say to yourself, "This is not an emergency. I feel uncomfortable, but I am not in danger. I can keep going even if I feel anxious."
- Be kind to your body:
  - Relieve tension by exercising or getting a massage.
  - Practise relaxation techniques. See page 386.
  - Get enough rest. If you have trouble sleeping, see Sleep Problems on page 376.
  - Avoid alcohol, caffeine, and nicotine. They can increase your anxiety level, cause sleep problems, or trigger a panic attack.
- Engage your mind:
  - Get out and do something you enjoy, such as going to a funny movie or taking a walk or a hike.
  - Plan your day. Having too much or too little to do can make you more anxious.
- Keep a record of your symptoms. Discuss your fears with a good friend or family member, or join a support group for people with similar problems. Confiding in others sometimes relieves stress.
- Get involved in social groups or volunteer to help others. Being alone sometimes makes things seem worse than they are.

When to Call a Health Professional

- If you are seriously considering harming yourself or someone else.
- If anxiety or irrational fear interferes with your daily activities.
- If sudden, severe attacks of fear or anxiety with physical symptoms (shaking, sweating) seem to occur for no reason.
- If symptoms of anxiety are still severe after 1 week of home treatment.
- If you suffer from nightmares or flashbacks to traumatic events.
- If you are unable to feel certain about things (for example, whether you unplugged the iron) no matter how many times you check, or if repetitive actions that you cannot control interfere with your daily activities.

Depression

Depression is a common problem that affects men and women of all ages, as well as children and teens. It is more than just the normal, temporary feelings of sadness and moodiness that come with the ups and downs of life. Depression can range from a minor problem to a major, life-threatening illness. Fortunately, effective treatments are available for most people who suffer from depression.

Depression is probably caused by a combination of factors, including the genetic traits that a person inherits from his or her parents. Most major depressions involve problems with the chemical messengers (neurotransmitters) in the brain. The amount of stress in a person's life and the way a person copes with stress also contribute to depression. Ongoing depression affects a person's body, mind, and social behaviour.

Many things can trigger depression, including:

- Drinking alcohol or using illegal drugs.
- Having a major illness or injury.
- Grieving the death of a family member or friend.
- Going through major life changes (loss of a job, divorce, children leaving home, retirement).
- Being under long-term stress, such as having a family member with a chronic illness.

Sadness or Depression?

People who are depressed:

- Have persistent feelings of sadness, anxiety, or hopelessness.
- Lose interest in or no longer enjoy their usual activities.

If you have also experienced 5 or more of the following symptoms nearly every day for more than 2 weeks, you may be suffering from depression:

- An unexplained change in your eating patterns that has caused weight gain or loss
- Restlessness or irritability
- Insomnia or excessive sleepiness
- Low energy or fatigue
- Feelings of worthlessness or guilt
- Inability to concentrate, remember, or make decisions
- Frequent thoughts of suicide or death

Home treatment may be all that is needed for mild depression. However, if you are feeling suicidal or if home treatment doesn't help lift your mood within 2 weeks, contact a health professional. With counselling, medication, and continued home treatment, you can overcome most cases of depression.

- Taking certain medications or having certain health conditions.
- Having recently had a baby (post-partum depression).

Reduced daylight during the winter seems to cause a form of depression called seasonal affective disorder in some people. See page 374.

Everyone gets sad. Gauging how deep and pervasive your sad feelings are can help you decide what to do. See Sadness or Depression? on page 372 to help determine if you are depressed.

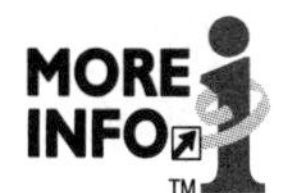

Because many things can contribute to depression, combining self-care and professional treatment is often most effective. The most common form of treatment combines counselling (psychotherapy) with medication. In-patient treatment is sometimes needed in severe cases.

Do You Feel Suicidal?

Call 1-800-SUICIDE (784-2433) for confidential help.

Home Treatment

For some people, self-care alone can improve symptoms of mild depression. For more serious depression, self-care can add to the benefits of professional treatment.

- Consider what might be causing or adding to your depression:
  - Are medications causing it? Review your prescription and non-prescription medications with a pharmacist or doctor.
  - If it's wintertime or you haven't been out in the sun for a while, read the information about seasonal affective disorder on page 374.
- Pace yourself according to your energy level. Choose what is most important to get done and do those things first.
- Do not make major life decisions when you are depressed. If you must make a major decision, ask someone you trust to help you.
- Do not drink alcohol or use medications that have not been prescribed by your health professional.
- Spend time with other people. Do things you usually enjoy, even if you don't feel like doing them.
- Get enough sleep. If you are having difficulty sleeping, see Sleep Problems on page 376.
- Eat a healthy diet (see Nutrition starting on page 351). If you don't feel like eating, try small snacks rather than large meals.
- Exercise regularly. Getting 20 to 30 minutes of exercise each day is good for your body and your mind. Go for a walk. Take the stairs instead of the elevator. Dance.

Seasonal Affective Disorder

Seasonal affective disorder (SAD), sometimes called the winter blues, is a mental health problem that usually occurs in the months when there is less sunlight. There is no known cure, but it can be controlled, and it improves in the spring when there are more hours of daylight. The main symptoms include depressed mood, decreased energy, and food cravings. If you notice such a pattern developing during the winter, try one or more of the following:

- Go out into the sun as often as possible. Protect your skin—it's your eyes' exposure to the sun that will help.
- Take a vacation to a sunny place.
- Get regular exercise, either outdoors or indoors near a window that lets in sunlight.

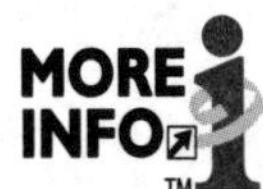

Light therapy (phototherapy) is sometimes successful in treating SAD. It involves sitting, working, or reading in front of special high-intensity lights for up to several hours a day. Medication and counselling can also be helpful.

- Believe that this mood will pass. Then look for signs that it is ending.
- Give yourself time to heal. Do not expect too much from yourself too soon.

When to Call a Health Professional

- If you are planning to hurt yourself or someone else.
- If you hear voices.
- If your behaviour changes suddenly or you start to do things that you wouldn't usually do (especially impulsive, irresponsible behaviour).
- If symptoms of depression (see Sadness or Depression? on page 372) last longer than 2 weeks despite home treatment.
- If grieving continues without improvement for more than 4 weeks. See Grief on page 379.

Eating Disorders

In a society where "thin is in," many of us have tried skipping meals or going on diets to lose weight. Unlike typical dieters, people who have eating disorders have medical problems that cause disturbances in their eating behaviour.

Anorexia nervosa is a disorder of severe self-imposed dieting. It most often affects teenage girls. Symptoms include refusing to eat;

extreme weight loss; loss of menstrual periods; a distorted body image (thinking you're fat when you're actually very thin); a preoccupation with food; low self-esteem; and excessive exercise.

Bulimia nervosa is an eating disorder characterized by eating large amounts of food (binge eating) and then purging the body of that food by forced vomiting, abuse of laxatives and diuretics, or excessive exercise. The binges are usually triggered by emotional upset, not hunger. Other symptoms include dry skin and brittle hair; swollen glands under the jaw from vomiting; depression and mood swings; a distorted body image; and secrecy to keep others from discovering the abnormal behaviour.

People who have anorexia usually look starved, but most people who have bulimia maintain a normal weight and look healthy. Most people with anorexia deny to themselves that they have a problem; people with bulimia know they have a problem, but they keep it a secret.

Compulsive overeating is characterized by binging on food. An overeater will consume thousands of calories at a time, quickly and without pleasure. Because there is no purging, a compulsive overeater becomes obese.

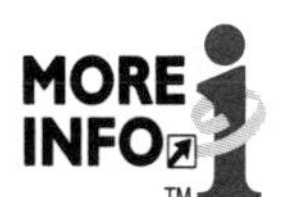

Eating disorders appear to be caused by emotional and psychological factors. They tend to run in families, so there may be a genetic link. Eating disorders require professional treatment. If untreated, they can lead to major health problems or even death. Treatment usually involves nutritional counselling, individual psychotherapy, family therapy, and medication. A hospital stay may be required in extreme cases.

Prevention

- Teach and model healthy eating and exercise habits at home and at school.
- Help young people develop confidence and self-esteem. Accept them for who they are, not how they look.
- Be careful about encouraging a young person to lose weight. Communicate that you love and care for the person regardless of how much he or she weighs.
- Don't set unrealistic expectations for your child. Striving to live up to them may lead to an eating disorder.
- Be alert to the stress in your child's life. Be available to talk over any problems.

When to Call a Health Professional

Call if you recognize any of these warning signs of an eating disorder:

- Unrealistic body image or an unreasonable fear of gaining weight

- Extreme weight loss in a short period of time
- Forced vomiting or excessive use of laxatives
- Excessive dieting or preoccupation with food
- Excessive, rigid exercise routines
- Loss of menstrual periods in a young woman
- Withdrawal from family and friends

Sleep Problems

The term **insomnia** can mean:

- Trouble getting to sleep (taking more than 45 minutes to fall asleep).
- Frequent awakenings with inability to fall back asleep.
- Early morning awakening.

None of these are problems unless they make you feel chronically tired. If you are less sleepy at night or wake up early in the morning, but still feel rested and alert, there is usually little need to worry. (Not feeling any need to sleep night after night is not normal and needs to be evaluated.)

Short-term insomnia, lasting from a few nights to a few weeks, is usually caused by worry over a stressful situation. Long-term insomnia, which can last months or even years, is often caused by general anxiety, medications, chronic pain, depression, or other physical disorders.

Sleep apnea is a sleep disorder that is usually caused by a blockage in the upper airways. When airflow through the nose and mouth is blocked, breathing repeatedly stops for 10 to 15 seconds or longer. People who have sleep apnea usually snore loudly and are very tired during the day. They are not aware of waking up at night but do have very restless sleep. Sleep apnea can affect children and adults.

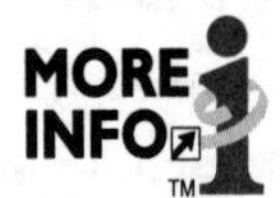

Mild sleep apnea may be cured by changing some of your pre-bedtime habits. More severe sleep apnea may require medical treatment.

Prevention

- Get regular exercise, but avoid strenuous exercise within 2 hours before bedtime.
- Avoid alcohol and smoking before bedtime. Drink caffeine in moderation and not after noon.
- Avoid foods that upset your stomach.
- Drink a glass of warm milk at bedtime. (But don't drink more than one glass of fluid before going to bed.)
- Make sure your sleeping conditions are comfortable and quiet.

Home Treatment

- Prescription and non-prescription sleep medications may provide rapid relief of insomnia. However, it's best to use these only for a short time and to stop taking them as soon as you can. They can cause daytime confusion, memory loss, and dizziness. Continued use of sleeping pills actually increases sleeplessness in many people.
- Try the following seven-step formula for 2 weeks:
  1. Engage in relaxing activities in the evening. For example, take a warm bath, read, or do some slow, easy stretches.
  2. Use your bed for sleeping and sex only. Don't eat, watch TV, read, or work in bed.
  3. Sleep only at bedtime. Don't take naps, especially in the late afternoon and evening.
  4. Go to bed only when you feel sleepy.
  5. If you lie awake for more than 15 minutes, get up, leave the bedroom, and do something relaxing.
  6. Repeat steps 4 and 5 until it is time to get up.
  7. Get up at the same time every day.
- Keep your bedroom dark, quiet, and cool. Try using a sleep mask and earplugs.
- Review the sleeping tips for snorers on page 206.
- Review all your prescription and non-prescription medications with a pharmacist to rule out drug-related sleep problems.
- Read about anxiety on page 370 and depression on page 372. Either condition can cause sleep problems.

When to Call a Health Professional

- If you regularly take sleeping pills and are unable to stop taking them.
- If you suspect medication or a health problem is causing sleep problems.
- If you or your partner snores loudly and feels excessively sleepy during the day.
- If you, your partner, or your child has many episodes of sleep apnea (stops breathing, gasps, and chokes during sleep).
- If your child snores, has difficulty breathing while asleep, sleeps restlessly and awakens frequently, or is very sleepy during the day.
- If you wake up frequently because your legs move or get cramps.
- If a full month of self-care doesn't solve the problem.

Suicide

If you are very depressed or feel overwhelmed, you may sometimes think of taking your own life. Occasional, fleeting thoughts of death are not a problem. However, if thoughts of suicide continue, or if you have made suicide plans, it becomes a very serious matter.

People who are considering suicide are often undecided about choosing life or death. With compassionate help, they may choose to live.

Prevention

When there are significant life crises, when you are depressed, or when someone you know is depressed, be alert to the warning signs for suicide:

- Verbal warning. Most people who commit suicide mention their intentions to someone.
- Preoccupation with death. A suicidal person may talk, read, draw, or write about death.
- Previous suicide attempt. Failed attempts are often followed by a completed attempt.
- Giving away prized possessions.
- Depression and social isolation.

If you are troubled by suicidal thoughts, avoid alcohol and illegal drugs. Alcohol and drugs can impair your judgment, which may make you more likely to do things you would not do when sober. Talk about your thoughts with someone you trust—a friend or family member, a clergyperson, or a health professional.

Home Treatment

- Use your common sense and a direct approach to determine if the suicide risk is high. Ask yourself or the person who you feel is at risk:
  - Do you feel there is no other way?
  - Do you have a suicide plan?
  - How and when do you plan to do it?
- Ask someone you trust to stay with you or the suicidal person until the crisis has passed.
- Encourage the person to seek professional help immediately. Follow up to find out how the treatment is going.
- Don't ignore warning signs, thinking that you or another person will "snap out of it."
- Talk about the situation as openly as possible. Show understanding and compassion. Don't argue with or challenge the person who is thinking of suicide.

When to Call a Health Professional

Call 911 or other emergency services if you or someone you know is about to attempt or is attempting suicide.

Call your health professional or 1-800-SUICIDE (784-2433):

- If you are considering suicide.
- If you suspect that someone has made suicide plans.

Grief

Grieving is a natural healing process that helps you adjust to a major change or loss. Grief may be expressed physically or emotionally and may have some of the same symptoms as depression (see page 372). The following tips may help you move through the grieving process.

- Take as much time as you need to grieve. Don't fight the emotions you feel.
- Take care of yourself. Get enough rest, and eat nourishing foods. Exercise to help release pent-up emotions.
- Discuss your feelings with friends who will support you while encouraging you to reconnect with the world. Join a support group, or talk to your clergyperson or a counsellor.
- Write down your thoughts in a journal or paint or draw your grief. Or write letters to the person you lost.
- Try to cut back on some of your usual responsibilities until your grieving period is past. Postpone any major decisions.
- As you begin to move beyond your grief, renew old interests and pursue new ones. Do things that give you a sense of control and hope.

There is no easy formula for getting over grief. It can take weeks, months, or years. Ask your friends, family, and doctor for help if you are having trouble moving through your grief.

Violent Behaviour and Abuse

Anger and disagreements are normal parts of healthy relationships. However, anger that leads to threats or violence, such as hitting or hurting, is not normal or healthy. Physical, verbal, or sexual abuse is not an acceptable part of any relationship. There is no excuse for it. No one deserves to be abused.

Violent behaviour and abuse are common problems. They often begin with verbal threats or relatively minor incidents, but over time they can become more serious, involving physical harm. Every year thousands of people are hurt or killed by their partners, spouses, or other family members.

Violent behaviour is learned behaviour. It is important to teach your children that violence is not a healthy solution to conflict and that it's not okay to hurt people or to let other people hurt them.

If you are unsure whether your relationship is abusive, there are signs to look for. This can be the first step in solving the problem.

Ask yourself, does my partner:

- Limit where I can go, what I can do, and whom I can talk to?
- Call me names or tell me that I'm crazy?
- Criticize what I do and say, or criticize how I look?

- Unexpectedly check up on me at work, home, school, or elsewhere?
- Hit, shove, slap, kick, punch, or choke me?
- Blame me for the abuse he or she commits?
- Force me to have sex against my will?
- Hurt my pets or destroy things that are special to me?
- Threaten to hurt or kill me?
- Apologize and tell me it will never happen again (even though it already has)?

If you answered yes to any of these questions or your partner could answer yes, you may be in an abusive relationship. Know that there are people who can help you—friends, family members, neighbours, health professionals, social workers, clergy. Everyone has the right to be in a safe relationship.

Prevention

- Seek non-violent ways to resolve conflicts. Disagreeing is fine, even healthy, so long as it does not turn violent. See page 369 for more information about controlling anger.
- Teach your children that violence is not a solution to conflicts. Do not use physical discipline such as spanking. If you need help with discipline, consider taking a course on parenting skills.
- Do not keep firearms or other weapons in your home if someone with a drug or alcohol problem, suicidal urges, or a tendency toward violent behaviour lives there.
- Be alert to warning signs, such as threats or drunkenness, so you can avoid dangerous situations. If you cannot predict when violence may occur, have an "exit plan" for use in an emergency.

When to Call a Health Professional

Call 911 or other emergency services:

- If you feel you or someone you know is in immediate danger.
- If you or someone in your family has just been physically or sexually abused or has been the victim of violence. Physical or sexual abuse is a crime, no matter who does it.

Call a health professional:

- If you are concerned about violent behaviour (such as physical, verbal, or sexual abuse) in your own relationship or that of a family member, friend, or co-worker.
- If you suspect abuse, neglect, or maltreatment of a child or if a child reports this kind of treatment to you. You may also call local child protective services or the police.

Check the phone directory for hotlines and other resources for victims of abuse, or call the BC NurseLine (see the back cover for phone numbers).

The Mind-Body Connection

Medical science is making remarkable discoveries about the relationship between your state of mind and your mental and physical health. Researchers have found that one function of the brain is to produce substances that can improve your health. Your brain can create endorphins, which are natural painkillers; gamma globulin for fortifying your immune system; and interferon for combatting infections, viruses, and even cancer. Your brain can combine these and other substances into a vast number of tailor-made prescriptions for whatever ails you.

The substances that your brain produces depend in part on your thoughts, feelings, and expectations. If your attitude about an illness (or life in general) is negative and you don't have expectations that your condition will get better, your brain may not produce enough of the substances your body needs to heal. On the other hand, if your attitude and expectations are more positive, your brain is likely to produce sufficient amounts of the substances that will boost your body's healing power.

Your physical health also has an impact on your brain's ability to produce substances that affect your mental well-being. An illness or injury that causes long-term physical stress can lead to chemical imbalances in the brain. These imbalances may lead to depression and other mental health problems.

Positive Thinking

People with positive attitudes generally enjoy life more, but are they any healthier? The answer is often yes. Optimism is a resource for healing. Optimists are more likely to overcome pain and adversity in their efforts to improve their medical treatment outcomes. For example, optimistic coronary bypass patients generally recover more quickly and have fewer complications after surgery than less hopeful patients do.

Your body responds to your thoughts, emotions, and actions. In addition to staying fit, eating right, and managing stress, you can use the following three strategies to help maintain your health:

1. Create positive expectations for health and healing.

Mental and emotional expectations can influence medical outcomes. The effectiveness of any medical treatment depends in part on how useful you expect it to be. The "placebo effect" proves this. A placebo is a drug or treatment that provides no medical benefit except for the patient's belief that it will help. Many patients who receive placebos report satisfactory relief from their medical problem, even though they received no actual medication.

Changing your expectations from negative to positive may enhance your physical health. Here's how to make the change:

- Stop all negative self-talk. Make positive statements that promote your recovery.
- Send yourself a steady stream of affirmations. An affirmation is a phrase or sentence that sends strong, positive statements to you about yourself, such as "I am a capable person" or "My joints are strong and flexible."
- Visualize health and healing. Add mental pictures that support your positive affirmations.
- Don't feel guilty. There is no value in feeling guilty about health problems. While there is a lot you can do to reduce your risk for health problems and improve your chances of recovery, some illnesses may develop and persist no matter what you do. Some things just are. Do the best you can.

2. Open yourself to humour, friendship, and love.

Positive emotions boost your health. Fortunately, almost anything that makes you feel good about yourself helps you stay healthy.

- Laugh. A little humour makes life richer and healthier. Laughter increases creativity, reduces pain, and speeds healing. Keep an emergency laughter kit that contains funny videotapes, jokes, cartoons, and photographs. Put it with your first aid supplies and keep it well stocked.
- Seek out friends. Friendships are vital to good health. Close social ties help you recover more quickly from illness and reduce your risk of developing diseases ranging from arthritis to depression.
- Volunteer. People who volunteer live longer and enjoy life more than those who do not volunteer. By helping others, we help ourselves.
- Plant a plant and pet a pet. Plants and pets can be highly therapeutic. When you stroke an animal, your blood pressure goes down and your heart rate slows. Animals and plants help us feel needed.

3. Appeal to a higher power.

If you believe in a higher power, ask for support in your pursuit of healing and health. Faith, prayer, and spiritual beliefs can play an important role in recovering from an illness. See Healing Touch on page 394.

Your sense of spiritual wellness can help you overcome personal trials and things you cannot change. If it suits you, use spiritual images in visualizations, affirmations, and expectations about your health and your life.

Dealing With Chronic Pain

Long-term, persistent pain (chronic pain) is a problem for many people, especially middle-aged and older adults. Chronic pain is associated with fatigue, sleep problems, irritability, stress, depression, anxiety, and withdrawal from daily activities. Arthritis, back problems, recurring sports injuries, nerve damage, cancer, and many other conditions can result in chronic pain. In many cases the cause of pain is not known. A variety of factors can contribute to it.

Your mind and body are important allies in your efforts to manage chronic pain. Pain often has a mental as well as a physical component. In other words, your thoughts and feelings about pain can affect how much pain you feel. Feeling anxious, angry, frustrated, or out of control about your pain may make the pain worse. If you can put your mind to work against the pain, you may find that you can manage pain better and that it interferes less with your life.

There is no magic solution for dealing with chronic pain, no matter what the cause. However, the following tips for dealing with both the mental and physical aspects of chronic pain may help:

- Take control of the pain. This may mean accepting that the pain is not going away but deciding to take active steps toward managing it.
- Practise positive thinking (see page 381). Recognize negative or self-defeating thoughts, such as "This pain will never get better" or "I'll never be able to play with the grandkids with this pain." Your thoughts can affect your perception of pain.
- Track how your moods, thoughts, and activities affect your pain. Record your pain level in relation to these factors several times a day for several days. You may find that your pain is worse during or after certain activities or when you are feeling a certain emotion.
- Try to relax. Chronic pain causes stress and tension, which may make the pain worse. Try the relaxation techniques on pages 386 to 388. Learning relaxation skills takes practice, so give each method a 2-week trial. If one doesn't work for you, try another.
- If your health professional has recommended or prescribed any pain medication, take it on schedule and in the correct dose.
- Exercise regularly. Try gentle, low-impact exercises that don't aggravate your pain, such as swimming, water aerobics, walking, or stationary cycling. Do the stretching exercises on page 348 every day. Ask your health professional about physical therapy too.
- Experiment with heat, cold, and massage. Find out what works best for you.

- Make sure you are getting enough sleep. See Sleep Problems on page 376. If pain frequently disrupts your sleep, talk to your health professional.
- Change the way you do daily activities so you can do them with less pain. Some people find assistive devices (such as canes, foot supports, or specially designed household tools) helpful.
- Consider complementary therapies such as biofeedback, acupuncture, or yoga in addition to your regular medical care (not as a substitute for it). See Complementary Medicine beginning on page 389.
- Join a support group. By being around others who share your problem, you and your family can learn skills for accepting and coping with pain. You may also feel less isolated. To find a group near you, contact the Chronic Pain Association of Canada at 1-780-482-6727, or go to www.chronicpaincanada.com.

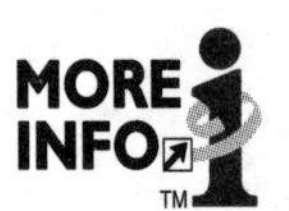

No one should have to suffer in uncontrolled pain. Call your health professional if chronic pain is affecting your quality of life. Although treatment will probably not be able to eliminate pain completely, it can help reduce the pain and its impact on your life.

Stress and Distress

Stress is the way you react physically, mentally, and emotionally to various conditions, changes, and demands in your life.

Stress is part and parcel of common life events, both large and small. It comes with all of life's daily hassles as well as with crises and life-changing events. Unless you can regularly release the tension that comes with stress, your risk for physical and mental illness may increase.

What Stress Does to the Body

At the first sign of alarm, chemicals released by the pituitary and adrenal glands and the nerve endings automatically trigger these physical reactions to stress:

- Your heart rate increases to move blood to your muscles and brain.
- Your blood pressure goes up.
- You start to breathe more rapidly.
- Your digestion slows down.
- You start to perspire more heavily.
- Your pupils dilate.
- You feel a rush of strength.

Your body is tense, alert, and ready for action and will stay this way until you feel that the danger has passed. Then your brain signals an "all clear" to your body, and your body stops producing the chemicals that caused the physical reaction and gradually returns to normal.

Problems with stress occur when your brain fails to give the "all clear" signal. If the alarm state lasts too long, you begin to suffer from the consequences of chronic stress. You may find it difficult to see the relationship between stress and physical health problems, because the long-term effects of stress are subtle and slow to develop. However, experts in every area of medicine are discovering links between stress, disease, and poor health. By changing the way you respond to stressful situations and finding ways to regularly relieve the tension caused by stress, you can decrease your risk for stress-related health problems.

Becoming More Stress-Hardy

Some people seem to be more resistant to stress, and studies indicate that these people are less likely to get sick. Certain characteristics stand out in stress-hardy people:

- They have a strong commitment to self, work, family, and other values.
- They have a sense of control over their lives.
- They generally see change in their lives as a challenge rather than a threat.
- They participate in activities that promote creativity and individuality.
- They have a strong network of support and close relationships.

It's never too late to develop a more stress-hardy personality. The first step is to believe that you can do it (remember, think positive!).

Approach one challenging area of your life at a time. Be committed to making things better for yourself and those around you. Identify the things you can control and those you cannot. Accept that changes will occur, and know that you will be able to deal with them. Call upon your support network to get the help you need, whether it's someone to watch your children for a few hours so you can run errands or someone who will just listen to your plans. As you begin to gain control over one challenging area of your life, you will find more time and energy for tackling additional areas.

Recognizing Stress

Classic signs of stress include headache, stiff neck, or a nagging backache. You may start to breathe rapidly or get sweaty palms or an upset stomach. You may become irritable and intolerant of even minor disturbances. You may lose your temper more often and yell at your family for no good reason. Your pulse rate may increase and you may feel jumpy or exhausted all the time. You may find it hard to concentrate.

When these symptoms appear, recognize them as signs of stress and find a way to deal with them. Just knowing why you're feeling the way you do may be the first step in coping with the problem. It is your attitude toward stress, not the stress itself, that affects your health the most.

Managing Symptoms of Stress

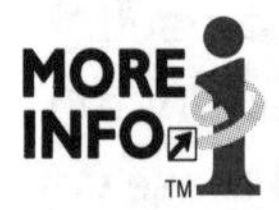

Some people try to relieve the symptoms of stress by smoking, drinking, overeating, using drugs, or just "shutting down." Some people become violent or abusive in response to stress. These methods of coping have harmful side effects. By learning other ways to deal with symptoms of stress, you can avoid those side effects and improve your overall quality of life.

- **Express yourself.** Stress and tension affect your emotions. By expressing those feelings to others, you may be able to understand and cope with them better. Talking about a problem with a spouse or a good friend is a valuable way to reduce tension and stress. Expressing yourself through writing, crafts, or art may also be a good tension reliever.
- **Cry.** Crying can relieve tension. It's part of your emotional healing process.
- **Get moving.** Regular, moderate physical activity may be the single best approach to managing stress. Walking briskly will take advantage of the rapid pulse and tensed muscles caused by stress and help you release your pent-up energy. After a long walk, your stress level is usually lower and more manageable.
- **Be kind to your body and mind.** Getting enough sleep, eating a nutritious diet, and taking time to do things you enjoy can help reduce stress and contribute to an overall feeling of balance in your life.

Relaxation Skills

Whatever you do to manage stress, you can benefit from the regular use of relaxation skills.

The following three methods of relaxation and meditation are among the simplest and most effective. They should be done once or twice a day for about 20 minutes each time. Pick a time and place where you won't be disturbed or distracted. Once you've trained your body and mind to relax, you'll be able to produce the same relaxed state whenever you want.

Roll Breathing

The way you breathe affects your whole body. Full, deep breathing is a good way to reduce tension and feel relaxed. The object of roll breathing is to develop full use of your lungs and get in touch with the rhythm of your breathing. It can be practised in any position, but it is best to learn it while lying on your back, with your knees bent.

1. Place your left hand on your abdomen and your right hand on your chest. Notice how your hands move as you breathe in and out.

2. Practise filling your lower lungs by breathing so that your left hand goes up when you inhale and your right hand remains still. Always inhale through your nose and exhale through your mouth.

3. When you have filled and emptied your lower lungs 8 to 10 times, add the second step to your breathing: inhale first into your lower lungs as before; then continue inhaling into your upper chest. As you do so, your right hand will rise and your left hand will fall a little as your abdomen falls.

4. As you exhale slowly through your mouth, make a quiet, whooshing sound as your left hand, and then your right hand, falls. As you exhale, feel the tension leaving your body as you become more and more relaxed.

5. Practise breathing in and out in this manner for 3 to 5 minutes. Notice that the movement of your abdomen and chest is like rolling waves rising and falling in a rhythmic motion.

Practise roll breathing daily for several weeks until you can do it almost anywhere. Then you'll have an instant relaxation tool anytime you need one.

CAUTION: Some people get dizzy the first few times they try roll breathing. If you begin to hyperventilate or become light-headed, slow your breathing. Get up slowly.

Progressive Muscle Relaxation

The body responds to stressful thoughts or situations with muscle tension, which can cause pain or discomfort. Deep muscle relaxation reduces muscle tension and general mental anxiety too. Progressive muscle relaxation is effective in combatting stress-related health problems and often helps people get to sleep.

Muscle Groups and Procedure

You can use a prerecorded audiotape to help you go through all the muscle groups, or you can do it by just tensing and relaxing each muscle group. Choose a place where you can lie down on your back and stretch out comfortably, such as a carpeted floor. Tense each muscle group (hard, but not to the point of cramping) for 4 to 10 seconds; then give yourself 10 to 20 seconds to release it and relax. At various points, check the muscle groups you've already done and relax each one a little more each time.

Hands: Clench them.

Wrists and forearms: Extend them and bend the hands back at the wrist.

Biceps and upper arms: Clench your hands into fists, bend your arms at the elbows, and flex your biceps.

Shoulders: Shrug them. (Check your arms and shoulders for tension.)

Forehead: Wrinkle it into a deep frown.

Around the eyes and bridge of the nose: Close your eyes as tightly as possible. (Remove contact lenses before beginning the exercise.)

Cheeks and jaws: Grin from ear to ear.

Around the mouth: Press your lips together tightly. (Check your facial area for tension.)

Back of the neck: Press the back of your head against the floor.

Front of the neck: Touch your chin to your chest. (Check your neck and head for tension.)

Chest: Take a deep breath and hold it; then exhale.

Back: Arch your back up and away from the floor.

Stomach: Suck it into a tight knot. (Check your chest and stomach area for tension.)

Hips and buttocks: Squeeze your buttocks together tightly.

Thighs: Clench them.

Lower legs: Point your toes toward your face, as if trying to bring your toes up to touch your head. Then point your toes away and curl them downward at the same time. (Check the area from your waist down for tension.)

When you are finished, return to alertness by counting backwards from 5 to 1.

Relaxation Response

The relaxation response is the exact opposite of the stress response. It slows your heart rate and breathing, lowers your blood pressure, and helps relieve muscle tension.

Technique (adapted from Herbert Benson, MD)

1. Lie down in a place where you can stretch out comfortably. Close your eyes.

2. Begin progressive muscle relaxation. See page 387.

3. Become aware of your breathing. Each time you exhale, say the word "one" (or any other word or phrase) silently or aloud. Concentrate on breathing from your abdomen, not from your chest.

Instead of focusing on a repeated word, you can fix your gaze on a stationary object. Any mental stimulus will help you clear your mind.

Continue this for 10 to 20 minutes. As distracting thoughts enter your mind, don't dwell on them. Allow them to drift away.

4. Sit quietly for several minutes, until you are ready to open your eyes.

5. Notice the difference in your breathing and your pulse rate.

Don't worry about becoming deeply relaxed. The key to this exercise is to remain passive, to let distracting thoughts slip away like waves on the beach.

For the times they are a-changin'.
Bob Dylan

21 Complementary Medicine

The term "complementary medicine" broadly describes any health approach that is not part of the conventional medical system of a particular society or culture. What is considered "complementary" or "alternative" varies from culture to culture. In British Columbia, many people use complementary therapies like acupuncture or herbal medicine along with mainstream medical treatments (medications or surgery, for instance) to help control pain, manage stress, and speed healing.

Complementary treatments are becoming more widely accepted. As with any other treatment option, the decision to try complementary medicine should be made only after you gather as much reliable information as possible, understand the benefits and risks, and consider your personal needs and preferences. For more information, see Making Wise Health Decisions starting on page 3.

Here are some important things to consider when deciding whether to try a complementary therapy:

- Think about what you want from complementary medicine. Are you looking for greater comfort and an improved quality of life? Or are you looking for a cure for illness? Seeking a cure through complementary medicine may be disappointing and, in rare cases, harmful to your health. Discuss your expectations with the practitioner and make sure they are realistic.

- Do you think that complementary medicine has something special to offer you, or are you seeking complementary treatment because you are fed up with conventional medicine? It is important to recognize the strengths and limitations of both conventional and complementary medicine.
- What is the practitioner's level of expertise? Check with provincial and local medical licensing agencies and departments of consumer affairs to see if the practitioner is licensed and in good standing. Talk to people who have had experience with the practitioner. Visit the practitioner and ask questions about his or her education, training, licences, certification, and insurance.
- What does the evidence show? Have studies been done on this therapy? Are they reliable studies? Do they apply to your situation?

Your primary care doctor may be able to help you make informed decisions about complementary medicine. Some people think their doctors don't want them to try complementary treatment. But more and more doctors are realizing that complementary therapies can work with conventional medicine to improve health and help people feel better. Your doctor may be able to refer you to some qualified complementary medicine practitioners.

If you do decide to try some form of complementary medicine, let your doctor know. Even if your doctor is not comfortable with your decision, it is important for your safety that he or she know what you are doing. Your complementary treatment should at least be safe and at best work in conjunction with your conventional medical treatment.

General Risks and Benefits of Complementary Medicine

All treatments, whether conventional or complementary, have risks and benefits. In general, the risks and benefits of complementary therapies are as follows.

Risks

Overlooking effective conventional medicine: Perhaps greater than the concern for risks of a specific complementary therapy is the concern that a person will forgo effective medical treatment or neglect to get an accurate diagnosis. Some practitioners of complementary therapies do not refer people to conventional doctors, even when it is possible that conventional medicine could help. And some people who choose complementary medicine refuse to consider conventional medicine for any problem. This can be dangerous. It is best to get as much information as possible and then make informed decisions, selecting from both conventional and complementary approaches for treatment of a specific health problem.

Potential dangers: Since many complementary therapies are not well studied, and the manufacture of complementary medicine products is not well regulated, you may be exposing yourself to unknown side effects or dangerous interactions. The lower level of regulation on products and practitioners may also expose you to additional health risks, especially if you have other medical conditions.

Many options and inadequate evidence: There are many different complementary treatments, and there is lots of information about them. Some of it is reliable. Relatively few complementary treatments have been studied for safety and effectiveness using traditional scientific methods. Unlike conventional medications, herbal medicines and nutritional supplements are regulated by Health Canada's Natural Health Products Directorate (NHPD) as dietary supplements, not as drugs. Little reliable information is available, which may make it difficult to reach an informed decision.

Cost: Many private health insurance companies cover the costs of complementary therapies. As with conventional medical treatments, you must decide whether a complementary therapy is working for you and whether its benefits are worth the time and money the therapy requires.

Health Fraud

People are taken in each year by medical fraud and worthless health products.

Cures lacking scientific proof that they really work are advertised for many chronic health problems, especially arthritis, cancer, baldness, obesity, and impotence. Unfortunately, many of these products may cause harmful side effects. It is wise to be suspicious of products that:

- Are advertised by testimonials.
- Claim to have a secret ingredient.
- Have not been evaluated in prominent medical journals.
- Claim benefits that seem too good to be true.
- Are available only by mail.

Be suspicious of any practitioner who:

- Prescribes medicines or gives injections at every visit.
- Promises a no-risk cure.
- Suggests something that seems unethical or illegal.

The best way to protect yourself from medical fraud is to be observant and ask questions. If you don't like what you see or hear, find another practitioner or get a second opinion.

Benefits

Holistic approach: Conventional visits to the doctor usually last about 10 to 15 minutes. Complementary medicine practitioners often take an hour or more to learn about your lifestyle and background, including information about your family, friends, diet, activities, and work. Many health problems, especially chronic ones, may respond best to treatment that considers the whole person and his or her environment and lifestyle.

Active listening and touch: People who provide complementary treatments are often taught to listen to and touch their patients. For many people, being listened to and touched in a caring way is helpful.

Mind-body connection: Science has shown that people's emotional states can affect their health. See The Mind-Body Connection on page 381. People who describe themselves as happy tend to be healthier than those who see themselves as unhappy. People who have a lot of stress in their lives are more likely to get sick. Conventional medicine offers little help for these kinds of problems. Complementary practices like meditation and tai chi can help ease stress and improve a person's sense of well-being, which may improve the person's health.

Empowerment: Many people find that having the freedom to try complementary therapies is empowering. It gives them a stronger sense of control over their bodies and their health.

Choosing the Right Therapy for You

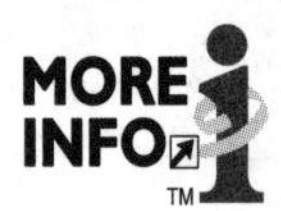

There are many types of complementary medicine. Choosing between different treatments can be confusing. This section describes several of the most widely available choices. Use this section to learn about different treatments and how they might work for you.

Acupuncture

Acupuncture is an ancient Chinese therapy based on the theory that there is energy called *chi* or *qi* (pronounced "chee") flowing through your body. Your *chi* flows along energy pathways called meridians. If the flow of *chi* is blocked or unbalanced at any point on a meridian, theoretically it may result in illness. Traditional practitioners believe acupuncture unblocks and balances the flow of *chi* to restore health. Western medical researchers who have studied acupuncture theorize that it reduces pain by acting on the biological mechanisms that control pain.

Traditional Chinese acupuncture is done by inserting very thin needles into the skin at certain points on the body to regulate energy flow along the body's energy pathways. Other types of acupuncture may use heat, pressure, or mild electric current.

Acupuncture may be used to relieve pain and treat certain health conditions, including addiction, asthma, headache, menstrual cramps, and joint and muscle problems. Promising results have been achieved by using acupuncture to relieve dental pain, pain after surgery, and nausea and vomiting related to chemotherapy.

Bodywork and Manual Therapy

Bodywork and manual therapy refer to a variety of body manipulation techniques used for relaxation and pain relief. Massage and chiropractic are well-known forms of manual therapy. Common forms of bodywork are the Alexander technique, the Feldenkrais method, the Trager approach, Rolfing, and deep tissue massage.

The idea behind bodywork is that people learn (or are forced into by injury or stress) unnatural ways of moving or holding their bodies. Theoretically, these unnatural movements or postures change the natural alignment of bones, which in turn causes discomfort and may contribute to health problems. The goal of bodywork is to realign and reposition the body to allow natural, graceful movement. Along with identifying possible contributing causes of unnatural movement and posture, bodywork is thought to reduce stress and ease pain.

There has not been extensive scientific testing of bodywork. A few studies suggest good results for people with arthritis, stress, or low back pain, and for children with cerebral palsy.

Chiropractic Treatment

Chiropractic is a manual therapy based on the theory that many medical disorders may be caused by misalignments in the spine. The main goal of chiropractic therapy is to help the body heal itself by correcting misalignments of the joints, particularly the bones of the spine (vertebrae).

Chiropractic treatments usually involve adjusting the joints and bones in the spine using twisting, pulling, or pushing movements. Some chiropractors use heat, electrical stimulation, or ultrasound to relax the muscles before doing an adjustment.

Chiropractic treatment has been shown to be helpful in treating low back pain, neck pain, and headaches.

Healing Touch

Healing touch, spiritual or energy healing, therapeutic touch, prayer, and distant healing are terms used to describe the conscious focus on another person to promote healing and well-being without physical intervention. Spiritual healing is widespread and may or may not have anything to do with an established religion. Therapeutic touch is taught in many nursing schools, and nurses may use it in conventional medical settings to help comfort their patients.

Like other complementary approaches, healing touch starts with the idea that people are naturally healthy. The way people live and think may disturb their natural health energy, and they become ill. The aim of healing touch is to focus or channel healing energy to restore natural health and balance. Some forms of healing touch use actual physical touch as part of the healing, but many do not.

There has been very little research on the effects of healing touch. It is a difficult form of therapy to study using traditional scientific methods. However, supporters of healing touch believe it is helpful in healing wounds, curing infection, and relieving pain. At the least, healing touch may help reduce anxiety and stress and provide comfort to a sick person.

The only known risk in using healing touch arises when people forgo effective medical treatment. Healing touch is not appropriate for acute, life-threatening situations or as a replacement for other treatments that are known to improve a disease. Prayer, healing, and therapeutic touch can always be used along with more conventional treatments.

Herbal Medicine

Plants and other natural products have been used for thousands of years to maintain health and treat illness. They are the basis for many conventional medications. For example, willow bark tea was used for centuries to control fever. Drug companies learned to copy the chemical makeup of willow bark to produce Aspirin.

Herbal medicines may do many of the same things that conventional drugs do. They may prevent illness. They may cure infection. They may soothe a fever or help wounds heal. They may keep your bowels regular or ease your pain. They may calm you down or perk you up.

Some herbal medicines may have no effect at all. Others may be harmful. Like conventional medicines, herbal medicines and natural supplements may cause side effects, trigger allergic reactions, or interact with other medications a person is taking.

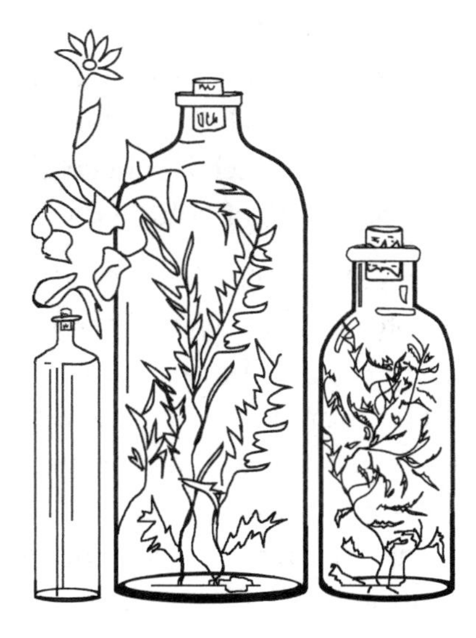

There have been thousands of studies on the effects of herbs. Most of the research has been done in Europe and Asia, where herbal medicine is more widely practised. In the United States, the analysis of this research began only recently, and many new studies are underway.

When shopping for herbal supplements, look for the NPN, or Natural Products Number. This number indicates that the product has complied with the manufacturing and safety standards set by Health Canada's Natural Health Products Directorate (NHPD). The NPN further indicates that the product has an NHPD-approved use. (NHPD regulation is being phased in over a 6-year period starting in 2004.)

Be sure to tell your doctor about any herbs or natural supplements you are taking. Pregnant and breast-feeding women and people with serious health problems should not use any herbal medicines or dietary supplements without first consulting their doctor.

Homeopathy

Like other complementary treatments, homeopathy is based on the idea that the body has the ability to heal itself. Sometimes the body needs to be stimulated to start the healing process. In homeopathy, a treatment is chosen because it can cause symptoms just like the ones that are troubling you. The treatment is given in a very small amount. In theory, it stimulates your body to heal the problem.

Homeopathy has been used to treat allergies, atopic dermatitis, rheumatoid arthritis, irritable bowel syndrome, and other chronic conditions. It is not considered appropriate for treatment of serious illnesses or emergencies.

Homeopathy is widely used in England and other European countries. It is not clear how or to what extent homeopathy works.

Massage Therapy

Massage therapy is based on the idea that physical manipulation and touch are healing. There are many different types of massage therapy. Some are gentle, while others are very active and intense. Typical treatments may include joint mobilization, hydrotherapy, and rehabilitative exercise such as stretching, strengthening, postural education, and home care.

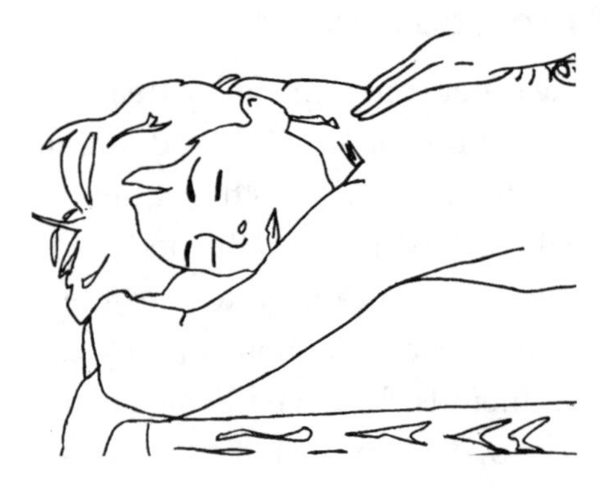

Massage therapy has been and continues to be widely studied. Many studies have shown that massage therapy decreases stress and helps control pain. Health problems that are caused by or made worse by stress (such as depression and inflammatory bowel disease) may also improve with massage treatment.

Current research is focusing on the effects of massage in treating conditions such as arthritis, multiple sclerosis, high blood pressure, behavioural problems, eating disorders, and fibromyalgia.

Naturopathy

Naturopathy blends many traditions of conventional and complementary medicine. Schools of naturopathy teach anatomy, cell biology, pharmacology, and other sciences studied in conventional medical schools. They also teach herbal medicine, acupuncture, and bodywork. The goal of naturopathy is to help you become and stay well, which is believed to be the natural state of your body.

Naturopathic medicine is used to promote health, prevent disease, and treat all kinds of health problems. Most naturopaths can treat earaches, allergies, and other common medical problems. A properly trained naturopath refers people to other practitioners for diagnosis or treatment when appropriate.

Fasting and recommendations for immunization are two controversial elements of naturopathic medicine. Fasting puts your body under stress and can be dangerous, especially if you have a disease like diabetes. Talk with your conventional doctor before you try fasting. If you start to feel sick while fasting, break your fast with small amounts of fruit or juice and then return to your normal diet.

Some naturopaths do not believe that immunization is necessary. This philosophy is very controversial. Before vaccinations were available, childhood illnesses caused large numbers of deaths and long-term health problems. Talk with your conventional doctor before deciding about immunization.

Tai Chi and Qi Gong

Tai chi and qi gong (pronounced "chee goong") are traditional Chinese exercises. They are based on the idea that gentle, graceful, repeated movements, deep concentration, and focused breathing can increase and improve the flow of energy (*chi* or *qi*) through the body and improve health.

Tai chi and qi gong are also founded on the Chinese belief that nature consists of opposing forces called yin and yang. This belief suggests that good health results when yin and yang are balanced. Tai chi and qi gong movements are done in an attempt to help restore the body's balance of yin and yang.

Tai chi is a series of movements done in a rhythmic pattern, either very slowly or very quickly. Qi gong is a lot of different movements that can be done in any order. Qi gong is useful to know because you can do it anywhere, anytime, even if you are unable to sit up or stand. Some common qi gong movements include raising and lowering your arms, moving your head from side to side, and rubbing your ears, feet, and hands.

Both tai chi and qi gong can be done by people of all ages. Their primary benefits are improved muscle strength, balance, coordination, posture, and flexibility. They may help increase stamina, lower blood pressure, and relieve stress. Possible muscle strains and sprains are their only harmful side effect. Gentle stretching before a tai chi or qi gong session can prevent most injuries.

Tai chi and qi gong can usually be used safely alongside conventional medical treatments for health problems, but they should not replace effective conventional treatment. Talk with your health professional so you can choose the tai chi or qi gong program that best suits your needs.

Yoga

Yoga is a meditation program that includes exercises to help improve flexibility and breathing, decrease stress, and maintain health. It has been practised in India for centuries and is based on the principle of mind-body unity.

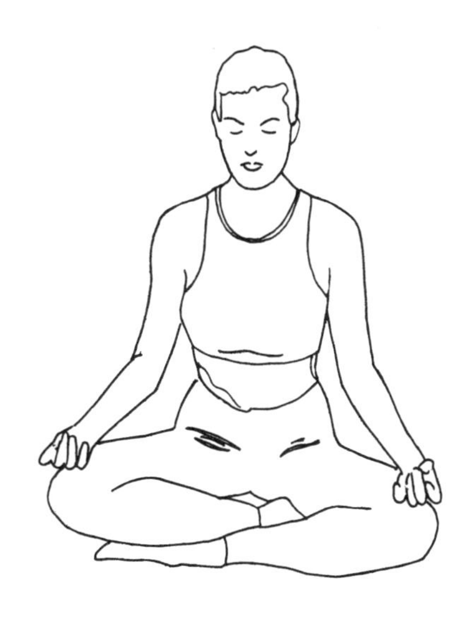

Two basic components of yoga are proper posture and breathing. There are many different yoga exercises or positions, called postures. These may be done while standing, lying down, or sitting in a chair; some are done in a headstand position. While practising a posture, which stretches the body, a person does breathing exercises to help relax muscles, maintain the posture, and focus the mind.

Most people who try yoga find that it improves flexibility and reduces stress. Several studies have shown that yoga helps lower blood pressure and improves a person's sense of well-being. Research has also shown that yoga can help people who have asthma learn to breathe more easily. People with chronic medical conditions like migraine headaches, heart disease, arthritis, or cancer may benefit from combining yoga and their conventional medical treatment.

Be prepared.
Boy Scout motto

22
Your Home Health Centre

More of your health care takes place in your home than anywhere else. Having the right tools, medicines, supplies, and information on hand will improve the quality of your self-care.

Store all your self-care tools and supplies in one central location, such as a large drawer in the bedroom or family room. Use the charts about tools and supplies in this chapter as checklists for keeping your home health centre well stocked.

Note: If small children are around, keep your supplies out of reach or stored in containers or cabinets with childproof safety latches.

Be familiar with the disaster preparation and response plan for your area. Keep the appropriate supplies on hand. See Disasters and Public Health Threats starting on page 51 for more information.

Self-Care Tools

Self-care tools are the basic equipment of your home health centre.

Cold Pack

A cold pack is a plastic envelope filled with gel that remains flexible at very cold temperatures. Buy two cold packs and keep them in the freezer. Use them for bumps, bruises, back sprains, turned ankles, sore joints, or any other health problem that calls for ice. A cold pack is more convenient than ice and may become the self-care tool you use the most.

You can make your own cold pack:

- Put 0.5 litre of rubbing alcohol and 1.5 litres of water in a 4-litre, heavy-duty, plastic freezer bag.
- Seal the bag, and then seal it in a second bag. Mark it "Cold pack: Do not eat," and place it in the freezer.

A bag of frozen vegetables will also work as a cold pack.

Self-Care Tools

For every household:

- Blood pressure cuff*
- Cold pack*
- Dental mirror
- Eyedropper
- Heating pad
- Humidifier or vaporizer*
- Medicine spoon*
- Nail clippers
- Penlight*
- Scissors
- Stethoscope*
- Digital thermometer
- Tweezers

For children younger than 6, add:

- Bulb aspirator/syringe
- Otoscope*

*Described in text

Humidifier and Vaporizer

Humidifiers and vaporizers add moisture to the air, making it less drying to your mouth, throat, and nose. A humidifier produces a cool mist, and a vaporizer puts out hot steam.

Cool mist from a humidifier may be more comfortable to breathe than hot steam. However, humidifiers are noisy, produce particles that may be irritating to some people, and need to be cleaned and disinfected regularly. This is especially important for people who have mould allergies.

A vaporizer's hot steam does not contain any irritating particles, and you can add medications such as Vicks VapoRub to ease breathing. Steam may feel good when you have a cold, but the hot water can burn anyone who gets too close to the vaporizer or overturns it.

Medicine Spoon

Medicine spoons are transparent tubes with marks that indicate typical dosage amounts. A medicine spoon makes it easy to give the right dose of liquid medicine. While the spoons are convenient for anyone, they are particularly helpful for young children. The tube shape and large lip get most of the medication into a child's mouth without spilling. Buy one at your local pharmacy.

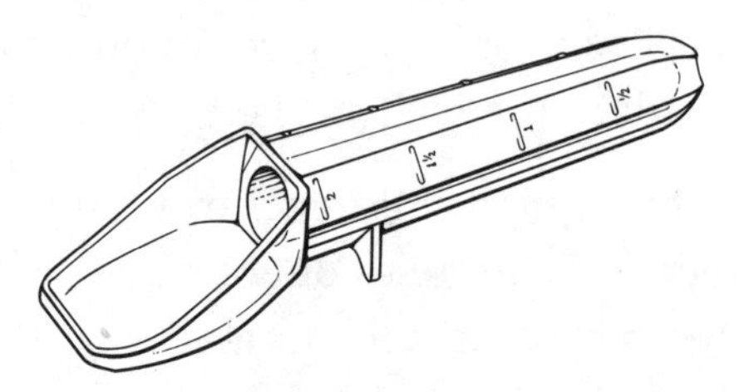

Medicine spoon

Otoscope

An otoscope is a flashlight with a special attachment for looking into the ear. With training, you can use an otoscope to help you decide if an ear infection is present. Inexpensive consumer-model otoscopes are available, but they do not illuminate the ear canal and eardrum as well as the one your doctor uses. They can also be used as high-intensity penlights.

Penlight

A penlight has a small, intense light that can be easily directed. It is useful for looking into the mouth or throat or examining the skin, and it is easier to handle than a flashlight.

Stethoscope and Blood Pressure Cuff

If you have heart disease or high blood pressure, it's a good idea to have both a stethoscope and a blood pressure cuff (sphygmomanometer) to monitor your blood pressure regularly.

Purchase a flat diaphragm-model stethoscope rather than a bell-shaped one. The flat surface makes it easier for you to hear.

Blood pressure cuffs come in many models. If you have difficulty reading the gauge on a regular cuff, look for a model that uses an upright mercury column, or buy an electronic digital model. Ask your pharmacist to recommend a blood pressure kit and show you how to use it.

Thermometer

Because of safety concerns, mercury-containing glass thermometers are no longer recommended. If you have one in your home, consider replacing it with a digital electronic thermometer.

Digital thermometers are accurate, easy to read, and durable. In BC, they are recommended for use in babies and children, using the armpit. Temperature strips are very convenient and safe but are not as accurate as digital thermometers and should only be used to measure axillary (armpit) temperature. They are inaccurate when used on the forehead. Thermometers that measure the temperature in the ear are fast, easy to use, and quite accurate, but they are expensive.

Rectal thermometers are no longer recommended for use in babies or young children.

Self-Care Supplies

The supplies listed below are useful to keep on hand in your home health centre. The products are inexpensive, easy to use, and generally available in any drugstore or pharmacy.

- Adhesive bandages in assorted sizes
- Adhesive tape, 2.5 cm wide
- Butterfly bandages
- Sterile gauze pads, 5 cm square
- Elastic ("Ace") bandage, 7.5 cm wide
- Roll of gauze bandage, 5 cm wide
- Cotton balls
- Safety pins

How to Take a Temperature

A normal oral temperature ranges from 36.4° to 37.5°C and for most people is 37°C. Temperature varies with time of day and other factors, so don't worry about minor changes.

Whenever a person feels hot or cold to your touch, it is a good idea to take and record his or her temperature. If you have to call your doctor during an illness, knowing your exact temperature will be very helpful.

There are four places where a thermometer can be placed to take a temperature:

1. In the mouth (oral)
2. In the anus (rectal)
3. Under the armpit (axillary)
4. In the ear (tympanic)

Unless otherwise specified, all temperatures in this book are oral Celsius readings. If you take a rectal or axillary temperature, adjust it accordingly (see below).

Oral thermometers are recommended for people age 6 and older.

- Do not drink hot or cold liquids before taking your temperature.
- Clean the thermometer with soapy water or rubbing alcohol.
- If you are using an alcohol or mercury thermometer, hold it firmly at the end opposite the bulb and shake it down to 35°C or lower.
- Place the bulb under your tongue and close your lips around it. Do not bite down. Breathe through your nose and don't talk.
- Wait 3 to 5 minutes (or until a digital thermometer beeps).

Rectal thermometers may be used if an older child or adult cannot hold an oral thermometer in the mouth. Do not use rectal thermometers in babies or young children. Use only a rectal thermometer to take a rectal temperature. Rectal temperature is 0.3° to 0.6°C higher than oral temperature. Rectal temperatures are the most accurate.

- Clean the thermometer. If you are using an alcohol or mercury thermometer, shake it down to 35°C or lower.
- Put Vaseline or another lubricant on the bulb.
- Have the person lie on his or her side with the upper leg slightly bent.
- Hold the thermometer 2.5 cm from the bulb and gently insert it into the rectum no more than 2.5 cm. Do not let go. Hold the thermometer right at the anus so it cannot slip in farther.
- Wait for 3 minutes (or until a digital thermometer beeps).

Axillary temperatures are less accurate and are about 0.3° to 0.6°C lower than oral temperatures. Axillary readings under the armpit are safest for babies and small children who will not hold still.

- Use an oral thermometer. If it is an alcohol or mercury thermometer rather than a digital one, shake it down below 35°C.
- Place the thermometer in the armpit and cross the child's arm over the chest to hold the opposite upper arm.
- Wait 5 minutes, or until a digital thermometer beeps.

How to Read a Thermometer

To read a thermometer that does not have a digital readout:

- Roll the thermometer between your fingers until you can see the thin ribbon of mercury (silver) or alcohol (red). Note that the thermometer is marked from 33° to 42°C.
- Each large mark indicates 0.5°C of temperature. Each small mark indicates 0.1°C.

Non-prescription Medications and Products

A non-prescription medication (sometimes called an over-the-counter or OTC medication) is any drug that you can buy without a doctor's prescription. However, don't assume that all non-prescription drugs are safe for you. These drugs can interact with other medications and can sometimes cause serious health problems.

Some medications should only be used by adults or older children. Be sure to read the package instructions carefully, or ask a pharmacist before giving any product to an infant or young child.

Carefully read the label of any non-prescription drug you use, especially if you also take prescription medications for other health problems. Ask your pharmacist for help in finding a non-prescription drug best suited to your needs. If you are concerned about side effects, call your community pharmacist, your doctor, or the BC NurseLine.

Some common non-prescription medications include:

- Antacids and acid reducers.
- Bulking agents and laxatives.
- Antidiarrheals.
- Cold and allergy remedies.
- Pain relievers.

These drugs can be very helpful when used properly but can also cause serious problems if used incorrectly. The following tips will help you use common non-prescription drugs wisely and safely. In some cases, you may find that you don't need to take them at all.

Antacids and Acid Reducers

Antacids are taken to relieve heartburn or indigestion caused by excess stomach acid. While they are safe if used occasionally, antacids may cause problems if taken regularly. There are several kinds of antacids.

Learn what ingredients are in each type so you can avoid any adverse effects.

- Sodium bicarbonate antacids (such as Alka-Seltzer and Bromo Seltzer) contain baking soda. Avoid these antacids if you have high blood pressure or are on a salt-restricted diet.
- Calcium carbonate antacids (such as Tums and Rolaids) are sometimes used as calcium supplements (see page 359). However, these products may cause constipation.
- Aluminum-based antacids (such as Amphojel) are less potent and work more slowly than other products do. They may also cause constipation. Some may cause calcium loss and should not be taken by post-menopausal women. If you have kidney problems, check with your doctor before using aluminum-based antacids.
- Magnesium compounds (such as Phillips' Milk of Magnesia) may cause diarrhea.
- Aluminum-magnesium antacids (such as Maalox, Mylanta, and Almagel) are less likely to cause constipation or diarrhea than aluminum-only or magnesium-only antacids are.

Acid reducers decrease the amount of acid produced by the stomach. There are several types of non-prescription acid reducers on the market. Each has slightly different cautions for use. Read and carefully follow the instructions included with the package.

Antacid and Acid Reducer Precautions

- Try to eliminate the cause of frequent heartburn instead of taking antacids regularly. See Heartburn on page 121.
- Consult your doctor or pharmacist before taking an antacid if you take other medications. Antacids may interfere with the absorption and action of some prescription medications. Also consult your doctor if you have ulcers or kidney problems.
- If you have a problem with the function of your kidneys or liver, you should be careful in using acid reducers. All drugs are broken down and removed from the body by the combined action of the liver and kidneys. If your liver or kidneys are not working correctly, it is possible that too much of the acid-reducing drug will build up in your body.

Bulking Agents and Laxatives

There are two types of products to prevent or treat constipation: bulking agents and laxatives.

Bulking agents, such as bran or psyllium (found in Metamucil, for example), ease constipation by increasing the volume of stool and making it easier to pass. Regular use of bulking agents is safe and helps make them more effective.

Laxatives (such as Correctol, Ex-Lax, Senokot, and Dulcolax) speed up the passage of stool by irritating the lining of the intestines. Regular laxative use is not recommended.

There are many other ways to treat constipation, such as drinking more water. See page 116.

Precautions

- Take laxatives or bulking agents with plenty of water or other liquids.
- Do not take laxatives regularly. Overuse of laxatives decreases tone and sensation in the large intestine, causing laxative dependence. If you need help keeping your bowels regular, use a bulking agent.
- Regular use of some laxatives (such as Correctol or Ex-Lax) may interfere with your body's ability to absorb vitamin D and calcium; this can lead to weakened bones.

Antidiarrheals

There are two types of antidiarrheal drugs: those that thicken the stool and those that slow intestinal spasms.

The **thickening** mixtures (such as Kaopectate) contain clay or fruit pectin and absorb bacteria and toxins in the intestine. They are safe because they do not go into the blood, but these products also absorb the bacteria needed for digestion. Long-term use is not advised.

Antispasmodic antidiarrheal products slow the spasms of the intestine. Loperamide (the active ingredient in products such as Imodium A-D and Pepto Diarrhea Control) is an example of this type of preparation. Some products (such as Donnagel and Parepectolin) contain both thickening and antispasmodic ingredients.

Antidiarrheal Precautions

- Diarrhea helps rid your body of an infection, so try to avoid using antidiarrheal medications for the first 24 hours. After that, use them only if cramping and pain continue and there are no other signs of illness, such as fever.
- Be sure to take a large enough dose. Take antidiarrheal preparations until your stools thicken; then stop immediately to avoid constipation.
- Replace lost body fluids. Dehydration can develop when someone, especially an infant, child, or older adult, has diarrhea. See Rehydration Drinks on page 119.

Cold and Allergy Remedies

In general, whether you take medications for your cold or not, you'll get better in about a week. Rest and liquids are the best treatment for a cold (see page 194). Antibiotics will not help. However, medications help relieve some cold symptoms, such as nasal congestion and cough.

Allergy symptoms, especially runny nose, often respond to antihistamines. Antihistamines are also found in many cold medications, often together with a decongestant. However, the value of antihistamines in treating cold symptoms is under debate.

Decongestants

Decongestants make breathing easier by shrinking swollen mucous membranes in the nose, allowing air to pass through. They also help relieve runny nose and post-nasal drip, which can cause a sore throat.

> **Saline Nose Drops**
>
> Non-prescription saline nasal sprays (such as Rhinaris and Salinex) are convenient, inexpensive, and sterile. They will keep nasal tissues moist so the tissues can filter the air. Saline nasal sprays will not cause mucous membranes in the nose to swell.
>
> Saline nose drops can also be easily made at home. Mix 5 g (1 tsp) salt in 470 ml (1 pint) of body temperature water (too much salt will dry nasal membranes). Place the solution in a clean bottle with a dropper (available at drugstores). Use as necessary. Make a fresh solution every 3 days.
>
> Insert the drops while lying on your back on a bed, with your head hanging over the side. This will help the drops get farther back. Try to keep the dropper from touching your nose.

Decongestants can be taken orally or used as nose drops or sprays. Oral decongestants (pills) are probably more effective and provide longer relief, but they cause more side effects. Pseudoephedrine (the active ingredient in products such as Sudafed) is an oral decongestant.

Sprays and drops provide rapid but temporary relief. Nasal sprays containing phenylephrine (such as Neo-Synephrine) are effective. Sprays and drops are less likely to interact with other drugs than oral decongestants are.

Decongestant Precautions

- Do not give cold medicines or oral decongestants to infants under 6 months of age. Non-prescription cold medicines have not been proven effective for preschool children.
- Do not use medicated nasal sprays or drops more than 3 times a day or for more than 3 days in a row. Continued use may cause a "rebound effect," in which your mucous membranes swell up more than before you used the spray.
- Drink extra fluids when taking cold medications.
- Decongestants can cause problems for people who have certain health problems, such as heart disease, high blood pressure, glaucoma, diabetes, or an overactive thyroid. Decongestants may also interact with some drugs, such as certain antidepressants and high blood pressure medications. Read the

package carefully or ask your pharmacist or doctor to help you choose one.

Cough Preparations

Coughing is your body's way of getting foreign substances and mucus out of your respiratory tract. Coughs are often useful, and you shouldn't try to eliminate them. Sometimes, though, coughs are severe enough to impair breathing or prevent rest.

Water and other liquids, such as fruit juices, are probably the best cough syrups. They help soothe the throat and also moisten and thin mucus so it can be coughed up more easily.

You can make a simple and soothing cough syrup at home by mixing 1 part lemon juice with 2 parts honey. Use as often as needed. This can be given to children older than 1 year of age.

There are two kinds of cough medicines: expectorants and suppressants. **Expectorants** help thin the mucus and make it easier to cough mucus up when you have a productive cough. Look for expectorants containing guaifenesin, such as Robitussin and Vicks 44E.

Suppressants control or suppress the cough reflex and work best for a dry, hacking cough that keeps you awake. Look for suppressant medications containing dextromethorphan, such as Robitussin-DM.

Don't suppress a productive cough too much (unless it is keeping you from getting enough rest).

Cough Preparation Precautions

- Cough preparations can cause problems for people with certain health problems, such as asthma, heart disease, high blood pressure, or an enlarged prostate. Cough preparations may also interact with sedatives, certain antidepressants, and other medications. Read the package carefully or ask your pharmacist or doctor to help you choose one.
- Cough suppressants can stifle breathing. Use them with caution if you give them to someone who is very old or frail or if you have chronic respiratory problems.
- Read the label so you know what the ingredients are. Some cough preparations contain a large percentage of alcohol; others contain codeine. There are many choices. Ask your pharmacist to advise you.

Antihistamines

Antihistamines dry up nasal secretions and are commonly used to treat allergy symptoms and itching.

If your runny nose is caused by allergies, an antihistamine will help. For cold symptoms, home treatment and perhaps a decongestant (see page 406) will probably be more helpful. It is usually best to take only single-ingredient allergy or cold preparations, instead of those containing many active ingredients.

Products such as Chlor-Tripolon (chlorpheniramine) and Benadryl (diphenhydramine) are single-ingredient antihistamine products.

Products such as Dristan, Coricidin, and Triaminic contain both a decongestant and an antihistamine.

Antihistamine Precautions

- Do not give antihistamines to infants younger than 4 months of age. For children between 4 months and 1 year, ask your doctor first.
- Use of antihistamines to treat the stuffiness of a cold will often thicken the mucus, making it harder to get rid of.
- Drink extra fluids when taking antihistamines.
- Antihistamines can cause problems for some people with conditions such as asthma, glaucoma, epilepsy, or an enlarged prostate. Antihistamines may also interact with certain antidepressants, sedatives, and tranquilizers. Read the package carefully or ask your pharmacist or doctor to help you choose one that will not cause problems.
- The drowsiness that antihistamines often cause usually lessens with continued use. If it continues, or if the medication isn't helping your allergies after 1 week, call your doctor for advice.
- Some antihistamines do not make you drowsy. Ask your health professional if these are appropriate for you.

Pain Relievers

There are dozens of pain reliever products. Most contain either acetylsalicylic acid (ASA, or Aspirin), ibuprofen, or acetaminophen. These three drugs, as well as ketoprofen and naproxen sodium, relieve pain and reduce fever. Aspirin, ibuprofen, ketoprofen, and naproxen sodium also relieve inflammation. They belong to a class of drugs called non-steroidal anti-inflammatory drugs (NSAIDs).

When purchasing pain relievers, keep in mind that generic products are chemically equivalent to more expensive brand-name products, and they usually work equally well.

Aspirin

Aspirin is widely used for relieving pain and reducing fever in adults. It also relieves minor itching and reduces swelling and inflammation. Most tablets contain 325 mg of Aspirin. Although it seems familiar and safe, Aspirin is a very powerful drug.

Aspirin Precautions

- Keep all Aspirin, especially baby Aspirin, out of children's reach.
- Aspirin increases the risk of Reye's syndrome in children (see page 268). Do not give Aspirin to anyone younger than 20 unless your doctor tells you to do so.
- Aspirin can irritate the stomach lining, causing bleeding or ulcers. If it upsets your stomach, try a

coated brand. Talk with your doctor or pharmacist to determine what will work best for you.

- Some people are allergic to Aspirin. They may also be allergic to ibuprofen.
- Throw Aspirin away if it starts to smell like vinegar.
- Do not take Aspirin if you have gout or if you take blood thinners (anticoagulants).
- Do not take Aspirin for a hangover. Aspirin used with alcohol increases your risk for stomach irritation.
- High doses may result in Aspirin poisoning. Stop taking Aspirin and call a health professional if any one of these symptoms occurs:
  - Ringing in the ears
  - Visual disturbances
  - Nausea
  - Dizziness
  - Rapid, deep breathing

Other Aspirin Uses

In addition to relieving pain and inflammation, Aspirin is effective against many other ailments. Because of the danger of side effects and the interactions Aspirin may have with other medications, do not try these uses of Aspirin without a doctor's supervision.

- **Heart attacks and strokes**: Aspirin in low but regular doses helps prevent heart attacks and strokes in certain people, including people with diabetes. Doses as low as 30 mg per day have helped. Aspirin may also help as a first aid measure for heart attacks. Chewing ½ tablet may be enough to help. See Heart Attack on page 86.
- **Stomach and colon cancer**: Some studies have shown that taking 1 Aspirin tablet per day can reduce the risk of cancers in the digestive system.
- **Migraines**: Regular, low-dose Aspirin use may reduce the frequency of migraines.

Other Pain Relievers

Ibuprofen (the active ingredient in products such as Advil and Motrin), **ketoprofen** (in products such as Orudis and Rhodis), and **naproxen sodium** are other non-steroidal anti-inflammatory drugs (NSAIDs). Like Aspirin, these drugs relieve pain and reduce fever and inflammation. Also like Aspirin, they can cause nausea, stomach irritation, and heartburn. People who take blood thinners (anticoagulants) should use these drugs with caution.

Acetaminophen (the active ingredient in products such as Tylenol) reduces fever and relieves pain. It does not have the anti-inflammatory effect of NSAIDs, such as Aspirin and ibuprofen, but it also does not cause stomach upset and other side effects.

The product's package label will tell you how many milligrams (mg) of medicine are in each pill; how much you should take; and how often you should take it. Do not exceed the dosage limits, and follow the instructions on the package if you have health problems that may make it unsafe for you to take the usual dosage of a product.

Medication Guidelines

The following are basic guidelines for taking prescription and non-prescription medications:

- Use medications only if non-drug approaches are not working.
- Know the benefits and side effects of a medication before taking it.
- Take the minimum effective dose.
- Never take a drug prescribed for someone else.
- Follow the prescription instructions exactly or let your doctor know why you didn't.
- Keep medications tightly capped in their original containers, and store them as directed.
- Do not take medications in front of small children. Children are great mimics. Don't oversell the "candy" taste of children's medicines or leave children's vitamins accessible to children.
- Call the BC NurseLine to speak with a pharmacist if you are concerned about side effects. This service is available between 5 p.m. and 9 a.m. every day.

Prescription Medications

There are thousands of different prescription medications used to treat hundreds of different medical conditions. Your doctor and your pharmacist are your best sources of information about your prescription medications.

Guidelines for taking every kind of prescription medication could fill several books. Common types covered here include antibiotics, minor tranquilizers, and sleeping pills.

Antibiotics

Antibiotics are drugs that kill bacteria. They are effective against bacteria only and have no effect on viruses. Therefore, antibiotics will not cure the common cold, flu, or any other viral illness. Unless you have a bacterial infection, it's best to avoid the possible adverse effects of antibiotics, which may include:

- **Side effects**, including **allergic reactions**. Common side effects of antibiotics include nausea, diarrhea, and increased sensitivity to sunlight. Most side effects are mild, but some, especially allergic reactions, can be severe. A severe allergic reaction usually causes shortness of breath and can be life-threatening. If you have any unexpected reaction to an antibiotic, tell your health professional before another antibiotic is prescribed.

- **Secondary infections**. Antibiotics kill most of the bacteria in your body that are sensitive to them, including the bacteria that help your body. Antibiotics can destroy the bacterial balance in your body, leading to stomach upset, diarrhea, vaginal infections, or other problems.
- **Bacterial resistance**. When antibiotics are used too often, bacteria change so that the antibiotics are no longer effective against them. This makes bacterial infections more difficult to treat.

When you and your health professional have decided that an antibiotic is necessary, carefully follow the instructions for taking the prescription.

- Take the whole dose for as many days as prescribed, unless you have unexpected side effects (in which case, call your health professional). Antibiotics kill off many bacteria quite quickly, so you may feel better in a few days. However, if you stop taking the antibiotic too soon, the weaker bacteria will have been eliminated, but the stronger ones may survive and flourish.
- Be sure you understand any special instructions about taking the medication. The instructions should be printed on the label, but double-check with your doctor and pharmacist.
- Store antibiotics in a cool, dry place. Check carefully to see if they need refrigeration.
- Never give an antibiotic prescribed for one person to someone else.
- Do not save leftover antibiotics, and do not take an antibiotic prescribed for another illness without a health professional's approval.

Adverse Drug Reactions

Side effects, drug-drug and food-drug interactions, overmedication, and addiction may cause:

- Nausea, indigestion, and vomiting.
- Constipation, diarrhea, or problems with urination.
- Dry mouth.
- Headache, dizziness, ringing in the ears, or blurred vision.
- Confusion, forgetfulness, disorientation, drowsiness, or depression.
- Difficulty sleeping, irritability, or nervousness.
- Difficulty breathing.
- Rashes, bruising, and bleeding problems.

Don't assume any symptom is a normal side effect that you have to suffer with. Call your doctor, your pharmacist, or the BC NurseLine anytime you suspect that your medicines are making you sick.

Minor Tranquilizers and Sleeping Pills

Minor tranquilizers (such as Valium, Xanax, and Ativan) and sleeping pills (such as Dalmane and Restoril) are widely prescribed. However, these drugs can cause problems, including memory loss, addiction, and injuries from falls caused by drug-induced unsteadiness.

Minor tranquilizers can be effective for short periods of time. However, long-term use is often of limited value and introduces the risk of addiction and mental impairment.

Sleeping pills may help for a few days or a few weeks, but using them for more than a month generally causes more sleep problems than it solves. For other approaches, see page 376.

If you have been taking minor tranquilizers or sleeping pills for a while, talk with your doctor about re-evaluating your need for the medication or reducing your dosage. If you have experienced any unsteadiness, dizziness, or memory loss, tell your doctor.

Medication Problems

Several kinds of adverse medication reactions can occur:

Side effects. Side effects are predictable but unpleasant reactions to a drug. They are usually mild, but they can be inconvenient. In some cases, they are more serious.

Allergies. Some people have severe, sometimes life-threatening reactions (called anaphylaxis) to certain medications. See When to Call a Health Professional on page 183 for signs of an allergic reaction.

Drug-drug interactions. These occur when two or more prescription or non-prescription drugs or herbal supplements mix in a person's body and cause an adverse reaction. The symptoms can be severe and may be improperly diagnosed as a new illness.

Drug-food interactions. These occur when medications react with food. Some drugs work best when taken with food, but others should be taken on an empty stomach. Some drug-food reactions can cause serious symptoms.

Overmedication. Sometimes the full adult dose of a medication is too much for small people and those over age 60. Too much of a drug can be very dangerous.

Addiction. Long-term use of some medications can lead to dependency, and severe reactions may occur if the medications are withdrawn suddenly. Narcotics, tranquilizers, and barbiturates must be taken very carefully to prevent addiction. See page 366.

Save Money on Medications

Non-prescription and prescription medications can be very expensive. Here are some ways to cut your medication costs:

- Buy generic non-prescription products. They are chemically equivalent to brand-name drugs but are usually cheaper. Ask your doctor if generic forms of your prescription medications are available and appropriate for you.
- Shop around and compare prices at several pharmacies. Prices can vary widely. It may be worth paying a little more if you know and trust the pharmacist.
- Ask your doctor for samples of newly prescribed medications, or ask your pharmacist to fill only the first week's worth of pills. If the medication has to be changed later, you will have saved paying for the full prescription.

Home Medical Tests

Many common medical tests are now available in home kits. Combined with regular visits to your health professional, home tests can help you monitor your health and, in some cases, detect problems early.

Home medical tests must be very accurate to be approved by Health Canada. However, they must be used correctly to give such accurate results. Follow the package directions exactly. If you have questions, ask your pharmacist or call the toll-free phone number on the product label.

Home medical tests are especially helpful if you have a chronic condition that requires frequent monitoring, such as diabetes, asthma, or high blood pressure. Ask your doctor which home medical tests are appropriate for you. Some common tests are described next.

Blood Sugar Monitoring

If you have diabetes, you may already monitor your blood sugar levels using a finger prick and a test strip or an electronic monitor.

This test should always be used under a doctor's supervision. Never adjust your insulin dose in response to a single abnormal test, unless your doctor has specifically instructed you to do so.

Check with your doctor if you have symptoms of abnormal blood sugar levels, even if the test is normal. See When to Call a Health Professional on page 289.

Blood Pressure Monitoring

If you have high blood pressure, it is important to monitor your blood pressure frequently. With a little instruction, you can easily monitor your blood pressure at home.

By checking your blood pressure at home, when you are relaxed, you will be able to track changes resulting from your home treatment and medications.

- Do not make any changes to your medications based on your home blood pressure readings without consulting your doctor first.
- Check your blood pressure at different times of day to see how rest and activities affect it. For regular readings, check it at the same time every day. Blood pressure is usually lowest in the morning and rises during the day.
- For the most accurate reading, sit still for 5 minutes before taking your blood pressure.
- Have your blood pressure cuff device adjusted (calibrated) yearly.

Tests for Blood in Stool

The fecal occult blood test can detect hidden blood in your stools, which may indicate colon cancer or other problems. This test is inexpensive and easy to do, but it does not detect colon cancer as well as other screening tests can. Your doctor may recommend a more accurate screening test for colon cancer, such as flexible sigmoidoscopy or colonoscopy. See page 131.

Home Pregnancy Tests

If you become pregnant, it is important that you know right away. The quickest way to find out is with a home pregnancy test. Home pregnancy tests are inexpensive and very reliable when done correctly. Some tests can show positive results within a few days of the first missed period. Use a test that has simple instructions and follow them exactly. Mistakes can lead to false results.

If the result is positive, schedule an appointment with your doctor to confirm the result.

Even if the pregnancy test result is negative, it is a good idea to see your doctor to confirm the results. Treat yourself as if you are pregnant until you know for sure.

Home Medical Records

Your home health centre is a good place to keep your family's medical records. A 3-ring binder or wire-bound notebook with dividers for each member of the family is helpful. Each person's section should have a cover sheet listing:

- Diagnosed chronic conditions (arthritis, asthma, diabetes, high blood pressure).
- Any known allergies to drugs, foods, or insects.
- Information that would be vital in an emergency, such as whether the person has a pacemaker or a hearing aid, has diabetes or epilepsy, or has impaired hearing or vision.
- Name and phone number of primary doctor.

You may also want to include:

- An up-to-date list of medications that includes name of drug, purpose, dose, instructions, name of doctor who prescribed the drug, and date prescribed.

- An immunization record with dates of childhood immunizations, tetanus boosters, flu shots, and pneumococcal vaccine.
- Health screening results for blood pressure, cholesterol, vision, and hearing.
- Results from cancer screenings, such as Pap tests, mammograms, colonoscopy, and PSA (prostate-specific antigen) tests.
- Records of major illnesses and injuries, such as pneumonia, bronchitis, and broken bones.
- Records of any major surgical procedures and hospitalizations.
- A list of major diseases in your family (such as heart disease, stroke, cancer, or diabetes).
- A copy of a Representation Agreement that deals with health care and any written instructions for medical emergencies.

Health Information at Home

Getting the right health information at the right time is the key to making good health decisions. If the information you need is not in this book, keep looking. Here's how:

On the Internet. Follow the instructions on the back cover of this book to get to BC HealthGuide OnLine, which contains the Healthwise® Knowledgebase. With over 100 times the information in the book, the Healthwise Knowledgebase has accurate, unbiased, and regularly updated information on almost all health problems. It is written in language most people can understand. And, it is free. If you have Internet access, go to this site first.

If you don't find everything you need in the Healthwise Knowledgebase, don't give up. There is plenty of reliable information out there if you know where and how to look for it. See Five Tips for Finding Good Web Sites on page 416.

On the phone. The BC NurseLine can respond to your health questions 24 hours a day, 7 days a week. (See the back cover for phone numbers.) Local offices of national organizations like the Canadian Cancer Society, Heart and Stroke Foundation, Arthritis Society, or Canadian Diabetes Association can also help connect you with information resources in your area. Check your phone book.

At your library or bookstore. Research librarians at public libraries spend a good part of their time helping people find information. Ask for their help if you are trying to learn more about a health problem. Libraries can also be a good place to use the Internet if you don't have a computer at home. Be aware that the information found in books and magazines is not guaranteed to be any more accurate than that found on the Internet. Use some of the tips for finding good Web sites as a guide for finding helpful books.

Health information you find on the Internet or in books or magazines should never replace the medical expertise and experience of a health professional. Discuss what you find with your doctor to learn if and how it relates to your particular situation.

Five Tips for Finding Good Web Sites

As a source of health information, the Internet has two major drawbacks. First, there is little or no regulation of what gets published. Misleading, contradictory, inaccurate, and even fraudulent health information is all over the Internet. Second, the amount of information available on the Internet can make your search overwhelming and time-consuming.

With so much information available, how do you separate the good from the bad? For starters, try these guidelines for finding information you can trust:

1. Don't rely on search engines. Instead, go to trusted sources recommended by your health professional or hospital. You can also rely on the information on BC HealthGuide OnLine at www.bchealthguide.org. If you have to use a search engine, be sure to follow the other four tips closely.

2. Don't trust the information on a health Web site unless the site clearly indicates:

- Who wrote and reviewed the information.
- When the information was last updated.
- What sources and references the information is based on. (Look for a bibliography or reference list.)

If information is missing, be skeptical of the site's reliability.

3. Check the site's privacy policy. It should tell you that your personal information will not be given to any third party without your explicit permission. Web sites displaying the URAC Health Web Site Accreditation seal should be safe.

4. Check the site ownership or sponsorship. Web sites displaying the URAC Health Web Site Accreditation seal should indicate any influence that the owner or sponsor has on the site's content.

5. Watch for these clues that a Web site is of questionable quality:

- Heavy use of personal testimonials without references to good research
- Unsupported claims of a "secret" or "revolutionary" cure
- Promotion of a specific drug, dietary supplement, medical device, or other product
- Requirement of a financial investment

Your final test should be the common sense test. If information doesn't make sense to you, don't trust it without first talking with your health professional. Never make a health care decision based solely on what you read on the Internet.

The role of government is to ensure that the citizens of British Columbia have access to appropriate and effective services and programs to improve their health and well-being.

Dr. Perry Kendall,
Provincial Health Officer,
British Columbia

23

Health Care in British Columbia

Before we had a publicly funded universal health care system, many people and their families could not afford medical care or faced bankruptcy with a serious illness.

Today, over 4 million British Columbians have access to quality health care. The Government of British Columbia (BC) funds a broad range of services, including acute care, ambulance, primary care, public health, home and community care, mental health, and addiction services. These services are delivered by health professionals across the province through hospitals, clinics, public health units, private offices, and residential and other care facilities.

Enquiry BC

Enquiry BC is a toll-free telephone service that can assist you in contacting any provincial program or service, with TDD service available for the deaf and hearing-impaired. Enquiry BC's telephone numbers are listed in your telephone directory's blue pages, under Government of BC. Detailed information about provincially funded health care services is also available through the BC Ministry of Health Web site at: www.gov.bc.ca/healthservices.

You can access public health, home and community care, mental health, and addiction programs directly in your area (see below for details). The regional health authorities in the BC health care system include: 5 health authorities that govern, plan, and coordinate services regionally; 16 health service delivery areas in which patients have a broad range of coordinated hospital and community-based health services; and one Provincial Health Services Authority that coordinates and/or provides provincial programs and specialized services such as cardiac care and transplants. To find out more about the services offered in your area, look in the blue pages of your local telephone directory.

Public health services provide community/public health nursing, health promotion, immunization, nutrition, audiology (hearing), speech and language pathology, and health inspection services. These are delivered in a variety of settings, such as at your home, public health units, child care facilities, schools, etc. Your local public health unit can provide information about the specific services available in your area.

Home and Community Care services include a range of health care and support services for eligible people who have acute, chronic, palliative, or rehabilitative health care needs. Home and Community Care services include case management, residential care, adult day centres, home support (including a self-managed option, home nursing, and community rehabilitation services), palliative care, and caregiver relief (respite). The type of assistance and support required varies from person to person, and the amount of service needed may change over time. Contact your local health authority to determine a person's eligibility for Home and Community Care services.

Community mental health teams provide free, confidential assessment and treatment services. Your local mental health office can assist you in obtaining these services. Alcohol, Drug, and other addiction services, such as the Problem Gambling Help Line, are also directly accessible and can be contacted through the numbers in your telephone directory's blue pages under Government of BC.

The Ministry of Health also offers an integrated self-care program called the BC HealthGuide Program. BC HealthGuide is designed to help British Columbians make better health decisions for themselves and their families. The Program empowers British Columbians to seek and access information to health information and advice, while helping them get the right care at the right time, in the right place.

BC HealthGuide has four components:

- *BC HealthGuide* handbook and *First Nations Health Handbook*
- BC NurseLine

- BC HealthGuide OnLine
- BC HealthFiles

The components work together by giving you access to high-quality, consistent health information wherever you are, whenever you need it.

To receive your copy of the *BC HealthGuide* handbook and *First Nations Health Handbook*, call 1-800-465-4911.

The BC NurseLine provides easy access to help for your health concerns, any time of the day or night. The BC NurseLine is a toll-free confidential health information line, staffed by knowledgeable, specially trained registered nurses who answer your questions 24 hours a day, 7 days a week. Pharmacist services are also available between 5 p.m. and 9 a.m., 7 days a week. Translation services are available in 130 languages.

The nurses help you know when you can safely treat a problem at home and when you need to see a doctor or go to the emergency room. The nurses use a comprehensive health information database in addition to their professional experience to provide accurate health information and answer questions about your health care concerns. They will help you decide when to seek medical assistance.

Call the BC NurseLine anytime toll-free:

- Within BC: 1-866-215-4700
- In Greater Vancouver: 604-215-4700
- Deaf/Hearing-Impaired: 1-866-889-4700

BC HealthGuide OnLine is an Internet site that links British Columbians with a world of up-to-date, reliable health information. The BC HealthGuide OnLine Web site has detailed information on more than 3,000 common health concerns. The site is based on sound medical information from leading medical and consumer publications that has been reviewed by BC doctors, nurses, and other health professionals.

It's a comprehensive source of health information that you can trust. Log in to www.bchealthguide.org.

The BC HealthFiles are a series of one- or two-page, easy-to-read fact sheets on a wide range of public and environmental health and safety issues. They provide information on many childhood and adult diseases, problems with pests, environmental health hazards, and safety and health tips. BC HealthFiles are updated regularly.

You can find BC HealthFiles at all local public health units or by visiting BC HealthGuide OnLine at www.bchealthguide.org.

For more information about the BC HealthGuide Program, see the outside back cover of this book.

The Medical Services Plan (MSP) of BC is the provincial health insurance plan that provides universal, comprehensive coverage for necessary medical care. MSP is a publicly administered, non-profit health care system, funded through public revenues and federal transfer funds. Like all provincial plans, MSP must meet the national standards set for medicare by Health Canada that guarantee universal access to medically required services for all Canadians.

We Can Help Keep Our Health Care System Strong

In recent years, the health care system in BC and the rest of Canada has come under increasing pressure: costs are rising, demand for services is increasing, the population is growing, and new technologies are creating new demands for funds. Provincial governments are struggling to keep pace with the changes. Health care is BC's biggest public expense, accounting for more than one-third of the province's total budget.

As a beneficiary of MSP, you have a very important role in helping to maintain a strong and responsive health care system in BC. The truth is, all the efforts taken by the government and the doctors of BC cannot equal the impact that you, the health care consumer, can have on your own health and the quality of our health care system—and it's easier than you think. Just by using this book as a tool to help you make decisions about your health care, you will be helping yourself and your health care system stay strong and healthy.

What You Need to Know

1. Enrollment in MSP is required by law. As a resident of BC, you must enroll yourself and your dependents in MSP. You are considered a resident of BC if you are a Canadian citizen or landed immigrant and you make your home in the Province of BC and stay in BC at least 6 months of each calendar year. Certain other groups are deemed to be residents, but tourists and visitors to BC are not. To be beneficiaries under your plan, your dependents must also qualify as residents of BC. Dependents include:

- Your spouse, either married or common-law (who may be of the same gender).
- Any unmarried child or legal ward who is supported by you and is either under the age of 19 or under the age of 25 and a full-time student.

Many BC residents—about 60% of the population—receive their MSP coverage through their employer, pension, social assistance, or union group plan. If this applies to you, your group plan administrator will coordinate the enrollment of you and your family in MSP.

A few British Columbians, for religious or other reasons, formally request to "opt out" of MSP, which means that they are ineligible for coverage of their medical care through *all* the province's health care programs.

How to enroll

Self-administered plan: If your employer, pension, social assistance, or union group plan does not cover you, you will have to enroll yourself in MSP. Applications can be obtained from MSP, any Government Agent office/BC Access Centre, or the MSP Web site. You will be asked to provide photocopies of documents to support the legal name and Canadian citizenship or immigration status of each person listed on your application.

New baby: You will be given a Baby Enrollment form in the hospital after your child's birth. Complete the form and submit it as soon as possible to your group plan administrator, if applicable, or send the form to MSP if you have a self-administered account.

Adding a family member to your MSP account: Contact your group plan administrator if you are covered under a group account. Otherwise, you can contact MSP or a Government Agent office/BC Access Centre. Contact information can be found at the end of this chapter. You will be requested to provide details of the person's name, personal health number (if the person is already enrolled under a separate account), and his or her relationship to you. If a name change is involved, you will be required to provide legal documentation of the name change, such as a marriage certificate.

Once enrolled, you and your family members will each receive a CareCard with a lifetime personal health number (PHN). This number enables you and your family to access all of BC's insured health services. Without it, none of your health care services will be paid for. It is a good idea to note each family member's PHN in your home medical files in case the cards are lost or stolen. When you turn 65, you will automatically be issued a gold CareCard. Show your card at your pharmacy when getting prescription drugs.

The first CareCard is issued without charge, but if you lose it and need a replacement, you may be asked to pay a small fee.

2. There is a waiting period before coverage begins. If you are a new resident or you are re-establishing residence in BC, you are eligible for benefits after completion of a waiting period—normally the balance of the month in which you arrived in BC plus 2 months. If absences from Canada exceed a total of 30 days during the waiting period, your eligibility for benefits may be affected. Coverage for medical care during the waiting period is your responsibility.

If a couple arrives separately from another part of Canada, the waiting period for family coverage begins on the date the second person arrives.

If you are moving from another province, you should arrange coverage from your former provincial insurance plan during the waiting period. If you are arriving from another country, you should arrange coverage with a private insurance company for the waiting period.

3. Premium payments are required for health insurance benefits in BC. MSP is based on a monthly premium payment system. Premium rates for MSP vary depending upon family size and income. If you are in financial need, you may qualify for assistance with partial or full payment of premiums. Further information about premium assistance is available from MSP. See contact information at the end of this chapter.

If your required premiums are not paid, the outstanding amount increases each month and becomes a debt owed to the province. If you are moving out of the province and want to cancel your MSP coverage, you can't simply stop paying your premiums. You must notify MSP of your departure and need to cancel. Otherwise, you may continue to be billed for premiums.

4. You must report any changes that affect your coverage with MSP. If you change your name, move within BC, or otherwise change your contact information, you must report this change to MSP as soon as possible. Other changes such as marriage, the birth of a child, or a change in family size, should also be reported.

If you are planning to move outside BC or are no longer a resident of BC, you must notify MSP to cancel your coverage. You will be asked to provide the date you are leaving and a forwarding address. Otherwise, you may continue to be billed for premiums.

Special conditions apply for students and others who are temporarily outside BC. For students, provincial health care benefits may be available for the time period of the studies within Canada. If you are studying outside Canada, benefits may be available for up to 5 years. Again, contact MSP before you leave.

5. BC provides the most comprehensive coverage in Canada. In BC you are entitled to the following benefits:

- Medically required services and surgical procedures provided by a physician.
- Maternity care provided by a physician or registered midwife.
- Diagnostic services, including X-rays and laboratory services, when ordered by a physician, podiatrist, dental or oral surgeon, or midwife.
- Dental and oral surgery, when medically required to be performed in hospital.
- Orthodontic services related to severe facial abnormalities that are present from birth (congenital).
- Acute hospital services.

- Home Nursing, Community Rehabilitation Services, and Case Management for BC residents of all ages with chronic, acute, palliative, or rehabilitative health care needs.
- Palliative Benefits for people nearing the end of their life that include most medications free of charge and access to necessary medical supplies and equipment. Enrollment for benefits is through your physician, and approved medications can be obtained through a local pharmacy.

BC also covers some supplementary health care services provided within BC with certain limits and restrictions. Benefits include:

- Eye examinations. Routine eye examinations are a benefit only for MSP beneficiaries 18 years of age and younger and 65 years of age and older. Medically required eye examinations are a benefit for all MSP beneficiaries. Your optometrist or ophthalmologist is qualified to determine if your eye examination is medically required.
- Chiropractic, massage therapy, naturopathy, physical therapy, and non-surgical podiatry. Only MSP beneficiaries receiving premium assistance are eligible for a combined limit of 10 visits for these services. MSP pays practitioners a subsidy for each visit; however, patients may be required to pay an additional amount.
- Surgical Podiatry. This service is a benefit for all MSP beneficiaries when performed in BC by a practitioner who is enrolled with MSP.
- Home and Community Care services, including home support, adult day centres, assisted living, respite care, and residential care, are available based on assessed need. Clients are charged a client rate, based on after-tax income, for home support, assisted living, and residential care. Client charges for respite and hospice are set at the lowest residential care rate, and a nominal fee is charged for adult day centres.

6. Some services you may obtain from your health care provider are not covered by your insurance. Some services you may wish to obtain from your doctor are not insured benefits under MSP. Your doctor or health care provider should inform you when a service is not covered and let you know what it will cost before the service is rendered. These may include:

- Services that are not medically required, such as cosmetic surgery, varicose vein treatment (for cosmetic reasons), wart removal, tattoo removal, routine circumcision of a newborn, and acupuncture.
- Annual or routine checkups where no disease or symptoms are present.
- Medical advice by telephone or letter when not related to a previous visit.

- Medical examinations, forms, or letters requested by a third party, such as for adoption, driver's licence, school, sports, camp, insurance, or legal requirements.
- Transfer of medical records.
- Most dental services.
- Routine eye examinations.
- Eyeglasses, hearing aids, and other health equipment or appliances.
- Services of counsellors and psychologists.

7. You may be required to pay for services received from a practitioner who has "opted out" of MSP. Some supplementary health care providers, such as chiropractors and massage therapists, have "opted out" of MSP. If you obtain services from them, you may be required to pay for these services yourself. If you are eligible, you can then request repayment directly from MSP by mailing in a form. Costs will be paid back to you at MSP rates. Practitioners who are "opted out" may charge you a fee greater than what would be paid back by MSP for the same insured service. This only applies to services provided by supplementary health care practitioners. Virtually all physicians who provide medical care in BC are enrolled with MSP.

8. If you get sick outside BC, you may be covered—but not always to the full amount. If you are outside BC and you become ill or have an accident, MSP will pay for your medical services under these conditions:

- You are a resident of BC and are enrolled with MSP.
- The services are medically required.
- A licensed physician provides the services.
- The services are normally insured by MSP.

In Canada, the cost of your medical care will be covered by the health insurance plan of the province you are visiting (except Quebec) if you present a valid BC CareCard. However, certain health care benefits that *may* be covered when provided in BC are not covered outside the province, including prescription drugs and supplementary health services such as chiropractic care and massage therapy.

Some medical services are also excluded from coverage by your BC health insurance when provided in another province. These include:

- Routine periodic health examinations, including routine eye exams.
- Services requested by a third party.
- Team conferences.
- Surgery for alteration of appearance (cosmetic surgery).
- Treatment of port-wine stains other than on face and neck.
- Sex-reassignment surgery.

- Surgery for reversal of sterilization.
- Therapeutic abortion.
- In vitro fertilization and artificial insemination.
- Genetic screening and other genetic investigations.
- Lithotripsy for gallstones.
- Acupuncture, acupressure, transcutaneous electro-nerve stimulations (TENS), moxibustion, biofeedback, and hypnotherapy.
- Anaesthetic services and surgical assistant services associated with all the above excluded services.
- Ambulance services.

When travelling in Quebec or outside Canada, you will be required to pay for the service and obtain repayment later from MSP. Claims for repayment must be submitted within 90 days of receiving medical care and, for hospital claims, 6 months from the date of hospital discharge.

Outside Canada, your coverage will only pay up to the amount the same service would cost in BC. It is important to purchase additional insurance when travelling outside BC, as the cost of services obtained outside the country can be very high. For example, the amount BC pays for emergency in-patient care in a hospital does not exceed $75 per day. In the United States, the average cost of a hospital stay exceeds $1,000 a day. This is a huge difference, and you will be responsible for paying for the service in a foreign country. Be sure you understand the extent of coverage provided under the extra insurance you purchase, as it often does not cover services related to a pre-existing condition.

You are advised to purchase additional insurance if you are travelling anywhere outside BC, including other areas of Canada, to help pay for any costs not covered by the Ministry of Health.

9. Obtain approval from MSP before planning medical care outside of BC. If you decide you want to seek medical care outside Canada, the medical specialist looking after you in BC must get written approval for a referral outside the country before MSP will pay for the out-of-country care. MSP will grant approval only if it is determined that no appropriate treatment options are available in BC or Canada and the proposed treatment is not considered experimental or under development (research). Without MSP preapproval, you are responsible for all costs of medical services obtained outside Canada.

10. MSP's Travel Assistance Program can help you obtain necessary medical care. A number of transportation companies participate in MSP's Travel Assistance Program (TAP) by offering travel discounts to eligible BC residents who must travel elsewhere in BC to receive medical services not available in their own community. To qualify, your travel expenses must be ineligible for coverage by third-party insurance or other government programs.

To be eligible for TAP, you must be a BC resident and be enrolled in MSP. You also must have a physician's referral for medical services that are not locally available. Escorts are also eligible if travelling with patients who are either under the age of 16 or incapable of independent travel for medical reasons.

A physician must indicate on the TAP form that an escort is required.

Participating transportation partners are Air Canada, Air Canada Jazz (Air BC), Central Mountain Air, BC Ferries, BC Rail/VIA Rail, Harbour Air, Angel Flight, Pacific Coach Lines, Malaspina Coach Lines, and Greyline Victoria.

Your physician's office will complete and sign a TAP form confirming your need to travel to receive necessary medical care. You will need to call the TAP program to verify your eligibility and obtain a confirmation number a few days in advance of travelling. Discounts must be obtained at the time of travel, as there is no repayment after travelling occurs.

11. MSP routinely monitors claims for services. Services paid by MSP are regularly checked to ensure that they were provided, appropriately billed, and properly recorded. On occasion, you may be randomly selected to participate in a service verification survey. The survey form asks if you received the service(s) as listed on the form. A return-addressed, prestamped envelope is provided for you to return the form. This important confirmation program helps ensure that services are being provided as billed. By completing this form, you are helping MSP do its job.

12. How to contact MSP. MSP is improving its services and all inquiries are being centralized to two numbers. Please check your telephone directory for local numbers, or call the following toll-free numbers:

- For 24/7 beneficiary information, including how to enroll, update your information, obtain forms, or get information on the Travel Assistance Program, call: 1-800-663-7100.
- For information on medical claims, call: 1-800-663-7206.
- **MSP Web site.** Visit the MSP Web site at www.healthservices.gov.bc.ca/msp/ for more information about MSP programs.
- **Visit one of the Government Agent offices / BC Access Centres** located throughout the province. Through these offices you can apply for coverage, pay your premiums, request a replacement CareCard, and get information about your MSP account. Check the blue pages of your telephone directory to find the location nearest to you.

By mail
Send your question or request to:
P.O. Box 9035 Stn Prov Govt
Victoria, BC V8W 9E3

Please note:
The information in this chapter provides a general outline of the Medical Services Plan of BC. All information is subject to change in accordance with the provisions of the *Medicare Protection Act* and Regulations and the *Hospital Insurance Act* and Regulations. If a discrepancy exists between this information and the legislation, the legislation will prevail.

BC PharmaCare

What is PharmaCare?

PharmaCare is British Columbia's drug insurance program. PharmaCare is designed to provide financial assistance to BC residents for eligible prescription drugs and designated medical supplies. The program provides reasonable access to drug therapy and is an integral part of the health care system that serves British Columbians.

PharmaCare was announced by the Government of British Columbia in 1973 and began operation on January 1, 1974. PharmaCare is funded by the Government of British Columbia and is not governed by the *Canada Health Act*.

Fair PharmaCare

BC's Fair PharmaCare plan started on May 1, 2003. Fair PharmaCare focuses financial assistance on BC families who need it most, based on their net income. In order to receive benefits under Fair PharmaCare, families must complete a one-time registration and sign a consent form allowing PharmaCare to retrieve income information annually from the Canada Revenue Agency.

How Fair PharmaCare works

Each Fair PharmaCare family is assigned an annual deductible and an annual maximum, both of which are calculated as a percentage of annual net family income. Families with a net family income of less than $15,000 (or less than $33,000 if one or more members were born before 1940) are assigned a $0 deductible. PharmaCare immediately assists these families with eligible drug purchases.

Families with incomes higher than $15,000 (or higher than $33,000 if one or more family members were born before 1940) are assigned a deductible based on their income. The deductible ranges from 1 to 3% of their annual net income. These families must pay 100% of their eligible drug costs until they pay this amount. Once the deductible is met (or immediately, for families with a $0 deductible), PharmaCare then pays the majority of the family's eligible drug costs, with the family responsible for "co-paying" either 25% (for families with one or more members born before 1940) or 30% (for all other families) until they reach their maximum.

Once a family's out-of-pocket expenses (deductible plus co-payments) equal their maximum, PharmaCare pays the full amount on eligible prescription costs for the remainder of the year. The annual maximum ranges from 1.25 to 4% of net family income, depending on income level.

Monthly Deductible Payment Option

Beginning in 2005, PharmaCare now offers an option for families to pay their annual deductible in monthly payments. **Enrollment in this payment plan is optional.** It is designed to make paying the deductible easier.

Families who choose to enroll will make monthly payments throughout the year and get PharmaCare assistance from the time they enroll. They are then responsible for co-paying either 25 or 30% for eligible drugs (depending on the age of family members), until their out-of-pocket expenses equal their annual maximum.

Eligible families are those who meet all of the following:

- Are registered for Fair PharmaCare,
- Do not have private health insurance with a drug benefit plan, and
- Have a deductible greater than $0.

PharmaCare Registration and Enrollment in Monthly Deductible Payment Option

- **Monthly Deductible Payment Option:** For more information on the Monthly Deductible Payment Option, or to enroll, please contact the Fair PharmaCare Registration Desk toll-free from anywhere in BC at 1-800-663-7100.
- **Fair PharmaCare:** New BC residents or BC families who have not yet registered for Fair PharmaCare can register online at https://pharmacare.moh.hnet.bc.ca/ or call toll-free in BC 1-800-663-7100.

What Does PharmaCare Cover?

PharmaCare covers:

- Eligible prescription drugs prescribed by a physician, dentist, midwife, or podiatrist.

  Certain medications require prior approval (an approved Special Authority) for PharmaCare coverage. Coverage exceptions granted via a Special Authority are not retroactive and must be requested before the medication is dispensed.
- Insulin, needles, and syringes for diabetics.
- Blood sugar test strips for diabetics for whom blood sugar testing is deemed medically necessary and who have a valid *Certificate of Training* from an approved Diabetic Teaching Centre.
- Certain ostomy supplies.

- Designated permanent prosthetic appliances and children's orthotic devices (braces).
- Selected digestive enzymes and nutritional supplements for cystic fibrosis patients.

PharmaCare does not cover:

- Eyeglasses.
- Hearing aids or hearing aid batteries.
- Bandages.
- Artificial sweeteners, antacids, laxatives or over-the-counter drugs.
- Wheelchairs, walkers, or other medical devices.
- Drug costs that have been fully reimbursed by another plan.
- Drugs or supplies obtained while outside of BC.
- Mail-order prescriptions requested from companies located outside BC.
- Greater than 100 days' supply of medications at any one time (for example, vacation supplies) or repeat prescriptions filled when more than 14 days' supply remains in the existing prescription.

PharmaCare Plans

PharmaCare provides assistance to British Columbia residents for the purchase of eligible prescription drugs and selected medical devices. To be eligible for PharmaCare benefits, individuals must be registered with the BC Medical Services Plan (MSP). Most BC residents will receive PharmaCare benefits under Fair PharmaCare. However, some patients will be eligible for coverage under different plans as described below.

Fair PharmaCare

All BC residents registered with MSP are eligible for Fair PharmaCare. In order to enroll in Fair PharmaCare, families must complete a one-time registration via the Internet, telephone, or facsimile.

Plan B (Long-Term Care)

Residents of designated Licensed Long-Term Care Facilities receive PharmaCare benefits at no charge.

Plan C (Income Assistance)

All BC residents receiving income assistance from the Ministry of Human Resources receive full funding for PharmaCare benefits through Plan C.

For information on Income Assistance through the Ministry of Human Resources, visit their Web site at www.mhr.gov.bc.ca/bcea.htm.

You may also call Enquiry BC, 7:30 a.m. to 5:00 p.m. PST, Monday through Friday at:
Victoria: 250-387-6121
Vancouver: 604-660-2421
Elsewhere in BC: 1-800-663-7867
Outside British Columbia:
604-660-2421

E-mail address:
EnquiryBC@gems3.gov.bc.ca

Telephone Device for the Deaf (TDD)
Vancouver: 604-775-0303
Elsewhere in BC: 1-800-661-8773

Plan D (Cystic Fibrosis)

Individuals who have cystic fibrosis who are registered with a provincial cystic fibrosis clinic receive digestive enzymes free of charge through this plan when prescribed by a physician at the clinic. The enzymes are dispensed through community pharmacies. Other products are covered under the patient's regular PharmaCare plan. Patients on Plan D may also be eligible to receive PharmaCare coverage through their regular PharmaCare plan for certain nutritional supplements, vitamins, and minerals, subject to regular plan rules.

Plan F (At-Home Children Program)

Plan F provides 100% financial assistance for eligible prescription drugs to children under the age of 19 who are eligible for benefits under the At-Home Program of the Ministry of Children and Family Development. Eligibility for this plan is determined through the Ministry of Children and Family Development.

For more information on PharmaCare's drug benefit program for at-home children (Plan F), clients should contact the Fair PharmaCare Registration Desk toll-free in BC at 1-800-663-7100.

For more information on the At-Home Program, contact the Ministry of Children and Family Development online at www.mcf.gov.bc.ca/at_home/

Plan G (No-Charge Psychiatric Medication)

PharmaCare provides 100% coverage for designated psychiatric medications for clients of mental health service centres who qualify for MSP Premium Assistance. Plan G patients should also register for Fair PharmaCare in order to receive coverage for other medications.

The BC Centre for Excellence in HIV/AIDS

HIV-positive individuals living in BC receive antiretroviral drugs free of charge from the BC Centre for Excellence. The Centre operates out of St. Paul's Hospital in Vancouver, and the drug program is fully supported and funded by PharmaCare.

Index

A

B

D

E

F

G

I

N

O

P

Q

R

S

T

U

V

W

Y

NOTES

NOTES

NOTES

NOTES